MW01181899

ADVANCES IN

Pediatrics

Editor-in-Chief
Michael S. Kappy, MD, PhD

Professor of Pediatrics, University of Colorado
School of Medicine, Children's Hospital Colorado,
Aurora, Colorado

PHILADELPHIA   LONDON   TORONTO   MONTREAL   SYDNEY   TOKYO

ADVANCES IN
Pediatrics

VOLUMES 1 THROUGH 59 (OUT OF PRINT)

Vice President, Global Medical Reference: Mary Gatsch
Editor: Kerry Holland
Developmental Editor: Donald Mumford

© 2014 Elsevier Inc. All rights reserved.

This periodical and the individual contributions contained in it are protected under copyright by Elsevier and the following terms and conditions apply to their use:

Photocopying
Single photocopies of single articles may be made for personal use as allowed by national copyright laws. Permission of the Publisher and payment of a fee is required for all other photocopying, including multiple or systematic copying, copying for advertising or promotional purposes, resale, and all forms of document delivery. Special rates are available for educational institutions that wish to make photocopies for non-profit educational classroom use.
For information on how to seek permission visit www.elsevier.com/permissions or call: (+44) 1865 843830 (UK)/(+1) 215 239 3804 (USA).

Derivative Works
Subscribers may reproduce tables of contents or prepare lists of articles including abstracts for internal circulation within their institutions. Permission of the Publisher is required for resale or distribution outside the institution. Permission of the Publisher is required for all other derivative works, including compilations and translations (please consult www.elsevier.com/permissions).

Electronic Storage or Usage
Permission of the Publisher is required to store or use electronically any material contained in this periodical, including any article or part of an article (please consult www.elsevier.com/permissions). Except as outlined above, no part of this publication may be reproduced, stored in a retrieval system or transmitted in any form or by any means, electronic, mechanical, photocopying, recording or otherwise, without prior written permission of the Publisher.

Notice
No responsibility is assumed by the Publisher for any injury and/or damage to persons or property as a matter of products liability, negligence or otherwise, or from any use or operation of any methods, products, instructions or ideas contained in the material herein. Because of rapid advances in the medical sciences, in particular, independent verification of diagnoses and drug dosages should be made.

Although all advertising material is expected to conform to ethical (medical) standards, inclusion in this publication does not constitute a guarantee or endorsement of the quality or value of such product or of the claims made of it by its manufacturer.

Reprints: For copies of 100 or more of articles in this publication, please contact the Commercial Reprints Department, Elsevier Inc., 360 Park Avenue South, New York, NY 10010-1710. Tel: 212-633-3874; Fax: 212-633-3820; E-mail: reprints@elsevier.com.

Printed in the United States of America.

Editorial Office:
Elsevier
1600 John F. Kennedy Blvd,
Suite 1800
Philadelphia, PA 19103-2899

International Standard Serial Number: 0065-3101
International Standard Book Number: 13: 978-0-323-26461-7

ADVANCES IN
Pediatrics

Editor-in-Chief

MICHAEL S. KAPPY, MD, PhD, Professor of Pediatrics, University of Colorado School of Medicine, Children's Hospital Colorado, Aurora, Colorado

Associate Editors

LEWIS A. BARNESS, MD, DSci(hc), DPH(hc), Distinguished University Professor Emeritus, Department of Pediatrics, University of South Florida College of Medicine, Tampa, Florida

LESLIE L. BARTON, MD, Professor Emerita, Department of Pediatrics, Steele Memorial Children's Research Center, University of Arizona, Tucson, Arizona

CAROL D. BERKOWITZ, MD, Executive Vice Chair, Department of Pediatrics, Harbor-UCLA Medical Center; Distinguished Professor of Pediatrics, David Geffen School of Medicine at UCLA, Torrance, California

ENID GILBERT-BARNESS, AO, MD, MBBS, FRCPA, FRCPath, DSci(hc), MD(hc), Professor, Departments of Pathology and Cell Biology, Pediatrics, and Obstetrics and Gynecology, University of South Florida College of Medicine, Tampa General Hospital, Tampa, Florida

JANE CARVER, PhD, MS, MPH, Professor, Department of Pediatrics and Molecular Medicine, University of South Florida College of Medicine, Tampa, Florida

MORITZ ZIEGLER, MD, Retired Surgeon-in-Chief, Pediatric Surgery, Children's Hospital Colorado, Retired, Professor of Surgery, University of Colorado School of Medicine, Denver, Colorado

ADVANCES IN
Pediatrics

CONTRIBUTORS

P. DAVID ADELSON, MD, Barrow Neurological Institute at Phoenix Children's Hospital, Phoenix, Arizona

KIMBERLEE ALLRED, RN, NNP-BC, Barrow Neurological Institute at Phoenix Children's Hospital, Phoenix, Arizona

SUSAN D. APKON, MD, Director, Associate Professor, Rehabilitation Medicine, Seattle Children's Hospital, University of Washington, Seattle, Washington

JO APPLEBAUM, MPH, Children's Health Fund and Community Pediatric Programs, Montefiore Medical Center, Bronx, New York

JORGE I. ARANGO, MD, Barrow Neurological Institute at Phoenix Children's Hospital, Phoenix, Arizona

SANDRA AREVALO, MPH, RD, CDE, Center for Child Health and Resiliency, Montefiore Medical Center, Bronx, New York

DANIEL K. BENJAMIN Jr, MD, PhD, MPH, Duke Clinical Research Institute, Duke University Medical Center; Department of Pediatrics, College of Medicine, Duke University, Durham, North Carolina

STEPHEN BERMAN, MD, Professor of Pediatrics and Public Health, University of Colorado Denver, Center for Global Health-Colorado School of Public Health, Aurora, Colorado

JANET C. BERRY, RN, MBA, Nursing Administration and Perioperative Services; Nationwide Children's Hospital, Columbus, Ohio

RICHARD J. BRILLI, MD, FAAP, FCCM, Chief Medical Officer, Hospital Administration, Quality Improvement Services; Nationwide Children's Hospital; Professor, Pediatrics, The Ohio State University College of Medicine, Columbus, Ohio

LEE BUDIN, MD, Quality Improvement Services; Nationwide Children's Hospital; Clinical Assistant Professor, The Ohio State University College of Medicine, Columbus, Ohio

CRISTINA CARBALLO, MD, Barrow Neurological Institute at Phoenix Children's Hospital, Phoenix, Arizona

JANE CARVER, PhD, MS, MPH, Professor, Department of Pediatrics and Molecular Medicine, University of South Florida College of Medicine, Tampa, Florida

ROBERT C. CASKEY, MD, MSc, Resident, Department of Surgery, University of Pennsylvania School of Medicine, Philadelphia, Pennsylvania

MICHAEL COHEN-WOLKOWIEZ, MD, PhD, Duke Clinical Research Institute, Duke University Medical Center; Department of Pediatrics, College of Medicine, Duke University, Durham, North Carolina

LINDSEY COOPER, MD, Clinical Assistant Professor of Pediatrics, University of Colorado Denver, Center for Global Health-Colorado School of Public Health, Aurora, Colorado

WALLACE V. CRANDALL, MD, Quality Improvement Services; Nationwide Children's Hospital; Professor, Clinical Pediatrics, The Ohio State University College of Medicine, Columbus, Ohio

HEDA DAPUL, MD, FAAP, Attending Physician, Pediatric Critical Care Medicine; Maimonides Medical Center, Infants and Children's Hospital of Brooklyn, Brooklyn, New York

J. TERRANCE DAVIS, MD, Quality Improvement Services; Nationwide Children's Hospital; Professor Emeritus, Clinical Surgery, The Ohio State University College of Medicine, Columbus, Ohio

BRIAN DUNOSKI, MD, Instructor, Radiology, Wayne State University School of Medicine, Children's Hospital of Michigan, Detroit, Michigan; Children's Mercy Hospital, Kansas City, Missouri

KRISTINA N. FEJA, MD, MPH, Division of Allergy, Immunology and Infectious Diseases, The Children's Hospital at Saint Peter's University Hospital, New Brunswick, New Jersey

JAIME L. FRÍAS, MD, FAAP, FACMG, Emeritus Professor and Former Lewis A. Barness Professor and Chairman, Department of Pediatrics, University of South Florida

BEATRIZ LLAMOSAS GALLARDO, MD, Associate Professor of Pediatrics, Emergency Department, Instituto Nacional de Pediatria, Distrito Federal, México

ENID GILBERT-BARNESS, MBBS, MD, FRCPA, FRCPath, DSci(hc), MD(hc), Professor of Pathology and Cell Biology, Laboratory Medicine, Pediatric, Obstetrics and Gynecology, Department of Pathology, College of Medicine, Tampa General Hospital, University of South Florida Morsani, Tampa, Florida

DANIEL GONZALEZ, PharmD, PhD, Division of Pharmacotherapy and Experimental Therapeutics, UNC Eshelman School of Pharmacy, University of North Carolina at Chapel Hill, Chapel Hill; Duke Clinical Research Institute, Duke University Medical Center, Durham, North Carolina

SEAN P. GLEESON, MD, MBA, Quality Improvement Services; Nationwide Children's Hospital; Assistant Professor, Pediatrics-Practice, The Ohio State University College of Medicine, Columbus, Ohio

RICHARD GRADY, MD, Professor of Urology; Section of Pediatric Urology, Seattle Children's Hospital, University of Washington School of Medicine, Seattle, Washington

LARRY A. GREENBAUM, MD, PhD, Marcus Professor of Pediatrics and Division Director, Pediatric Nephrology, Emory University and Children's Healthcare of Atlanta, Atlanta, Georgia

HONGYAN GUAN, MD, PhD, Associate Professor of Pediatrics, Department of Early Childhood Development, Capital Institute of Pediatrics, Beijing, China

SOLVEIG HART, PT, MSPT, PCS, Rehabilitation Services, Seattle Children's Hospital, Seattle, Washington

ANA A. ORTIZ-HERNÁNDEZ, MD, Associate Professor of Pediatrics, Emergency Department, Instituto Nacional de Pediatria, Distrito Federal, México

JORDANA E. HOPPE, MD, Pediatric Pulmonary Fellow, Department of Pediatrics, Children's Hospital Colorado, University of Colorado Denver, Aurora, Colorado

HOPE T. JACKSON, MD, Surgical Resident, The George Washington University School of Medicine and Health Sciences, Washington, DC

SABAH KALYOUSSEF, DO, Division of Allergy, Immunology and Infectious Diseases, The Children's Hospital at Saint Peter's University Hospital, New Brunswick, New Jersey

TIMOTHY D. KANE, MD, FACS, Professor of Surgery and Pediatrics, The George Washington University School of Medicine and Health Sciences; Director, Surgical Residency Training Program; Chief, Division of Pediatric Surgery, Department of Surgery, Sheikh Zayed Institute for Pediatric Surgical Innovation, Children's National Medical Center, Washington, DC

MICHAEL S. KAPPY, MD, PhD, Department of Pediatrics, University of Colorado School of Medicine, Children's Hospital Colorado, Aurora, Colorado

KELLY J. KELLEHER, MD, Quality Improvement Services; Nationwide Children's Hospital; Professor, Pediatrics, Psychiatry, and Public Health, The Ohio State University College of Medicine, Columbus, Ohio

DANIELLE LARAQUE, MD, FAAP, Maimonides Medical Center, Infants and Children's Hospital of Brooklyn, Brooklyn, New York; Professor of Pediatrics, New York University School of Medicine, New York City, New York

AMY LEE, MD, Assistant Professor, Pediatric Neurosurgery, Seattle Children's Hospital, University of Washington, Seattle, Washington

BERTRAM LUBIN, MD, President and Chief Executive Officer, UCSF Benioff Children's Hospital Oakland, Oakland, California

HILDRED MACHUCA, DO, Center for Child Health and Resiliency, Montefiore Medical Center, Bronx, New York

STACEY L. MARTINIANO, MD, Assistant Professor of Pediatrics, Department of Pediatrics, Children's Hospital Colorado, University of Colorado Denver, Aurora, Colorado

PATRICIA J. McFEELEY, MD, Professor Emerita, Department of Pathology, Office of the Medical Investigator, University of New Mexico School of Medicine, University of New Mexico, Albuquerque, New Mexico

THOMAS McNALLEY, MD, MA, Assistant Professor, Rehabilitation Medicine, Seattle Children's Hospital, University of Washington, Seattle, Washington

GRANT MORROW III, MD, Professor Emeritus of Pediatrics, The Ohio State University, Columbus, Ohio; Medical Director, Research Institute at Nationwide Children's Hospital

MICHAEL L. NANCE, MD, Professor of Surgery; Director of Pediatric Trauma Program, Children's Hospital of Pennsylvania, Philadelphia, Pennsylvania

LEE NISWANDER, PhD, Department of Pediatrics, Section Head of Developmental Biology, Children's Hospital Colorado, Investigator, Howard Hughes Medical Institute, Professor, University of Colorado School of Medicine, Aurora, Colorado

JULIETTE PETERSEN, MS, Doctoral Candidate, Molecular Biology Program, University of Colorado Denver Anschutz Medical Campus, Aurora, Colorado

IAN M. PAUL, MD, MSc, Departments of Pediatrics and Public Health Sciences, College of Medicine, Penn State University, Hershey, Pennsylvania

SHERIDAN REMLEY, PT, DPT, Rehabilitation Services, Seattle Children's Hospital, Seattle, Washington

GENESIS RIVERA, MD, Assistant Professor of Pediatrics, St. Luke's College of Medicine, Quezon City, Philippines

KERRY ROSEN, MD, MBA, FACC, FAAP, Quality Improvement Services; Nationwide Children's Hospital; Associate Professor, Clinical Pediatrics, The Ohio State University College of Medicine, Columbus, Ohio

DEBORAH ROTENSTEIN, MD, Director, Pediatric Endocrinology, Endocrine Division, Pediatric Alliance, Pittsburgh, Pennsylvania

SCOTT D. SAGEL, MD, PhD, Associate Professor of Pediatrics, Department of Pediatrics, Children's Hospital Colorado, University of Colorado Denver, Aurora, Colorado

ALAN SHAPIRO, MD, Children's Health Fund and Community Pediatric Programs, Montefiore Medical Center, Bronx, New York

BENJAMIN SHULMAN, BA, Department of Biostatistics and Informatics, University of Colorado School of Public Health, Aurora, Colorado

HILLARY SHURTLEFF, PhD, Clinical Associate Professor, Department of Neurology, University of Washington School of Medicine; Department of Child Psychiatry, Seattle Children's Hospital, Seattle, Washington

THOMAS L. SLOVIS, MD, Professor Emeritus, Radiology, Wayne State University School of Medicine, Children's Hospital of Michigan, Detroit, Michigan

PARITA SONI, MD, Barrow Neurological Institute at Phoenix Children's Hospital, Phoenix, Arizona

LINDA STOVEROCK, RN, DNP, MSN, NEA-BC, Chief Nursing Officer, Nursing Administration; Nationwide Children's Hospital, Columbus, Ohio

RYAN STRADLEIGH, BS, Barrow Neurological Institute at Phoenix Children's Hospital, Phoenix, Arizona

ALTAGRACIA TOLENTINO, MD, Center for Child Health and Resiliency, Montefiore Medical Center, Bronx, New York

REMY WAHNOUN, PhD, Barrow Neurological Institute at Phoenix Children's Hospital, Phoenix, Arizona

WILLIAM O. WALKER Jr, MD, Chief, Division of Developmental Medicine, Seattle Children's Hospital, Robert A. Aldrich Endowed Professor of Pediatrics, University of Washington School of Medicine, Seattle, Washington

MOLLY WARNER, PhD, ABPP-CN, Clinical Associate Professor, Department of Neurology, University of Washington School of Medicine; Neuropsychologist, Neuropsychology Consult Service, Department of Psychiatry, Seattle Children's Hospital, Seattle, Washington

JOSEPH WATHEN, MD, Associate Professor of Pediatrics, University of Colorado Denver, Center for Global Health-Colorado School of Public Health, Aurora, Colorado

EDITH T. ZEMANICK, MD, MSCS, Assistant Professor of Pediatrics, Department of Pediatrics, Children's Hospital Colorado, University of Colorado Denver, Aurora, Colorado

ADVANCES IN
Pediatrics

CONTENTS VOLUME 61 • 2014

Advances in the Care of Children with Spina Bifida

Susan D. Apkon, Richard Grady, Solveig Hart, Amy Lee, Thomas McNalley, Lee Niswander, Juliette Petersen, Sheridan Remley, Deborah Rotenstein, Hillary Shurtleff, Molly Warner, and William O. Walker Jr

Update in Pediatric Imaging
Brian Dunoski and Thomas L. Slovis

Conduction Defects/Cardiomyopathies
Enid Gilbert-Barness

Advances in Minimally Invasive Surgery in Pediatric Patients
Hope T. Jackson and Timothy D. Kane

A Patient/Family-Centered Strategic Plan Can Drive Significant Improvement

Richard J. Brilli, Wallace V. Crandall, Janet C. Berry,
Linda Stoverock, Kerry Rosen, Lee Budin, Kelly J. Kelleher,
Sean P. Gleeson, and J. Terrance Davis

Hypothermia in Hypoxic Ischemic Encephalopathy: A 5-Year Experience at Phoenix Children's Hospital Neuro NICU

Jorge I. Arango, Kimberlee Allred, P. David Adelson,
Parita Soni, Ryan Stradleigh, Remy Wahnoun, and
Cristina Carballo

Advances in the Diagnosis and Treatment of Cystic Fibrosis
Stacey L. Martiniano, Jordana E. Hoppe, Scott D. Sagel, and Edith T. Zemanick

Pediatrics in Disasters: Evaluation of a Global Training Program
Lindsey Cooper, Hongyan Guan, Ana A. Ortiz-Hernández, Beatriz Llamosas Gallardo, Genesis Rivera, Joseph Wathen, Benjamin Shulman, and Stephen Berman

Prevention and Management of Pediatric Obesity: A Multipronged, Community-Based Agenda
Alan Shapiro, Sandra Arevalo, Altagracia Tolentino, Hildred Machuca, and Jo Applebaum

Management of Pediatric Mild Traumatic Brain Injury
Robert C. Caskey and Michael L. Nance

Foodborne Illnesses
Sabah Kalyoussef and Kristina N. Feja

Lead Poisoning in Children
Heda Dapul and Danielle Laraque

Atypical Hemolytic Uremic Syndrome
Larry A. Greenbaum

Advances in Pediatrics 61 (2014) xxiii

ADVANCES IN PEDIATRICS

Introduction

Michael S. Kappy, MD, PhD

The editors present volume 61 of *Advances in Pediatrics*, founded in 1952. We are saddened by the death of one of the prime developers of this journal, Dr Lewis Barness, and a tributory article in his memory begins this volume.

Our annual "Foundations of Pediatrics" honors Lula Lubchenco, a distinguished physician who greatly improved the care of neonates and who set the standards by which we estimate risk in the newborn period. The article was written by her daughter, PatriciaMcFeeley.

We include our biennial review of advances in pharmacology and toxicology, submitted this year by Daniel Gonzalez and others.

In addition, we begin a series of multidisciplinary clinical care topics with the article by Susan Apkon and others on the care of children with spina bifida.

A comprehensive review of advances in pediatric radiologic imaging is presented by Dunoski and Slovis, and, in keeping with the purpose of this journal, a wide variety of updates in many medical and surgical areas of pediatrics, including cystic fibrosis, heart disease, obesity, brain injury, lead poisoning, and others, are presented, including an update on patient safety by Brilli and others.

As always, we welcome comments about each volume of *Advances in Pediatrics*, as well as suggestions for future topics. These can be sent to:

Michael S. Kappy, MD, PhD
Department of Pediatrics
University of Colorado School of Medicine
Children's Hospital Colorado
13123 East 16th Avenue, B-265
Aurora, CO 80045, USA

E-mail address: michael.kappy@childrenscolorado.org

0065-3101/14/$ – see front matter
http://dx.doi.org/10.1016/j.yapd.2014.04.006   © 2014 Elsevier Inc. All rights reserved.

ADVANCES IN PEDIATRICS

In Memoriam: Lew Barness

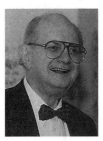

Lewis A. Barness, MD: 1921–2013

GRANT MORROW III, MD

When first asked to write some comments about one of the greatest pediatricians of his time, it seemed sad not to be able to talk with him and laugh about our past experiences. But, as I mulled the challenge over, I realized that solo reminiscing about Lewis A. Barness would be a wonderful trip through the past by itself and there would be no restrictions on which memories could be used to describe this great, caring human known by all of us as THE CHIEF.

He trained at exemplary places, Harvard for medical school and internship, followed by a research fellowship and pediatric residency at Boston Children's. From 1950 through 1972, he served as a faculty member at the University of Pennsylvania. In 1972, the University of South Florida wisely appointed him Chair of Pediatrics. In 1987, love moved him to the University of Wisconsin to join his distinguished wife, Dr Enid Gilbert-Barness, as an emeritus professor. In 1993, they both came back to the University of South Florida to finish their careers together.

Lew was one of the rare "triple-threat" academicians—a superb clinician, a superb researcher, and a superb teacher. He received almost all of the major pediatric academic awards during his career—a great testimony, by his peers, to his national and international prominence. His seminal work with children suffering with methylmalonic acidemia is only one example of his many innovative research studies that lasted throughout his entire career.

His true love was teaching. It was insightful, instructive, and flavored with good humor. But the most important characteristic of his effective teaching was that he loved students; he respected people, and he was optimistic about society. He kept that attitude throughout his entire life.

He loved to tell awful jokes. It was almost painful to hear the groans after his shaggy dog stories. A good example is the one about two snails walking down

0065-3101/14/$ – see front matter
http://dx.doi.org/10.1016/j.yapd.2014.04.005
© 2014 Elsevier Inc. All rights reserved.

the street. They went into a Jaguar car dealer and after some negotiations one snail said he'd buy the most expensive car if the dealer would paint large "S's" on both sides of the car. The other snail was perplexed and asked why. The answer: "So when I drive down the street everyone will watch me and say, look at that S car go." Typical but awful.

His bedside patient rounds with the students, residents, and staff were classic. He would go to the bedside, examine the patient, discuss issues, and then, most terrifying of all, he would become very Socratic by firing questions at someone in the group. They were thought-provoking and usually had a humorous flavor. Sometimes his water gun got the attention of a distracted student. Another wakeup alarm was that THE CHIEF had alternative names to call various faculty and students. Walter Tunnessen was one of the teaching staff and a great pediatrician. Lew would call him, "Tunafish," and if there was no quick answer, he'd call him "Tuna." It always got a smile. My appellation was "Edgar" due to the fact that Edgar R. Murrow, a well-known newsman, had died and Lew felt that some of my answers were dead wrong. Frank Oski, a great academician, was "Oscar," named for Oscar Mayer wieners. The unusual thing about his using alternative names was that no one felt they were the brunt of a joke or singled out for ridicule. It was just THE CHIEF having a good time on rounds. Somehow his brisk comments made the individual try harder, read up on the disease, and want to become a better physician. When I had written my first paper, I asked him if he'd review it. He did and said that it was fine except for two problems. I felt a sense of relief and said, "What are they?" He came back with, "Edgar, the science is pure $%#&" and "It needs to be rewritten in English." We finally got the paper published but I certainly learned a lot about how to write a manuscript. He was always very effective in supporting and cultivating the careers of his faculty.

Later in his career, when he was Chair of the Department of Pediatrics at the University of South Florida, he was able to build the Department, recruit excellent faculty, and produce a culture of camaraderie and excitement that made working there a privilege. Lew was well established nationally and internationally as an expert in nutrition and how it affects one's individual health. He never overate and, in fact, he never ate much at all. He usually had a Mr. Goodbar for lunch as he smoked his pipe, and he participated in absolutely no physical exercise whatsoever. What was the outcome of his not following his own advice? Were his arteries clogged? No, he didn't have one scintilla of calcium in any of his arteries and his intellect was perfectly intact. Being a geneticist, Lew knew that could trust his genetics more than his eating habits.

Even after he retired in 2007, he and Enid wrote many of the classic textbooks about nutrition, metabolic diseases, as well as physical and clinical diagnoses. One of his favorite quotes was by Socrates (ie, "The unexamined life is not worth living"). It was a true mantra for him and helped explain why he was so insightful and productive throughout his entire career.

Other flashes of memory are that he was humble for being so well-known and prominent. Throughout his career, he always bought his clothes from a Haband catalog. He had no need to flaunt his status.

In trying to express how people felt about Lew, the word Mensch seems most appropriate. It's perfect since it means a person of integrity and honor, a person to admire and emulate, and a person of noble character. Lew personified all of these traits.

The field of pediatrics, its pediatric institutions, and mostly the children, have benefited greatly because of Lew.

All of us hope that we could be remembered by as many people and with as much fondness as there is for THE CHIEF. All of us, particularly the family, will miss him.

Grant Morrow III, MD
Research Institute at Nationwide Children's Hospital
The Ohio State University
700 Children's Drive, Columbus, OH 43205-2696, USA

E-mail address: morrowg@ccri.net

BERTRAM LUBIN, MD

It is an honor for me to write a few paragraphs that will be included in a tribute to Dr Lewis Barness. Dr Barness was a friend, a mentor, the pediatrician for two of my children, and a role model whom I have cherished my entire career. He was truly a pediatrician's pediatrician. I first met Dr Barness when I was an intern at Children's Hospital of Philadelphia in 1964. He had assembled a staff at the University of Pennsylvania that included future leaders in pediatrics, among whom was Frank Oski, my friend, mentor, and colleague for life. I recall the first visit to Dr Barness' office, where stacks of journals were on his desk and on the floor, the content of which he had stored in his brain, ready to ask me and others to recall. He remembered details that proved to be pearls for all of us. I was petrified when I first met him as his reputation preceded him. However, within seconds, without receiving a squirt from his water pistol, which he concealed in his white coat, my heart was won over. Over the years, I appreciated that what I had experienced was something shared by many, and the warmth he had for his students was one of his shining characteristics.

Dr Barness was an enormous help to my family and me. When I was a fellow in Hematology/Oncology at Boston Children's Hospital, I sought his advice as to how my family could make a decision regarding our newborn son, who had Down syndrome. I will never forget his wise comments when I stated that we would get attached to Charlie if we brought him home. Dr Barness promptly responded that we had already been attached to him for nine months, and that both of us had the strength to raise him in a world that did not understand that not all of us can make a great contribution to society. Charlie is now 45 years old and has brought joy to many people.

Dr Barness was always willing to visit Children's Hospital in Oakland and give Grand Rounds. On one occasion, when the topic for his talk was "Pediatric Smells," he accidentally left his slides on the plane. You can imagine the challenge of giving a talk on metabolic disease without slides. This did not faze him. The talk was excellent and much was learned by the community doctors, our house staff, and me.

I have this wonderful picture of Dr Barness in my office, bowtie and all, and his great smile. I will always remember Dr Barness and will use the knowledge he passed on to me. I try to be like Dr Barness, always available, always willing to help, always engaging, always comforting, always caring, always ready to laugh. Dr Barness, I will never forget you.

Bertram Lubin, MD
Children's Hospital and Research Center
Oakland, CA, USA

E-mail address: blubin@mail.cho.org

JAIME L. FRÍAS, MD, FAAP, FACMG

Lew Barness was widely recognized and admired for his stature as a pediatrician and a scientist, his encyclopedic knowledge, his strong commitment to his patients and students, and his gentle demeanor. But sartorial elegance was definitely not one of his attributes, as he regularly purchased his clothing from Haband—a mail-order haberdasher. A frequently repeated story that forms part of the legend surrounding Lew tells that a few months after arriving in Tampa as the Founding Chairman of the Department of Pediatrics, and probably as a result of having ordered several new outfits befitting his new role, Haband executives contacted Lew to offer him a position as their local representative. He, obviously, did not accept the offer, but did continue to be their devoted customer.

Lew was also admired for his delightful sense of humor along with his quick and amusing comments and rejoinders. One example is a classic Lew Barness response during an interview for the Oral History Project of the American Academy of Pediatrics. While talking about Lew's days in medical school, the interviewer, Howard Pearson, asked him, "Your role models were General Practitioners, but you decided early to be a pediatrician. Why?" Lew responded, "I don't know why. I guess I felt that I would never grow up anyway." And, if keeping the curiosity and the positive and optimistic attitude of the young means not growing up, Lew indeed never did. Same as a child who loves without reservation, he loved his family, his friends, his colleagues, his students, and his patients. Same as a child, he ignored the imperfections of those of us who surrounded him. And, same as a child, he could laugh freely when he found that something was funny. In the dedication of *The Little Prince*, Saint-Exupéry writes, "All grown-ups were once children… but only few of them remember it." It is evident that Lew Barness never forgot.

Jaime L. Frías, MD, FAAP, FACMG
Department of Pediatrics
University of South Florida
Tampa, FL, USA

E-mail address: jfrias3540@gmail.com

JANE CARVER, PhD, MS, MPH

In 1980, I had the great fortune to be offered the opportunity to complete my graduate studies in Dr Barness' laboratory, where I worked under the guidance of him and Dr Susan Carlson. Those were exciting times in infant nutrition research. Considerable federal funding for research was available, and new analytical methods were revealing the unique components of human milk and their roles in infant nutrition and development. Dr Barness, a staunch advocate of breast-feeding, was convinced that "Mother Nature" knew best and was not wasteful. He accurately predicted that many human milk components considered to be artifacts did in fact play important roles in development. His insights led to improvements in infant formulas.

The atmosphere in Dr Barness' laboratory was one of hard work and dedication, tempered by fun, collegiality, and a stimulating intellectual atmosphere. Dr Barness was a very humble and light-hearted person, and he was quick to "correct" people who took themselves too seriously; he always did this in a kindly and amusing way. His birthday was a major event each year and we honored him in various ways, including having the entire lab wear T-shirts emblazoned with his picture, printing "Barness Bucks," and creating elaborate cakes themed after his favorite interests, including breast-feeding and baseball! One of Dr Barness' most endearing characteristics was the compassion he exhibited for colleagues, students, and employees. I often worked late in the lab, and it was not uncommon to find him in his office in the evening chatting with a member of the custodial staff, patiently listening to concerns they had about their children and families. Dr Barness made it clear to all of us that family interests came first. It's a lesson I have remembered over the years. His wisdom and guidance—both professional and personal—continue to guide me.

Jane Carver, PhD, MS, MPH
University of South Florida College of Medicine
Department of Pediatrics and Molecular Medicine
Tampa, FL, USA

E-mail address: jcarver@health.usf.edu

MICHAEL S. KAPPY, MD, PhD

Lew Barness was a giant in the field of pediatrics. He was the *only person in the long history of pediatrics* to be honored with all three of our most prestigious awards: the St. Geme Award (1991), the Jacobi Award (1991), and the Howland Award (1993).

He was born to Russian immigrants. His name, Barness, loosely translated from the Hebrew, as "Bar-Ness," means "son of a miracle." Whether or not this is accurate is not relevant, but he liked to mention it from time to time.

I once visited him and his wife, Enid, in Madison, Wisconsin, when he took a year's sabbatical from South Florida to be with her, a highly regarded professor of Pediatrics at the University of Wisconsin Medical School. He said, "It's too d*** cold here!"

He had a quality that drew people to him. In one of his tributes, it was stated that he was "one of the few remaining great clinicians, whose love for children, for his peers and students, and for advancing knowledge through research, and whose dedication to improving the human condition, have made him a 'legend in his own time'."

His list of publications numbers in the several hundreds. His trainees are also in the hundreds. His achievements were honored "officially" when he was Chief of Pediatrics at the University of South Florida Medical School, by the Mayor of Tampa's declaration of June 23, 1987 as "Lew Barness Day."

Finally, the American Academy of Pediatrics, in their Oral History Project in 1998, published a comprehensive interview of Lew by Dr Howard Pearson, a distinguished Professor of Pediatrics in his own right. When I asked Lew what he thought of the honor of being part of this project, he joked, "I fell asleep reading it."

It is fitting that we honor him in this volume of *Advances in Pediatrics*. He assumed the editor-in-chiefship of this journal in 1973—just the third person in this position since its founding in 1952. He served in that role for 30 years and remained on the Editorial Board along with Enid until he died. We miss him.

Michael S. Kappy, MD, PhD
Department of Pediatrics
University of Colorado School of Medicine
Children's Hospital Colorado
13123 East 16th Avenue
B-265, Aurora, CO 80045, USA

E-mail address: michael.kappy@childrenscolorado.org

Advances in Pediatrics 61 (2014) 1–6

ADVANCES IN PEDIATRICS

ELSEVIER
MOSBY

Foundations of Pediatrics
Lula Olga Lubchenco, MD (1915–2001); Scientist, Teacher, Mentor/Mother to Many

Patricia J. McFeeley, MD

Department of Pathology, Office of the Medical Investigator, University of New Mexico School of Medicine, MSC09 5040, 1 University of New Mexico, Albuquerque, NM 87131, USA

Keywords

• Lula Olga Lubchenco • Scientist • Teacher • Mentor

Lula Olga Lubchenco (Fig. 1) was born in Turkistan, Russia, in 1915. Her mother, an American doctor, had married a Russian agronomist whom she had met when he was in South Carolina studying cotton growing. Lula was the second of what eventually would be 5 children. She was, ironically, premature, (or maybe small for gestational age, she would later ponder). In 1917, the family fled war-torn Russia, escaping across Siberia to China, crossing the Pacific to San Francisco, and eventually arriving back at the family home and farm in South Carolina. In 1930, with the depression looming and the boll weevil destroying their cotton crop, the Lubchencos moved to northeast Colorado. Lula was 15 years old.

Following high school, Lula attended Denver University on a scholarship and graduated from University of Colorado School of Medicine in 1939. She did a rotating internship at Colorado General Hospital and then began her pediatric training at Strong Memorial Hospital in Rochester, New York; a position she had accepted and began before her decision to marry Carl Josephson, a Denver internist. She continued to use her maiden name professionally because at that time married women (or men) were not desirable candidates. Between 1941 and 1945 she returned to Denver Children's Hospital for her pediatric residency, a research fellowship, and a year in private practice. Her first publications were on polio and vitamin A absorption while she was a fellow with Dr Harold Palmer [1,2]. She became an associate in the Department of Pediatrics at the University of Colorado Medical Center in 1943 and moved through the academic ranks becoming Professor in 1969.

E-mail address: patricia.mcfeeley@gmail.com

0065-3101/14/$ – see front matter
http://dx.doi.org/10.1016/j.yapd.2014.04.002 © 2014 Elsevier Inc. All rights reserved.

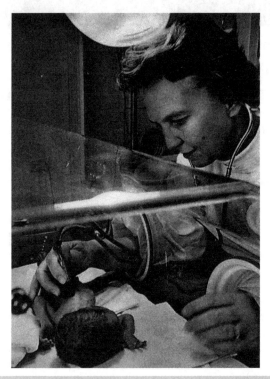

Fig. 1. Dr Lula Lubchenco.

When Colorado General Hospital under the direction of Drs Harry Gordon, Chair of Pediatrics, and E. Stewart Taylor, Chair of Obstetrics, established the Premature Infant Center in 1947, she became its first Medical Director. Lula said it was supposed to be a temporary position until they could find someone more suitable. She served as the director/codirector until her official retirement 30 years later. During the early years of the center she and Dr Taylor began the collaborative process of training pediatric and obstetrics residents together in neonatal resuscitation. Lula also recognized that, in order to ensure a good pregnancy outcome, prenatal care needed to encompass more than medical care, and she advocated for including social workers, nutritionists, and visiting nurses in the care of pregnant women. She published 2 prophetic articles: "Joint Responsibilities of Obstetrician and Pediatrician" in 1950 [3] and "Care of the Premature Infant" in 1951 [4]. Her research interests were always motivated by the challenges she met as a clinician.

Additional changes in care included advocating for transporting high-risk mothers to regional health care centers before delivery, suggesting that the mother was the best incubator for as long as possible for these tiny infants. She was also a staunch advocate for on-demand feeding, breast-feeding, and the associated rooming-in (in which a baby remains in the mother's room rather than the nursery). Although this was not well received by the nursing staff, which preferred the controlled environment of the nursery, she reportedly, and uncharacteristically, took a firm stand and gave them an ultimatum: it was either she or them in the nursery. When she thought a course of action was in the best interest of the baby and the mother, there was no compromise.

Perhaps the most distressing and anxious time in her career was in 1949, when the center had recently moved into the new and nearly state-of-the art nursery. The nursery was equipped with isolettes that had portholes for access, an oximeter to measure ambient oxygen, and facilities for the preparation of specific formulas with added vitamins, iron, and antibiotics. However, that was when she realized that, in spite of what they considered optimal care for these tiny babies, 8 of the first 12 babies in their nursery were blind from retrolental fibroplasia (RLF), now known as retinopathy of prematurity. In her own words, her reaction was a near panic. Her way of dealing with this was to conduct a scientific study. During the years 1943 to 1949 there had been a low incidence of RLF, so they went back to how they had cared for these tiny babies 5 years before: no isolettes; no water-soluble vitamins; no iron; no detergents; and, incidentally, low oxygen. Within 3 months blindness had significantly decreased. By exclusion, and supported by another study, they concluded that high oxygen was the cause. This was 1950. It took 6 years to convince colleagues in other centers that high oxygen concentrations were dangerous.

The natural extension of these studies was to examine the health and development of children who were graduates of the premature nursery as they returned to the so-called Crippled Children's clinic for care. There were no funds at first, so the faculty staff volunteered their time. The first study was focused on infants weighing less than 1500 g at birth and who had been admitted to the premature center from the opening of the center in 1947 to 1950. The results were published as "Sequelae of Premature Birth: Evaluation of Premature Infants of Low Birth Weights at 10 Years of Age" [5], and this was the beginning of many long-term follow-up studies for which she is well known.

Among her more than 52 published articles, 34 abstracts, 19 chapters in books, and her own book *The High Risk Infant*, her sentinel publication on intrauterine growth in 1963 [6] earned worldwide recognition. That publication and subsequent data from more than 40 years of practice has become known and recognized as the Lula Gram (Fig. 2).

The original article evaluated the intrauterine growth of nearly 6000 live-born infants admitted to Colorado General Hospital from 1948 to 1961. It was a landmark in that, for the first time, it provided data from live-born infants with known gestational duration. The curves divided the chart into 9 curvilinear zones based on birth weight and gestational age and delineated the differences, as an example, between small babies caused by prematurity and those caused by intrauterine growth retardation (now called growth restriction). "Dr Lubchenco was primarily responsible for the important new concept of the small-for-gestational-age

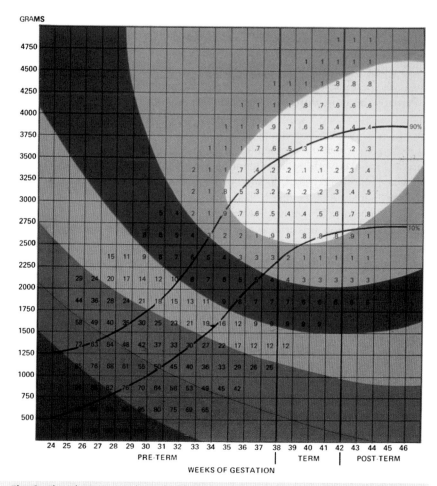

Fig. 2. The Lula Gram: newborn classification and neonatal mortality risk by birth weight and gestational age (1972).

(SGA) infant," said Henry Kempe, MD, former Chair of Pediatrics at the University of Colorado in a 1983 profile in *Perinatology-Neonatology*. Lula and her colleagues also recognized the relationship between high altitude and intrauterine growth, citing data from Lake County (Leadville), Colorado (altitude 3094 m [10,152 feet]), where term appropriate-for-gestational-age infants had a mean birth weight of 200 g less than appropriate-for-gestational-age infants at the lower altitude of Denver (1609 m [5280 feet]). In a recent analysis in the journal *Pediatrics* identifying the 100 most cited pediatric articles between 1945 and 2010, Lula was an author or coauthor of 3 of them [7].

Perhaps Lula's greatest contribution to medicine was her lasting influence on generations of medical students, pediatric residents, and neonatology fellows. In the words of Dr Richard Krugman, Dean, University of Colorado Medical

School: "For more than a half century she helped thousands of trainees overcome their fear of even touching tiny premature babies, and, in her remarkable quiet competence, helped our oversized awkward hands learn how to examine, treat, and comfort neonates." This characterized how she taught and how she lived. As Dr Krugman put it, "When something was going on with a baby we didn't understand, she would say with a little twinkle in her eye, 'let's see if we can figure this out.' It was rare that we didn't."

Although Dr Lu, as she was fondly known, was the recipient of numerous honors and awards, including the University of Colorado Alumni Silver and Gold Award, the Virginia Apgar Award in Perinatal Pediatrics, the naming of the Lubchenco Premature Infant and Family Center in her honor, and a second honorary Doctorate of Medicine Degree from the University of Colorado Medical School, you would never have known it or heard it from her.

Lula and her husband Dr Carl Josephson (Dr Joe) had 4 daughters, the first 2 of whom became physicians. The third was a graduate of the Colorado Child Health Associate Program (started by Dr Henry Silver) and is also a lawyer. Their youngest daughter, Gretchen, was born with Down syndrome. Thus started a less recognized but important aspect of her professional and personal life: her advocacy and leadership for children and adults with Down syndrome. Dr Lu and Dr Joe encouraged and supported their youngest daughter, at a time when there were few available resources, to gain the skills needed to become a national and international spokesperson and self-advocate for Down syndrome, as well as a published poet. Dr Lu was instrumental in the development of the Denver Adult Down Syndrome Clinic.

Although her full-time academic career spanned from 1943 to 1977, she continued to contribute to academic medicine and served on the admissions and ethics committees until her unexpected death in 2001 at 86 years of age.

Acknowledgments

I would like to thank my sisters Johanna Abernathy, MD, and Karen Josephson, PA-C, JD, for their input and support and my son Matthew McFeeley, MPP, JD for his excellent editing and advice. In addition, of course, I also thank Gretchen Josephson for her continued inspiration to us all. Deep thanks to Drs Lu-Ann Papile, Virginia Delaney-Black, Michael Kappy, and Richard Krugman, along with Perry Butterfield, MA, for giving me their time and significant input. Thanks also to our mother for keeping files of her correspondence, drafts, photographs, and hand-written notes that, although invaluable and enlightening, caused me many a tearful break from my writings.

References

[1] Lubchenco LO, Scandalis R, Palmer H, et al. Poliomyelitis 1943, Children's Hospital, Denver. Rocky Mt Med J 1944.

[2] Palmer HD, Danielson WH, Lubchenco LO, et al. Absorption of vitamin A following enteral use of prostigmine in cystic fibrosis of pancreas. Am J Clin Pathol 1946;10:535–49.

[3] Taylor ES, Lubchenco LO. Joint responsibilities of obstetrician and pediatrician. Am J Nurs 1950;50:275–7.

[4] Githens JH, Lubchenco LO. Care of the premature infant. Postgrad Med 1951;10:62.

[5] Lubchenco LO, Horner FA, Reed LH, et al. Sequelae of premature birth: evaluation of premature infants of low birth weights at 10 years of age. Am J Dis Child 1963;106:101–15.

[6] Lubchenco LO, Hansman C, Dressler M, et al. Intrauterine growth: a standard derived from liveborn infants 24 to 42 weeks of gestation. Pediatrics 1963;32:793–800.

[7] Quinn N, Hensey O, McDowell DT. A historical perspective of pediatric publications: a bibliometric analysis. Pediatrics 2013;132(3):406–12.

Advances in Pediatrics 61 (2014) 7–31

ELSEVIER
MOSBY

Advances in Pediatric Pharmacology, Therapeutics, and Toxicology

Daniel Gonzalez, PharmD, PhD[a,b], Ian M. Paul, MD, MSc[c,d],
Daniel K. Benjamin Jr, MD, PhD, MPH[b,e],
Michael Cohen-Wolkowiez, MD, PhD[b,e,*]

[a]Division of Pharmacotherapy and Experimental Therapeutics, UNC Eshelman School of Pharmacy, University of North Carolina at Chapel Hill, 301 Pharmacy Lane, Chapel Hill, NC 27599, USA; [b]Duke Clinical Research Institute, Duke University Medical Center, 2400 Pratt Street, Durham, NC 27705, USA; [c]Department of Pediatrics, College of Medicine, Penn State University, 500 University Drive, HS83, Hershey, PA 17033, USA; [d]Department of Public Health Sciences, College of Medicine, Penn State University, 500 University Drive, HS83, Hershey, PA 17033, USA; [e]Department of Pediatrics, College of Medicine, Duke University, T901/Children's Health Center, Durham, NC 27705, USA

Keywords

• Pediatrics • Pharmacology • Pharmacokinetics • Toxicology

Key points

• Pediatric research has expanded in the United States and Europe, largely because of legislation providing a framework for the design and execution of pediatric studies.
• Although much work remains, as a result of greater regulatory guidance more pediatric data are reaching product labels.
• The pharmacokinetic/pharmacodynamic properties of many drugs used to treat children have yet to be characterized.

INTRODUCTION

Significant advancements have been made in pediatric therapeutics over the last 2 years. Of note, the US Food and Drug Administration Safety and Innovation Act (FDASIA) was signed into law on July 9, 2012, making the Best

Disclosure: See last page of article.

*Corresponding author. Duke Clinical Research Institute, Duke University Medical Center, P.O. Box 17969, Durham, NC 27715. *E-mail address*: michael.cohenwolkowiez@duke.edu

0065-3101/14/$ – see front matter
http://dx.doi.org/10.1016/j.yapd.2014.03.005   © 2014 Elsevier Inc. All rights reserved.

Pharmaceuticals for Children Act (BPCA) and Pediatric Research Equity Act (PREA) permanent for the Food and Drug Administration (FDA), no longer requiring reauthorization every 5 years. BPCA, which was also authorized for the National Institutes of Health (NIH) for the next 5 years, provides a mechanism for off-patent drug development and a pediatric exclusivity incentive, encouraging manufacturers to perform pediatric studies in exchange for an additional 6 months of patent protection. PREA gives the FDA the authority to require that studies be performed if the indication being sought for approval in adults is relevant to child health. As a result of BPCA and PREA, pediatric labeling information has improved, but one analysis reported that as of 2009 only 46% of drugs had some labeling information related to pediatric use, an increase from the 22% estimated in 1975; also, 41% of new molecular entities had pediatric labeling, up from 20% in 1999 [1]. A summary of select labeling changes made by the FDA in 2012 and 2013 is presented in Table 1.

In Europe, the Pediatric Regulation went into effect in 2007 to promote the expansion of pediatric research in this region. The European Medicines Agency (EMA) highlighted successes over the first 5 years of the regulation, and reported that about 400 clinical trials including children (0–18 years) are performed each year. The EMA Pediatric Committee has agreed to more than 600 Pediatric Investigational Plans (PIPs) with pharmaceutical companies, and a large collaboration of pediatric research networks (Enpr-EMA) has been created [2]. More pediatric research has translated into more information in the Summary of Product Characteristics: 221 changes with regard to safety and efficacy, 89 additions of dosing information, and 77 other modifications related to new study data being added [2].

An important requirement in FDASIA and in the EMA Pediatric Regulation is that clinical trials also be performed in neonates when appropriate, because neonates historically have been excluded from drug trials far too often. If neonatal studies are not warranted or cannot be performed for logistical or ethical reasons, sponsors must provide justification. This provision is important, as limited pharmacokinetic (PK) and pharmacodynamic (PD) data are available in this vulnerable population. Between 1997 and 2012 only 31 drug products were studied in neonates, resulting in labeling changes for 27; these figures are relatively small when compared with pediatric studies performed in older age groups for more than 400 drug products [3]. A separate analysis indicated that approximately 54% of neonatal labeling changes resulted in addition of the following statement: "safety and efficacy have not been established" [4]. For the remaining 46% (4 human immunodeficiency virus [HIV] drugs, 3 anesthesia drugs, 4 drugs for other indications), an approval for use in neonates was obtained [4]. Therefore there is an overall lack of PK/PD data in neonates, in particular premature infants, and clinical trials are not being performed for widely prescribed medications in this population.

Another concern receiving considerable attention relates to drug shortages. Drug shortages can be problematic because they cause clinicians to alter drug treatment and, in some cases, prescribe less effective or more toxic medications. For example, for the treatment of Hodgkin lymphoma in children, one study reported less favorable outcomes when cyclophosphamide was prescribed in place of mechlorethamine as a result of a drug shortage [5]. One survey found that 83% of oncologists polled reported being unable to prescribe standard chemotherapy because of drug shortages [6]. In February 2012, the American Academy of Pediatrics (AAP) submitted testimony to the US House of Representatives Committee on Energy and Commerce Subcommittee on Health, stressing the impact of drug shortages for pediatricians [7]. Then, in March 2013, AAP provided comments on the establishment of an FDA Drug Shortages Task Force and Strategic Plan [8]. Pursuant to FDASIA, the FDA was asked to develop this task force to address drug shortages; as stated in the FDA's strategic plan, the goal of the task force will be to develop mitigation strategies when the agency is informed of a drug shortage and a long-term prevention plan [9].

In light of the aforementioned developments, the goal of this article is to highlight important advancements made in pediatric pharmacology, toxicology, and therapeutics from January 2012 to December 2013. Select articles were chosen to identify important developments within various therapeutic areas with the exception of oncology, for which only FDA label changes made over the last 2 years are highlighted.

ANESTHESIA
Pharmacokinetics

Etomidate is a hypnotic drug used for induction of general anesthesia. Because data are lacking, it is not currently recommended for use in children younger than 10 years [10]. With the goal of describing the drug's disposition in children, a population PK analysis was performed [11]. Forty-nine children with a median age of 4 years (range 0.53–13.21 years) undergoing elective surgery received an intravenous bolus dose of etomidate (0.3 mg/kg). After accounting for size-based differences (ie, body weight) in PK parameters, an increased clearance and central volume of distribution was observed for younger children (0.5 vs 4 years reported). Hemodynamic changes were stable, and only slight decreases in systolic blood pressure were noted. As a result, the investigators suggest that younger children may require higher bolus doses [11].

Sedation

Dexmedetomidine, an intravenous α_2-adrenergic agonist, is widely prescribed off-label as a sedative agent for children. Dexmedetomidine is currently not approved by the FDA or EMA for use in pediatric patients because efficacy and safety have not been established, but the lack of respiratory depression and relatively short half-life (~ 2 hours) are major advantages to the use of this agent. Unfortunately, few studies have evaluated the use of dexmedetomidine in children. A retrospective analysis evaluated the safety and efficacy of prolonged dexmedetomidine use in critically ill children with cardiovascular disease [12]. A total of 52 children (median age 10.5 months; interquartile range 5.8–20 months) received dexmedetomidine via continuous infusion for at least

Table 1
Select drug-label changes made by US Food and Drug Administration in 2012 and 2013

Generic name	Trade name	Indication studied	Summary of label change(s)
Azelastine	Astepro nasal spray	Treatment of perennial and seasonal allergic rhinitis	Expanded indication to include pediatric patients ≥6 y of age
Beclomethasone dipropionate	QNASL	Treatment of nasal symptoms associated with seasonal and perennial allergic rhinitis	Safety and efficacy established in pediatric patients ≥12 y of age
Dexmedetomidine hydrochloride	Precedex	Sedation in intubated and mechanically ventilated patients	Safety and effectiveness for procedural or intensive care unit sedation is not established in pediatric patients
Dolutegravir	Tivicay	Treatment of human immunodeficiency virus (HIV)-1 infection	Indicated in combination with other antiretroviral drugs in children ≥12 y of age and weighing ≥40 kg
Duloxetine hydrochloride	Cymbalta	Treatment of major depressive disorder (MDD)	Efficacy was not established in 2 10-week, placebo-controlled trials of 800 patients with MDD 7–17 y of age
Entravirine	Intelence	Treatment of HIV-1 in treatment-experienced patients with other antiretroviral drugs	Expanded indication to include pediatric patients ≥6 y of age
Eszopiclone	Lunesta	Attention-deficit/hyperactivity disorder (ADHD) associated with insomnia	Safety and effectiveness have not been established in pediatric patients
Fluticasone/ salmeterol	Advair HFA	Treatment of asthma	Safety and effectiveness have not been established in children <12 y of age
Fosamprenavir	Lexiva	Treatment of HIV-1 infection	Expanded indication to include pediatric patients 4 wk to <2 y of age
Iron sucrose	Venofer	Treatment of iron-deficiency anemia in patients with chronic kidney disease	Expanded indication from adults to pediatric patients ≥2 y of age
Ivermectin	Sklice	Topical treatment of head lice infestations	Safety and efficacy established in children ≥6 mo of age

Generic	Brand	Indication	Pediatric Labeling Update
Lisdexamfetamine	Vyvanse	Maintenance treatment of ADHD	Approved for treatment of ADHD in patients aged 6–17 y
Micafungin sodium	Mycamine	Treatment and prophylaxis of *Candida* infections	Safety and effectiveness demonstrated in pediatric patients ≥4 mo of age
Montelukast	Singulair oral granules, tablets, and chewable tablets	Prevention of exercise-induced bronchoconstriction	Expanded indication to include pediatric patients 6–14 y of age
Nevirapine	Viramune XR	Treatment of HIV-1 infection	Approved for use as treatment for HIV-1 infection with other antiretroviral agents in children ≥6 to <18 y of age
Olanzapine and fluoxetine	Symbyax	Treatment of depressive episodes associated with bipolar I disorder	Expanded indication to include pediatric patients age 10–17 y
Oxcarbazepine	Oxtellar XR	Adjunctive therapy for partial seizures	Safety and effectiveness for treatment of partial-onset seizures is established in pediatric patients 6–16 y of age
Perampanel	Fycompa	Treatment of partial-onset seizures with or without secondarily generalized seizures in patients with epilepsy	Safety and efficacy in pediatric patients 12–16 y of age established by 3 double-blind, placebo-controlled studies
Rabeprazole	Aciphex	Gastroesophageal reflux	Expanded indication to pediatric patients ≥1 y of age
Retapamulin	Altabax	Treatment of impetigo	Use not indicated in patients <9 mo of age
Sildenafil	Revatio	Treatment of pulmonary hypertension	Warning added: "Use of Revatio, particularly chronic use, is not recommended in children"
Tenofovir disoproxil fumarate	Viread	Treatment of chronic hepatitis B	Expanded indication from adults to include pediatric patients 12 to <18 y of age
Tenofovir disoproxil fumarate	Viread	Treatment of HIV infection in combination with other antiretroviral agents	Expanded indication from adults to include pediatric patients 2 to <12 y of age, weighing ≥17 kg, and who can swallow an intact tablet

Data from the FDA Pediatric Labeling Information Database. Available at: http://www.accessdata.fda.gov/scripts/sda/sdNavigation.cfm?sd=labelingdatabase. Accessed December 9, 2013.

96 hours. When compared with control patients who received conventional sedative agents (eg, midazolam), no differences were noted in mechanical ventilation, length of stay in the intensive care unit, heart rate, or blood pressure measurements between treatment groups. Moreover, dexmedetomidine use was associated with a shorter duration of continuous midazolam and morphine infusions. No serious safety concerns were reported. In a small sample of patients with heart failure, dexmedetomidine did not appear to affect heart rate, mean arterial pressure, or inotrope score when the drug infusion was stopped [13].

Another retrospective analysis evaluated outcomes of hypotension, hypertension, and bradycardia in a large sample (N = 669) of children (median age 4.5 years; range 0.1–22.5 years) who received dexmedetomidine for sedation during nuclear medicine imaging [14]. Hypotension, hypertension, and bradycardia, defined as a 20% or greater deviation from age-adjusted awake normal values, occurred in 58.7%, 2.1%, and 4.3% of children, respectively. Older children (age categories 3–6 and 6–12 years) experienced a significantly greater number of hypotensive and bradycardic events relative to younger peers. None of these events, however, required pharmacologic treatment.

In a prospective, randomized, double-blind, clinical trial, intranasal dexmedetomidine was compared with intranasal midazolam in 90 children (median age 6 years; interquartile range 2–9) undergoing adenotonsillectomy [15]. All patients also received general anesthesia with nitrous oxide, oxygen, and sevoflurane administered via a face mask. Midazolam and dexmedetomidine were found to be equally effective with regard to decreasing anxiety following separation from parents, but midazolam was superior in obtaining satisfactory mask induction (82.2% vs 60%, $P = .01$).

CARDIOLOGY
Pulmonary hypertension
Sildenafil is a phosphodiesterase-5 inhibitor used for the treatment of pulmonary arterial hypertension (PAH). In adults, sildenafil is labeled for the treatment of PAH, whereas in children it is used off-label. The Sildenafil in Treatment-Naïve Children With Pulmonary Arterial Hypertension trial (STARTS-1) was a randomized, double-blind, placebo-controlled, dose-ranging study designed to evaluate the safety and efficacy of sildenafil citrate administered to children (age 1–17 years weighing ≥ 8 kg) with PAH [16]. With regard to efficacy, percentage change in peak oxygen consumption reached only marginal significance for all dose groups combined, although improvements, including hemodynamics and functional class, were noted for the medium and high groups when compared with placebo. For safety outcomes, sildenafil was well tolerated over a 16-week period; however, in the STARTS-2 trial, long-term treatment (>2 years) with high doses resulted in greater mortality [16]. On August 30, 2012, the FDA issued a Drug Safety Communication informing clinicians of the STARTS-2 findings and reminding them that use in children is an off-label recommendation, not approved by the agency [17]. Moreover, the EMA revised its Summary of Product Characteristics to inform

clinicians that doses higher than those recommended by the agency should not be used in pediatric patients with PAH [18].

Hypertension

In obese children and adolescents, identifying and treating systemic prehypertension (systolic or diastolic blood pressure $\geq$90th and <95th percentile) is important, as this group of patients is at risk for progression to hypertension [19,20]. Some have hypothesized that uric acid may play an important role in hypertension and cardiovascular disease. A randomized, double-blind trial was performed to assess the impact of uric acid reduction in obese adolescents treated with allopurinol, probenecid, or placebo [20]. Patients treated with urate-lowering drugs had a significant reduction in systolic (−10.2 vs 1.7 mm Hg), diastolic (−9 vs 1.6 mm Hg), and systemic vascular resistance when compared with placebo. These results indicate that in prehypertensive obese adolescents, uric acid reduction may play a role in reducing blood pressure.

Few studies of antihypertensive agents in children have been conducted over the past 2 years. The PK and safety of the antihypertensive agent olmesartan medoxomil was evaluated in children and adolescents (age 12 months to 16 years) [21]. Olmesartan is an angiotensin II receptor blocker used in the treatment of hypertension. Although one of the goals of this study was to collect data in children 12 to 23 months of age, no patients in this age group were enrolled. In the older age groups, a total of 24 hypertensive patients were studied. Body size–adjusted oral clearance (CL/F) and volume of distribution (V/F) estimates were found to be similar to those in adults (CL/F 0.06–0.1 L/h/kg; V/F 0.32–0.49 L/kg). No serious adverse effects were reported. Another study evaluated the safety PK of the phosphodiesterase III inhibitor, milrinone, which is used off-label in the pediatric population for the treatment of pulmonary hypertension [22]. Eleven neonates with persistent pulmonary hypertension received milrinone as an intravenous loading dose (50 µg/kg) over 60 minutes, and a maintenance infusion (0.33–0.99 µg/kg/min) for 24 to 72 hours. When compared with a published study in older children (mean 4.7 years; range 0.7–15 years) [23], both clearance (0.11 vs 0.6 L/kg/h) and steady-state volume of distribution (0.6 vs 1.5 L/kg) were lower in neonates. In patients with a poor response to inhaled nitric oxide, improvements in pulmonary and systemic hemodynamics were noted.

Congenital heart disease

Systemic-to-pulmonary artery shunts are placed in some patients with cyanotic congenital heart disease. Because of the risk for shunt thrombosis, antiplatelet agents are frequently prescribed. A multicenter, double-blind, event-driven trial randomized infants to clopidogrel 0.2 mg/kg/day (n = 467) or placebo (n = 439) to assess whether addition of clopidogrel to conventional therapy improved shunt-related morbidity or all-cause mortality [24]. No differences were noted between the groups for the primary composite end point or in any subgroup analyses, or in bleeding rates. The results of this trial indicate that clopidogrel did not provide any additional benefit over conventional therapy alone.

DERMATOLOGY

The American Acne and Rosacea Society published guidelines, which were reviewed and endorsed by the AAP, that specifically address the management of pediatric acne [25]. The expert recommendations provide a framework for: classification of pediatric acne based on age and form of presentation; severity assessment; and treatment algorithms. Potential treatment options discussed include over-the-counter (OTC) use of topical benzoyl peroxide, topical retinoids, topical/oral antibiotics, isotretinoin, and hormonal therapy. Additional considerations such as medication adherence, selection of an appropriate formulation, impact of previous treatment and history, prevention of bacterial resistance, and psychological factors are also discussed.

GASTROENTEROLOGY

Crohn disease

Crohn disease is a chronic, systemic inflammatory condition that can affect any part of the gastrointestinal tract. Cases of Crohn disease in children can be of greater severity than those in adults, and approximately 18% of patients require surgery within 5 years of disease onset [26]. Initial treatment of the disease in children includes corticosteroids or enteral nutrition, with the latter favored in Europe, followed by use of immunomodulatory drugs (eg, azathioprine, 6-mercaptopurine) [27,28]. Thalidomide is an immunomodulatory drug that may be effective as an alternative treatment in some patients with Crohn disease [29]. A multicenter, randomized, double-blind, placebo-controlled clinical trial evaluated the use of thalidomide on clinical remission in 56 children (mean age ∼ 15 years, range 2–18 years) with active Crohn disease despite being on immunosuppressive treatment [26]. Clinical activity was assessed at predefined time points using a validated clinical activity index, the Pediatric Chronic Disease Activity Index (PCDAI) score. The primary study outcome was clinical remission at week 8, defined as a PCDAI score of 10 or less, and a reduction in the PCDAI score of at least 25% or 75% at weeks 4 and 8, respectively. Patients were administered thalidomide (1.5–2.5 mg/kg/d) or placebo for 8 weeks. In an open-label extension study, patients originally randomized to placebo and who were not in remission or did not have at least a 75% reduction in their PCDAI score were given thalidomide for an additional 8 weeks. Responders to treatment were followed for at least 52 weeks. Of 28 and 26 children administered thalidomide and placebo, respectively, greater clinical remission was observed with drug treatment (13 of 28 [46.4%] vs 3 of 26 [11.5%]; risk ratio 4.0; 95% confidence interval [CI] 1.2–12.5; $P = .01$). In the open-label phase, for patients initially randomized to placebo and then administered thalidomide, 11 of 21 (52.4%) had reached clinical remission at week 8 (risk ratio 4.5; 95% CI 1.4–14.1; $P = .01$). The most common serious adverse effect was peripheral neuropathy, with an incidence of 1 per 1000 patient-weeks for clinical manifestations (no electromyography alterations) to 2.7 per 1000 patient-weeks for electromyography alterations (no clinical manifestation). The results of this study showed that thalidomide resulted in greater clinical remission at 8 weeks and long-term maintenance of remission when compared with placebo [26].

Tumor necrosis factor (TNF) antagonists are also effective in the treatment of Crohn disease. Infliximab is approved by the FDA and EMA for treatment of moderate to severe Crohn disease in pediatric patients 6 years of age or older who fail to respond to conventional treatments (corticosteroids, enteral nutrition, and immunomodulators). In a phase 3, multicenter, randomized, open-label trial, the TNF antagonist adalimumab was studied in children with severe Crohn disease [30]. The percentage of patients in clinical remission at weeks 26 and 52 were 33.5% and 28.4%, respectively. No statistically significant differences were noted between high-dose and low-dose groups (38.7% vs 28.4%, $P = .075$). The safety profile was found to be comparable with that observed in adults.

Interestingly in a separate analysis, data collected from a large prospective, observational study (RISK: Risk Stratification and Identification of Immunogenetic and Microbial Markers of Rapid Disease Progression in Children with Crohn's Disease) was used to assess whether early (within 3 months of diagnosis) treatment with TNF antagonists improves 1-year outcomes when compared with early immunomodulatory monotherapy [28]. Immunomodulatory therapy included azathioprine, 6-mercaptopurine, and methotrexate. A propensity score analysis was performed to compare study outcomes between treatment groups. The investigators reported that early treatment with an anti-TNFα drug was associated with greater remission than early treatment with an immunomodulator (85.3% vs 60.3%; relative risk 1.41; 95% CI 1.14–1.75; $P = .0017$). With regard to early immunomodulator therapy versus no early immunotherapy, no differences were noted in achieving remission at 1 year (60.3% vs 54.4%; relative risk 1.11; 95% CI 0.83–1.48; $P = .49$). The investigators acknowledge that additional data are needed to identify which children would be most likely to benefit from treatment with anti-TNFα agents [28].

Constipation

When patients with autism spectrum disorder suffer from gastrointestinal discomfort such as diarrhea, constipation, and dyspepsia, identification, diagnosis, and treatment of these symptoms is challenging. The Gastroenterology Committee of the Autism Speaks Autism Treatment Network (ATN) performed a systematic review of the literature and field testing with the goal of generating a treatment algorithm useful for clinicians [31]. Using the North American Society of Pediatric Gastroenterology, Hepatology, and Nutrition (NASPGHAN) treatment guideline for constipation as an initial template, an optimized guideline for children with autism was developed, first by expert opinion and then by applying the optimized algorithm in 4 pilot sites where the feasibility was evaluated by autism health care providers. Atypical and in particular self-abusive behavior and posturing (eg, grimacing, holding abdomen), were noted as potential signs and symptoms of constipation. Field testing demonstrated that the algorithm was "readily applied and did not interrupt the clinic flow," and highlighted the importance of follow-up visits and identifying nonresponders early in treatment [31]. Treatment options and appropriate dosages were also noted. The investigators observed that children with autism may not respond as favorably to standard treatment because of "volume, texture, or taste sensitivities" [31].

Dyspepsia

Cyproheptadine, a serotonin and histamine antagonist, has been used in children as an appetite stimulant. One study sought to evaluate the use of cyproheptadine in children and adolescents with dyspeptic symptoms who were refractory to other treatment options (dietary changes, H_2-antagonists, and/or proton-pump inhibitors) [32]. A retrospective open-label study was performed with response to cyproheptadine treatment assessed at clinic visits. Patients with idiopathic disease and those with a known pathophysiologic cause for the dyspepsia (eg, fundoplication) were included in the analysis. Out of a total of 80 patients, 44 responded to treatment (33 had a "significant response"; symptoms resolved in 11). In a multivariate analysis, a superior response was noted in children younger than 12 years and in females. Moreover, the frequency of responders was higher (12 of 14 = 86%) in patients who received the drug following Nissen fundoplication. The most common side effects were somnolence (16%), irritability and behavioral changes (6%), weight gain (5%), and abdominal pain (2.5%).

INFECTIOUS DISEASES

Pharmacokinetics

Over the last 2 years, advancements have been made in characterizing drug disposition for several anti-infective agents (Table 2). Characterizing the PK of drugs in children is critical in accounting for physiologic and developmental changes that may affect drug exposure.

Pneumonia

Clinical practice guidelines (CPG) can provide a framework for clinicians to diagnose and treat medical conditions, and can potentially affect antimicrobial selection, costs, and outcomes. One study sought to evaluate the impact of institutional CPG for community-acquired pneumonia (CAP) on length of stay in hospital, readmission within 14 days of discharge, and antibiotic selection, among other outcomes [50]. A multicenter, retrospective cohort study was performed using data collected through the Pediatric Health Information Database. Data from 43 tertiary care children's hospitals were reviewed; a survey sent to each institution to query the availability of a CPG; and relevant outcomes compared between institutions with and without CPGs. Of 43 hospitals, 41 completed the survey (95%), and 13 (32%) indicated that they had an institutional CPG for nonsevere CAP. Significant between-institution variability in

Table 2
Recently published pediatric pharmacokinetic studies of anti-infective agents

Drug	Patient population	PK analysis approach	Dosing modifications recommended for studied population (yes/no)
Antimicrobials			
Daptomycin [33]	Infants	Noncompartmental	Yes
Daptomycin [34]	Infants and children	Descriptive	Yes
Metronidazole [35]	Preterm infants	Population	Yes
Tigecycline [36]	Children	Noncompartmental	Yes
Vancomycin [37]	Neonates	Population	Yes
Vancomycin [38]	Children <18 y	Population	Yes
Antifungals			
Fluconazole [39]	Infants	Individual, compartmental	Yes
Micafungin [40]	Infants, children, adolescents	Noncompartmental	No
Voriconazole [41]	Children, adolescents, adults	Population	Yes
Antivirals			
Abacavir [42]	Infants and toddlers	Population	Yes
Acyclovir [43]	Preterm and term infants	Population	Yes
Darunavir/ ritonavir [44]	Children	Noncompartmental	No
Etravirine [45]	Children and adolescents	Noncompartmental	Yes
Oseltamivir [46]	Neonates and infants	Population	Yes
Tenofovir [47]	Children and adolescents	Population	No
Valganciclovir [48]	Infants and children	Noncompartmental	Yes
Antimalarials			
Artesunate [49]	Infants and children	Population	Yes

the recommendations for diagnostic testing was noted by the investigators. For the 19,710 children included in the analysis, no differences were noted between institutions with and without CPGs for the following outcomes: length of stay in hospital, hospital readmissions at 14 days, hospital costs, and ordering patterns for most diagnostic tests. The exception to the latter was that institutions that recommended viral testing (eg, influenza or respiratory syncytial viral testing) were more successful in having this test performed. By contrast, antibiotic drug selection was associated with CPG recommendations. At institutions with a CPG, penicillins and aminopenicillins were more likely to be prescribed when recommended as first-line treatment (46.3% vs 23.9%). As a result, the investigators concluded that the availability of CPGs did not affect resource utilization, whereas antibiotic impact was notably different.

In a separate study, the impact of CPGs on antibiotic management of children with CAP was investigated [51]. A retrospective analysis was performed using medical records of patients discharged from Children's Mercy Hospital in Kansas City, Missouri, 12 months before and after the CPG was introduced. The impact of an antimicrobial stewardship program was also assessed. A total of 1033 patients were included in the analysis: 530 (51%) before and 503 (49%) after introduction of the CPG. The key recommendations in the CPG were use of empiric treatment with ampicillin, then use of amoxicillin on discharge, and treatment duration of 5 to 7 days [51]. The investigators reported that use of the CPG successfully led to an increased use of ampicillin (13% before vs 63% after) and a decrease in ceftriaxone prescribing (72% before vs 21% after). For discharge antibiotics, there was also a statistically significant increased use of amoxicillin (P <.001), whereas prescribing of cefdinir and amoxicillin-clavulanate was significantly lower (P <.001); the combined effect of the CPG and antimicrobial stewardship program resulted in decreases of 12% and 16%, respectively. In uncomplicated CAP, the use of a CPG and antimicrobial stewardship program successfully aided in changing antimicrobial prescribing patterns at one institution.

For the treatment of severe pneumonia, a randomized, double-blind, placebo-controlled clinical trial was performed to assess the benefit of zinc supplementation as adjuvant therapy in 610 children [52]. The primary outcome, time to cessation of severe pneumonia (defined using the Integrated Management of Childhood Illness algorithm), was assessed in a total of 580 children (2–35 months of age) who were enrolled in the study until recovery from the condition (288 zinc; 292 placebo). A standardized treatment algorithm was used for all patients, and zinc or placebo was administered as a single oral dose for up to 14 days. Neither the median time to cessation of severe pneumonia nor the risk of treatment failure was significantly different between the zinc and placebo groups, although marginal differences were noted. The results of this study do not provide compelling evidence to recommend the use of zinc as adjuvant therapy in young children with severe pneumonia.

Intra-abdominal infections

Meropenem is a broad-spectrum antibiotic currently approved by the FDA for the treatment of bacterial meningitis and/or complicated intra-abdominal infections in children 3 months of age and upward. The results of an open-label, 24-center, prospective, multidose, PK, safety, and effectiveness study in infants younger than 91 days treated with meropenem for suspected or confirmed intra-abdominal infection were recently published [53]. Dosing groups evaluated were based on gestational age (GA) and postnatal age (PNA): group 1 (GA <32 weeks, PNA <2 weeks), 20 mg/kg every 12 hours; groups 2 (GA <32 weeks, PNA ≥2 weeks) and 3 (GA ≥32 weeks, PNA <2 weeks), 20 mg/kg every 8 hours; and group 4 (GA ≥32 weeks, PNA ≥2 weeks), 30 mg/kg every 8 hours. Treatment duration lasted between at least 3 and up to 21 days. A total of 200 infants were enrolled in the study, 142 (71%) of whom were less than 32 weeks GA. In terms of efficacy, of 192 infants, therapeutic success was reported in 162 (84%). The lowest frequency of success

(29 of 39 [74%]) was observed for infants in group 1 (GA <32 weeks, PNA <2 weeks). Adverse events were reported for 99 infants (50%), of which 30 events in 21 infants were deemed to be possibly related to meropenem. Moreover, there were 36 serious adverse events in 34 infants (17%), of which 2 were deemed as possibly related to meropenem. The most common adverse effects were sepsis (6%), seizures (5%), elevated conjugated bilirubin (5%), and hypokalemia (5%). The study results demonstrate that most infants met the criteria for therapeutic success and that meropenem was generally well tolerated.

Hepatitis B
Adefovir dipivoxil and tenofovir disoproxil fumarate are both nucleotide analogues with activity against the hepatitis B virus. Moreover, both are FDA-approved for treatment against hepatitis infection in patients 12 years of age or older. Two separate studies were performed to study the safety and efficacy of these agents in the pediatric population. First, the results of a long-term (up to 240 weeks), open-label study evaluating adefovir use in 162 pediatric patients originally enrolled in a 48-week, double-blind, placebo-controlled trial were reported [54]. Following the original 48-week study, continued viral suppression and normalization of alanine aminotransferase was observed for patients on adefovir alone or in combination with lamivudine. Virologic failure was reported for 61 of 162 patients on adefovir; hepatitis B envelope antigen (HBeAg) and surface antigen seroconversion were reported in 55 and 5 subjects, respectively. Adefovir resistance was reported for 1 treatment-naïve child who was on monotherapy. Adefovir was generally well tolerated during long-term use.

A separate double-blind, placebo-controlled study evaluated the efficacy and safety of tenofovir disoproxil fumarate in adolescents (12 to <18 years of age) [55]. A total of 101 patients completed 72 weeks of tenofovir treatment, with the primary outcome being virologic response (<400 copies/mL hepatitis B DNA) at week 72. Patients were randomized to once-daily tenofovir disoproxil fumarate 300 mg (n = 52) or placebo (n = 54). In the tenofovir treatment group, 89% of patients (46 of 52) had a virologic response, compared with 0% (0 of 54) in the placebo group. No resistance development to tenofovir was observed. Tenofovir was well tolerated by patients, and only one serious adverse effect was reported (hepatitis) in this group.

HIV
HIV-infected children can suffer from neurodevelopmental delay or encephalopathy. To evaluate the impact of early versus delayed treatment with antiretroviral therapy (ART) in HIV-infected children, the Children with HIV Early Antiretroviral Therapy (CHER) trial prospectively enrolled and compared neurodevelopmental outcomes in 90 infants of median age 11 months (age range 10–16 months; 64 infants on early ART; 26 on deferred treatment) [56]. For infants in the delayed-treatment group, ART was deferred until clinical or immunologic progression was observed. In the early treatment arm, ART was limited to 40 or 90 weeks. A neurologic examination and the

Griffiths Mental Development Scales (GMDS) were performed at the study visit closest to 10 to 12 months of age and were used to assess neurodevelopmental outcomes. The median time to start ART in the early versus delayed treatment groups was 8.4 versus 31.4 weeks, respectively. Using the GMDS, all scores were found to be lower in the deferred-treatment group, and the general and locomotor scores, in particular, were significantly lower, indicating superior neurodevelopmental outcomes with early treatment. Moreover, scores in the early treatment group were found to be similar to those in HIV-uninfected infants (except on the locomotor subscale) who were exposed or unexposed to HIV.

The CHER trial also compared immunologic, clinical, and virologic outcomes between early time-limited ART (restricted to 40 or 96 weeks) and deferred treatment [57]. A total of 377 infants was enrolled (median age 7.4 weeks; interquartile range ~6.4–9 weeks). The primary outcome was time to failure of first-line ART (zidovudine, lamivudine, and lopinavir/ritonavir) or death. Infants were randomized to 1 of 3 treatment strategies: deferred therapy, early ART restricted to 40 weeks, and early ART restricted to 96 weeks. Treatment failure was defined as a CD4-positive T lymphocytes (%) decrease to less than 20% from week 24, CDC severe stage B or C events, or regimen-limiting toxicity. An HIV-RNA viral load of 10,000 copies per mm^3 was considered virologic failure. Relative to subjects in the deferred treatment arm, the hazard ratios for early therapy restricted to 40 and 96 weeks were 0.59 (95% CI 0.38–0.93; $P = .02$) and 0.47 (95% CI 0.27–0.76; $P = .002$), respectively [57].

A separate randomized trial performed in 6 African countries and India sought to compare nevirapine with ritonavir-boosted lopinavir plus zidovudine and lamivudine in 288 children 2 to 36 months of age with no prior exposure to nevirapine [58]. Because of its low cost, stability at high temperatures, acceptable safety profile, and the availability of fixed-dose combination, nevirapine is frequently an important treatment option for children in resource-limited settings [58]. For children younger than 2 years, the World Health Organization guidelines for ART currently recommend ritonavir-boosted lopinavir for children with previous nevirapine (maternal or infant) exposure, and nevirapine in the absence of previous antiretroviral exposure [59]. The primary end point in the trial was treatment failure, defined as virologic failure or discontinuation of nevirapine or ritonavir-boosted lopinavir component of the ART at 24 weeks. The percentage of children with treatment failure was significantly greater in the nevirapine group when compared with ritonavir-boosted lopinavir (40.8% vs 19.3%, $P < .001$). In addition, the time to a protocol-defined toxicity end point was significantly shorter for the nevirapine group. It is possible that resistance to nevirapine played a role in the poorer efficacy outcomes. Nineteen of 32 patients in the nevirapine group with resistance data available were reported as resistant at the time of treatment failure. The investigators concluded that in children with no prior exposure to nevirapine, more favorable outcomes were observed in patients treated with ritonavir-boosted lopinavir.

Influenza

Trivalent influenza vaccines contain 2 influenza A strains and 1 B strain. For influenza B, an important contributor to disease in children, there are 2 genetically distinct lineages of the hemagglutinin gene, which encodes a glycoprotein important for viral binding to cells [60]. Between 2001 and 2011, the correct B lineage was only selected 5 out of 10 times, suggesting there is a need for a quadrivalent vaccine that includes both [61]. A phase 3, randomized, double-blind study evaluated the immunogenicity and safety of a quadrivalent split virion influenza vaccine (QIV) versus a trivalent vaccine (TIV) in children 3 to 17 years of age [62]. A total of 2738 children received QIV, TIV-B/Victoria, or TIV-B/Yamagata in a 1:1:1 fashion. An additional 277 children aged 6 to 35 months were enrolled in an open-label group administered QIV. Blood samples were collected on day 0 (before vaccination) and 28 days after the last vaccine dose, after which antibody titers were assessed using a hemagglutination-inhibition assay. The investigators reported that QIV showed superior immunogenicity in comparison with TIV with regard to the additional B strain, and thus may offer improved protection against influenza B in children [62]. Safety of QIV was similar to that of TIV. Favorable immunogenicity was also shown against all 4 strains in the open-label group.

A separate randomized, multicenter study compared 2 trivalent live attenuated vaccines (T/LAIV), each containing a strain for each influenza B lineage, versus a quadrivalent live attenuated vaccine (Q/LAIV) [63]. A total of 2312 patients in 2 age groups (2–8 years, 9–17 years) were randomized to 1 of the 3 groups. The Q/LAIV was found to be noninferior to T/LAIV in terms of immunogenicity for children 2 to 17 years of age. As in the previous study, safety was also comparable between treatment groups.

NEUROLOGY

Migraines

Triptans are an important treatment option for migraine prevention in adults. Until recently, only almotriptan was indicated for use in adolescents (12–17 years), and none are approved for treatment in younger age groups. In late 2011, the FDA approved rizatriptan for use as migraine treatment in children as young as 6 years [64]. Since its approval the results of PK, safety, and efficacy studies performed in the pediatric population have been published.

First, to evaluate the PK and tolerability of rizatriptan, a randomized, double-blind, placebo-controlled, parallel-group, single-dose study was performed in patients 6 to 17 years of age with a history of migraines [65]. Rizatriptan oral disintegrating tablets (ODT) were administered using a weight-based dosing scheme: children weighing less than 40 kg received rizatriptan ODT 5 mg or placebo; those 40 kg or heavier received 10 mg ODT or placebo. When area under the concentration versus time curve from zero to infinity ($AUC0-\infty$) and maximal drug concentration (Cmax) were compared with adult historical data (rizatriptan ODT 10 mg), the ratios in the less than 40 kg group were 0.85 (90% CI 0.73–0.98) and 1.07 (90% CI 0.86–1.34), respectively. For those weighing greater than or equal to 40 kg group, AUC0–∞ and Cmax ratios were 1.17 (90% CI 1.02–1.34) and 1.06 (90% CI 0.87–1.30), respectively. Second, in terms of efficacy, rizatriptan was superior to placebo in patients 12 to 17 years of age and for the primary outcome, pain resolution at 2 hours (30.6% vs 22%, $P = .025$) [66]. In the age category of 6 to 11 years, greater response (2-hour pain freedom) was observed with rizatriptan, but did not reach statistical significance ($P = .269$). These results may be related to a small sample size in this age category, as the study was powered for the adolescent (12–17 years) and combined 6- to 17-year age groups [66]. When the 2 age groups were combined (6–17 years), rizatriptan was significantly superior to placebo in terms of 2-hour pain freedom (33% vs 24.2%, $P = .01$). The proven efficacy in the 6- to 17-year-old age group, with comparable efficacy between the 2 subgroups (6–11 years vs 12–17 years) and favorable safety profile served as the basis for regulatory approval [67].

Clinical trials evaluating migraine response to treatment in children are challenging because of a high placebo response rate that may result from inadequate study design and short duration of migraine attacks, among other factors [68]. A systematic analysis of trial data submitted to the FDA for approval as acute treatment of migraine attacks in the pediatric population was assessed to identify causes of study failures [69]. Clinical trial data for sumatriptan succinate, zolmitriptan, eletriptan hydrobromide, almotriptan malate, and rizatriptan benzoate were included in the analysis. A high placebo response rate was reported across trials: 53% to 57.5% for pain relief at 2 hours [69]. The investigators emphasized the benefit of using a double randomization strategy whereby patients with an early placebo response are not included in a second randomization phase. This strategy was used for rizatriptan, and resulted in a 6% reduction in the placebo response rate compared with a previous trial [69].

A separate meta-analysis evaluated evidence of effectiveness for prophylactic treatment of migraines in the pediatric population (<18 years) [70]. Data for 21 clinical trials were included: 13 placebo-controlled and 10 active-comparator trials (2 comparator trials also included placebo). Drugs found to be more effective than placebo were topiramate (difference in headaches per month, −0.71; 95% CI −1.19 to −0.24) and trazodone (−0.6; 95% CI −1.09 to −0.11), whereas clonidine, flunarizine, pizotifen, propranolol, and valproate were ineffective [70]. A significant placebo response was reported: a reduction in headaches from 5.5 (95% CI 4.52–6.77) to 2.9 (95% CI 1.66–4.08) per month. The investigators noted only limited data are available that evaluate the use of pharmacologic agents for prevention of migraine headaches in children [70].

Seizures

Topiramate (Topamax) is an antiepileptic drug approved for use as monotherapy or adjunctive therapy in children 2 years of age or older treated for partial-onset or primary generalized tonic-clonic seizures. A phase 1, safety and PK study sought to evaluate topiramate use in infants (n = 55, 1–24 months of age) with refractory partial-onset seizures [71]. A total of 4 dose groups

(3, 5, 15, or 25 mg/kg/d) were evaluated, with infants stratified into a dose group based on age category (1–6, 7–12, and 13–24 months). Oral liquid or sprinkle capsule formations were administered. In subjects with complete PK profiles (n = 35), linear PK and dose proportionality were observed across all dose groups [71]. Drug clearance values on a per-kilogram basis were higher in infants (1–24 months) relative to published values in children and adolescents [71]. Patients receiving enzyme-inducing antiepileptic drugs had 2-fold higher clearance values. The most commonly reported adverse effects were upper respiratory tract infection (15%), fever (15%), vomiting (13%), somnolence (11%), and anorexia (11%).

A recent study sought to characterize the PK of lorazepam following single-dose administration to pediatric patients (aged 5 months to 17 years) in status epilepticus (n = 48) or patients with a history of seizures recruited as part of an elective cohort (n = 15) [72]. The population estimates for clearance, half-life, and volume of distribution were 1.2 mL/min/kg, 16.8 hours, and 1.5 L/kg, respectively. Lorazepam clearance values normalized by body weight reported in this study approximately 20% higher than those in adults. The investigators report that a 0.1 mg/kg dose would be expected to achieve lorazepam concentrations of approximately 100 ng/mL and stay in the range of 30 to 50 ng/mL for 6 to 12 hours, whereby the latter concentration is expected to provide anticonvulsant effects while minimizing the drug's sedative effects. In terms of efficacy, of the 48 patients with status epilepticus, 42 were successfully treated with 1 or 2 doses while 6 patients required 3 doses.

In a double-blind, randomized, noninferiority trial, intravenous lorazepam was compared with intramuscularly administered midazolam for the treatment of status epilepticus in both pediatric and adult patients [73]. Subjects who experienced convulsions for longer than 5 minutes and were still convulsing at the time paramedics arrived on the scene were administered a study medication. The primary outcome, absence of seizures before arriving to the emergency department and in the absence of rescue therapy, was compared between treatment groups. In the intramuscular midazolam group, 329 of 448 (73.4%) patients were no longer convulsing on arrival to the emergency department, compared with 282 of 445 (63.4%) in the intravenous lorazepam group. As a result, the investigators reported that intramuscular midazolam was at least as effective as intravenous lorazepam when administered by paramedics before arrival at the hospital [73].

ONCOLOGY

Four label changes were made for oncology drugs between 2012 and 2013 [64]. First, for palifermin (Kepivance), based on a phase 1 study in 27 pediatric patients, use is now indicated in children ages 1 to 16 years with acute leukemia undergoing hematopoietic stem cell transplant. Second, for patients 1 year of age and upward with tuberous sclerosis complex, everolimus (Afinitor Disperz) is now approved for treatment of subependymal giant-cell astrocytoma. For bendamustine hydrochloride (Treanda) and temsirolimus (Torisel), label changes include a statement informing clinicians that effectiveness has not been established in pediatric patients.

PULMONARY AND ALLERGY

Asthma

It is hypothesized that asymptomatic gastroesophageal reflux can be a contributor to poor asthma control in children. In The Study of Acid Reflux in Children with Asthma, investigators compared the impact of lansoprazole, a proton-pump inhibitor, on asthma control in 306 pediatric patients (range 6–17 years of age) [74]. A randomized, double-masked, placebo-controlled, parallel study in children with poor asthma control and no symptoms of gastroesophageal reflux disease showed no statistically significant differences in the Asthma Control Questionnaire and in secondary outcomes, including forced expiratory volume after 1 second and quality of life after 24 weeks of treatment. In addition, in a subgroup analysis (n = 115) where esophageal pH study results were available, 49 patients were found to have positive results indicating gastroesophageal reflux. When compared with patients with normal esophageal pH, lansoprazole did not appear to affect any study outcomes. With regard to toxicity, a greater number of upper respiratory tract infections, sore throats, and episodes of bronchitis were reported in patients receiving lansoprazole. These results demonstrate that in patients with poorly controlled asthma and no symptoms of gastroesophageal reflux, addition of lansoprazole did not improve treatment outcomes.

In a genetic substudy, 279 of the 306 aforementioned participants provided DNA for analysis [75]. The frequency of adverse events with lansoprazole was evaluated in children with single-nucleotide polymorphisms in *CYP2C19*, as this gene may affect lansoprazole clearance and exposure. Patients were classified as poor metabolizers if they carried at least 1 *CYP2C19*2*, **3*, **8*, or **9* allele, whereas extensive metabolizers were those patients with 2 wild-type alleles. The frequency of upper respiratory tract infections was highest in poor metabolizers when compared with extensive metabolizers (69% vs 60%), and both groups had higher frequencies that than that observed with placebo (48%, $P = .0039$; Cochran-Armitage test for trend). Likewise, the frequency of sore throat was higher in poor metabolizers (66%) when compared with extensive metabolizers (45%) or placebo (38%, $P = .0015$; Cochran-Armitage test for trend). Blood samples were collected in some patients (2–3 hours after final dose) for measurement of lansoprazole concentration. Mean plasma concentrations were significantly higher in poor (n = 23, 207 ± 179 ng/mL) versus extensive (n = 33, 132 ± 141 ng/mL) metabolizers ($P = .04$). If these findings are replicated in an independent sample the results may be clinically meaningful, as a dosage adjustment may be performed to mitigate the occurrence of these side effects in patients classified as poor metabolizers [75].

Inhaled glucocorticoids are the mainstay of therapy for most children with asthma. When inhaled glucocorticoids are administered to prepubertal children, a reduction in growth velocity can occur. However, the relationship between chronic use of inhaled glucocorticoids and attainment of adult height is not well understood [76]. The Childhood Asthma Management Program (CAMP) was a clinical trial that enrolled 1041 children 5 to 13 years of age and compared the safety and efficacy of budesonide, nedocromil, and placebo [77]. Children in this study were followed long term, and adult height was assessed at a mean (standard deviation) age of 24.9 (2.7) years [76]. Budesonide, an inhaled glucocorticoid, resulted in a 1.2 cm lower adult height (95% CI −1.9 to −0.5) when compared with placebo (P = .001). By contrast, patients administered nedocromil, a mast-cell stabilizer, had a 0.2 cm lower adult height (95% CI −0.9 to 0.5), though not statistically significant. The reduction observed in the budesonide group was similar to that reported after 2 years of treatment (−1.3 cm; 95% CI −1.7 to −0.9). Moreover, in the first 2 years of treatment a larger daily budesonide dose was associated with a lower adult height (−0.1 cm for each microgram per kg body weight). The investigators concluded that although the reduction in growth velocity observed in the first 2 years of treatment persisted into adulthood, the benefits of these drugs in persistent asthma is well established. The use of the lowest effective dose is encouraged to minimize the impact on growth velocity.

For asthma, a notable drug-label change was reported by the FDA for montelukast (Singulair), which is now indicated for the treatment of exercise-induced bronchoconstriction in children as young as 6 years of age (previously 15 years or older) [64].

Allergic rhinitis

Drug-label changes or approvals were made for 3 drugs indicated to treat allergic rhinitis: the combination product azelastine hydrochloride and fluticasone propionate; azelastine; and beclomethasone dipropionate. The combination product azelastine hydrochloride 0.1%/fluticasone propionate 0.037%, which is administered as a nasal spray, was approved for the treatment of allergic rhinitis in children older than 12 years who require both an H_1-antagonist and a corticosteroid for symptomatic relief. The age category for which azelastine is indicated for treatment of seasonal and perennial allergic rhinitis was expanded to include 6 to 12 years (previously >12 years). Beclomethasone dipropionate, an intranasal corticosteroid, is now indicated for the treatment of nasal symptoms associated with seasonal and perennial allergic rhinitis in children older than 12 years. QNasl is formulated as a nonaqueous-based formulation, and thus may be less susceptible to adverse reactions that result from postnasal drip [78].

Cystic fibrosis

A significant advancement was made in the treatment of cystic fibrosis with the approval of the new chemical entity ivacaftor. Ivacaftor is approved for the treatment of cystic fibrosis in patients 6 years and upward with the *G551D* mutation in the cystic fibrosis transmembrane conductance regulator (*CFTR*) gene. This new drug potentiates the action of the CFTR protein, a chloride-ion channel, by affecting the "channel-open probability" and facilitating ion transport [79].

SYMPTOMATIC CARE
Analgesia
To investigate the opioid-sparing effects of intravenous acetaminophen in neonates and infants undergoing major noncardiac surgery, a randomized, double-blind, single-center study was performed [80]. A total of 71 neonates or infants (age <1 year) were enrolled and followed for 48 hours following major thoracic or abdominal surgery. Patients were randomized to receive morphine (age $\leq$10 days: 2.5 μg/kg$^{1.5}$ per hour; age 11 days to 1 year: 5 μg/kg$^{1.5}$ per hour) or paracetamol (30 mg/kg/d in 4 doses). For patients randomized to paracetamol, a placebo normal saline infusion was used, whereas normal saline was administered in 4 separate doses for patients randomized to morphine. Morphine was also administered as needed ($\leq$10 days: 10 μg/kg; 11 days to 1 year: 15 μg/kg) to patients in both groups when pain scales (Numeric Rating Scale-11 and COMFORT-Behavior Scale) indicated pain. Following 3 rescue doses, if the patient was still in pain, a continuous morphine infusion was initiated. The primary outcome was cumulative morphine dose (study and rescue), and secondary outcomes were pain scores and adverse effects. The cumulative morphine dose during the first 48 postoperative hours was 357 μg/kg (n = 38; interquartile range 220–605) and 121 μg/kg (n = 33; interquartile range 99–264) in the morphine and paracetamol groups, respectively (P <.001). No significant differences were noted in pain scores or adverse effects between groups. The investigators concluded that intermittent use of paracetamol lowered the 48-hour cumulative morphine dose when compared with use of a continuous morphine infusion [80].

SUMMARY
In the United States, passage of the FDASIA legislation made BPCA and PREA permanent, no longer requiring reauthorization every 5 years. This landmark legislation also stressed the importance of performing clinical trials in neonates when appropriate. In Europe the Pediatric Regulation, which went into effect in early 2007, also provides a framework for expanding pediatric clinical research. Although much work remains, as a result of greater regulatory guidance more pediatric data are reaching product labels.

Acknowledgments
D. Gonzalez is funded by training grant T32GM086330 from the National Institute of General Medical Sciences. I.M. Paul receives support from the United States government through HHSN275201000003I. D.K. Benjamin Jr. receives support from the United States government for his work in pediatric and neonatal clinical pharmacology (1R01HD057956-05, 1K24HD058735-05, UL1TR001117, and NICHD contract HHSN275201000003I) and the nonprofit organization Thrasher Research Fund for his work in neonatal

candidiasis (www.thrasherresearch.org); he also receives research support from industry for neonatal and pediatric drug development (www.dcri.duke.edu/research/coi.jsp). M.C. Cohen-Wolkowiez receives support for research from the National Institutes of Health (NIH) (1K23HD064814), the National Center for Advancing Translational Sciences of the NIH (UL1TR001117), the Food and Drug Administration (1U01FD004858-01), the Biomedical Advanced Research and Development Authority (BARDA) (HHSO100201300009C), the nonprofit organization Thrasher Research Fund (www.thrasherresearch.org), and from industry for drug development in adults and children (www.dcri.duke.edu/research/coi.jsp).

Research reported in this publication was also supported by the National Center for Advancing Translational Sciences of the National Institutes of Health under award number UL1TR001117. The content is solely the responsibility of the authors and does not necessarily represent the official views of the National Institutes of Health or the National Institute of General Medical Sciences.

References

[1] Sachs AN, Avant D, Lee CS, et al. Pediatric information in drug product labeling. JAMA 2012;307(18):1914–5.

[2] European Medicines Agency. Successes of the paediatric regulation after 5 years: August 2007-December 2012. Available at: http://www.ema.europa.eu/docs/en_GB/document_library/Other/2013/06/WC500143984.pdf. Accessed December 18, 2013.

[3] U.S. Food and Drug Administration Office of Pediatric Therapeutics and Pediatric & Maternal Health Staff. Studies of drugs in neonates challenging but necessary. AAP News 2012;33(6):7. Available at: www.aapsnews.org. Accessed December 16, 2013.

[4] Laughon MM, Avant D, Tripathi N, et al. Drug labeling and exposure in neonates. JAMA Pediatr 2014;168(2):130–6.

[5] Metzger M, Billett A, Link M. The impact of drug shortages on children with cancer—the example of mechlorethamine. N Engl J Med 2012;367(26):2461–3.

[6] Emanuel E, Shuman K, Chinn D, et al. Impact of oncology drug shortages. J Clin Oncol 2013;31(Suppl) [abstract CRA6510].

[7] American Academy of Pediatrics. Testimony for the record: on behalf of the American Academy of Pediatrics before the Energy and Commerce Committee Health Subcommittee. Available at: http://www.aap.org/en-us/advocacy-and-policy/federal-advocacy/Documents/TestimonyforRecordDrugShortages_Feb2012.pdf. Accessed December 16, 2013.

[8] American Academy of Pediatrics. American Academy of Pediatrics comments to FDA Task Force on Drug Shortages. Available at: http://www.aap.org/en-us/advocacy-and-policy/federal-advocacy/Documents/FDADrugShortagesTaskForceComments_03_13_13.pdf. Accessed December 16, 2013.

[9] Food and Drug Administration. Strategic plan for preventing and mitigating drug shortages. Available at: http://www.fda.gov/downloads/Drugs/DrugSafety/DrugShortages/UCM372566.pdf. Accessed December 16, 2013.

[10] Hospira. Etomidate injection package insert. Available at: http://www.hospira.com/Images/EN-2864_32-5792_1.pdf. Accessed December 19, 2013.

[11] Lin L, Zhang JW, Huang Y, et al. Population pharmacokinetics of intravenous bolus etomidate in children over 6 months of age. Paediatr Anaesth 2012;22(4):318–26.

[12] Gupta P, Whiteside W, Sabati A, et al. Safety and efficacy of prolonged dexmedetomidine use in critically ill children with heart disease. Pediatr Crit Care Med 2012;13(6):660–6.

[13] Lam F, Ransom C, Gossett JM, et al. Safety and efficacy of dexmedetomidine in children with heart failure. Pediatr Cardiol 2013;34(4):835–41.

[14] Mason K, Robinson F, Fontaine P, et al. Dexmedetomidine offers an option for safe and effective sedation for nuclear medicine imaging in children. Radiology 2013;267(3): 911–7.

[15] Akin A, Bayram A, Esmaoglu A, et al. Dexmedetomidine vs midazolam for premedication of pediatric patients undergoing anesthesia. Paediatr Anaesth 2012;22(9):871–6.

[16] Barst RJ, Ivy DD, Gaitan G, et al. A randomized, double-blind, placebo-controlled, dose-ranging study of oral sildenafil citrate in treatment-naive children with pulmonary arterial hypertension. Circulation 2012;125(2):324–34.

[17] U.S. Food and Drug Administration. FDA drug safety communication: FDA recommends against use of Revatio (sildenafil) in children with pulmonary hypertension. 2012. Available at: http://www.fda.gov/Drugs/DrugSafety/ucm317123.htm. Accessed December 19, 2013.

[18] European Medicines Agency. Revatio: summary of product characteristics. Available at: http://www.ema.europa.eu/docs/en_GB/document_library/EPAR_-_Product_Information/human/000638/WC500055840.pdf. Accessed December 19, 2013.

[19] National High Blood Pressure Education Program Working Group on High Blood Pressure in Children and Adolescents. The fourth report on the diagnosis, evaluation, and treatment of high blood pressure in children and adolescents. Pediatrics 2004;114(2): 555–76.

[20] Soletsky B, Feig DI. Uric acid reduction rectifies prehypertension in obese adolescents. Hypertension 2012;60(5):1148–56.

[21] Wells TG, Blowey DL, Sullivan JE, et al. Pharmacokinetics of olmesartan medoxomil in pediatric patients with hypertension. Paediatr Drugs 2012;14(6):401–9.

[22] McNamara PJ, Shivananda SP, Sahni M, et al. Pharmacology of milrinone in neonates with persistent pulmonary hypertension of the newborn and suboptimal response to inhaled nitric oxide. Pediatr Crit Care Med 2013;14(1):74–84.

[23] Lindsay C, Barton P, Lawless S, et al. Pharmacokinetics and pharmacodynamics of milrinone lactate in pediatric patients with septic shock. J Pediatr 1998;132(2):329–34.

[24] Wessel DL, Berger F, Li JS, et al. Clopidogrel in infants with systemic-to-pulmonary-artery shunts. N Engl J Med 2013;368(25):2377–84.

[25] Eichenfield LF, Krakowski AC, Piggott C, et al. Evidence-based recommendations for the diagnosis and treatment of pediatric acne. Pediatrics 2013;131(Suppl):S163–86.

[26] Lazzerini M, Martelossi S, Magazzù G, et al. Effect of thalidomide on clinical remission in children and adolescents with refractory Crohn's disease: a randomized clinical trial. JAMA 2013;310(20):2164–73.

[27] Wilson DC, Thomas G, Croft NM, et al. Systematic review of the evidence base for the medical treatment of paediatric inflammatory bowel disease. J Pediatr Gastroenterol Nutr 2010;50(Suppl 1):S14–34.

[28] Walters TD, Kim M, Denson L, et al. Increased effectiveness of early therapy with anti-tumor necrosis factor-α vs. an immunomodulator in children with Crohn's disease. Gastroenterology 2014;146(2):383–91.

[29] Plamondon S, Ng SC, Kamm M. Thalidomide in luminal and fistulizing Crohn's disease resistant to standard therapies. Aliment Pharmacol Ther 2007;25(5):557–67.

[30] Hyams JS, Griffiths A, Markowitz J, et al. Safety and efficacy of adalimumab for moderate to severe Crohn's disease in children. Gastroenterology 2012;143(2):365–74.

[31] Furuta GT, Williams K, Kooros K, et al. Management of constipation in children and adolescents with autism spectrum disorders. Pediatrics 2012;130(Suppl):S98–105.

[32] Rodriguez L, Diaz J, Nurko S. Safety and efficacy of cyproheptadine for treating dyspeptic symptoms in children. J Pediatr 2013;163(1):261–7.

[33] Cohen-Wolkowiez M, Watt KM, Hornik CP, et al. Pharmacokinetics and tolerability of single-dose daptomycin in young infants. Pediatr Infect Dis J 2012;31(9):935–7.

[34] Antachopoulos C, Iosifidis E, Sarafidis K, et al. Serum levels of daptomycin in pediatric patients. Infection 2012;40(4):367–71.

[35] Cohen-Wolkowiez M, Ouellet D, Smith PB, et al. Population pharmacokinetics of metronidazole evaluated using scavenged samples from preterm infants. Antimicrob Agents Chemother 2012;56(4):1828–37.

[36] Purdy J, Jouve S, Yan JL, et al. Pharmacokinetics and safety profile of tigecycline in children aged 8 to 11 years with selected serious infections: a multicenter, open-label, ascending-dose study. Clin Ther 2012;34(2):496–507.

[37] Zhao W, Lopez E, Biran V, et al. Vancomycin continuous infusion in neonates: dosing optimisation and therapeutic drug monitoring. Arch Dis Child 2013;98(6):449–53.

[38] Stockmann C, Sherwin CM, Zobell JT, et al. Population pharmacokinetics of intermittent vancomycin in children with cystic fibrosis. Pharmacotherapy 2013;33(12):1288–96.

[39] Watt KM, Benjamin DK, Cheifetz IM, et al. Pharmacokinetics and safety of fluconazole in young infants supported with extracorporeal membrane oxygenation. Pediatr Infect Dis J 2012;31:1042–7.

[40] Benjamin DK Jr, Deville JG, Azie N, et al. Safety and pharmacokinetic profiles of repeated-dose micafungin in children and adolescents treated for invasive candidiasis. Pediatr Infect Dis J 2013;32:e419–25.

[41] Friberg LE, Ravva P, Karlsson MO, et al. Integrated population pharmacokinetic analysis of voriconazole in children, adolescents, and adults. Antimicrob Agents Chemother 2012;56(6):3032–42.

[42] Zhao W, Cella M, Della Pasqua O, et al. Population pharmacokinetics and maximum a posteriori probability Bayesian estimator of abacavir: application of individualized therapy in HIV-infected infants and toddlers. Br J Clin Pharmacol 2012;73(4):641–50.

[43] Sampson MR, Bloom BT, Lenfestey RW, et al. Population pharmacokinetics of intravenous acyclovir in preterm and term infants. Pediatr Infect Dis J 2014;33(1):42–9.

[44] Chokephaibulkit K, Prasitsuebsai W, Wittawatmongkol O, et al. Pharmacokinetics of darunavir/ritonavir in Asian HIV-1-infected children aged ≥7 years. Antivir Ther 2012;17(7):1263–9.

[45] Königs C, Feiterna-Sperling C, Esposito S, et al. Pharmacokinetics and short-term safety and tolerability of etravirine in treatment-experienced HIV-1-infected children and adolescents. AIDS 2012;26(4):447–55.

[46] Standing JF, Nika A, Tsagris V, et al. Oseltamivir pharmacokinetics and clinical experience in neonates and infants during an outbreak of H1N1 influenza A virus infection in a neonatal intensive care unit. Antimicrob Agents Chemother 2012;56(7):3833–40.

[47] Baheti G, King JR, Acosta EP, et al. Age-related differences in plasma and intracellular tenofovir concentrations in HIV-1-infected children, adolescents and adults. AIDS 2013;27(2):221–5.

[48] Villeneuve D, Brothers A, Harvey E, et al. Valganciclovir dosing using area under the curve calculations in pediatric solid organ transplant recipients. Pediatr Transplant 2013;17(1):80–5.

[49] Hendriksen IC, Mtove G, Kent A, et al. Population pharmacokinetics of intramuscular artesunate in African children with severe malaria: implications for a practical dosing regimen. Clin Pharmacol Ther 2013;93(5):443–50.

[50] Neuman MI, Hall M, Hersh AL, et al. Influence of hospital guidelines on management of children hospitalized with pneumonia. Pediatrics 2012;130(5):e823–30.

[51] Newman RE, Hedican EB, Herigon JC, et al. Impact of a guideline on management of children hospitalized with community-acquired pneumonia. Pediatrics 2012;129(3):e597–604.

[52] Basnet S, Shrestha PS, Sharma A, et al. A randomized controlled trial of zinc as adjuvant therapy for severe pneumonia in young children. Pediatrics 2012;129(4):701–8.

[53] Cohen-Wolkowiez M, Poindexter B, Bidegain M, et al. Safety and effectiveness of meropenem in infants with suspected or complicated intra-abdominal infections. Clin Infect Dis 2012;55(11):1495–502.

[54] Jonas M, Kelly D, Pollack H, et al. Efficacy and safety of long-term adefovir dipivoxil therapy in children with chronic hepatitis B infection. Pediatr Infect Dis J 2012;31(6):578–82.

[55] Murray KF, Szenborn L, Wysocki J, et al. Randomized, placebo-controlled trial of tenofovir disoproxil fumarate in adolescents with chronic hepatitis B. Hepatology 2012;56(6): 2018–26.

[56] Laughton B, Cornell M, Grove D, et al. Early antiretroviral therapy improves neurodevelopmental outcomes in infants. AIDS 2012;26(13):1685–90.

[57] Cotton MF, Violari A, Otwombe K, et al. Early time-limited antiretroviral therapy versus deferred therapy in South African infants infected with HIV: results from the children with HIV early antiretroviral (CHER) randomised trial. Lancet 2013;382(9904):1555–63.

[58] Violari A, Lindsey J. Nevirapine versus ritonavir-boosted lopinavir for HIV-infected children. N Engl J Med 2012;366(25):2380–9.

[59] World Health Organization. Antiretroviral therapy for HIV infection in infants and children: towards universal access: recommendations for a public health approach—2010 revision. Available at: http://apps.who.int/medicinedocs/en/m/abstract/Js18809en/. Accessed January 3, 2014.

[60] Belshe RB, Coelingh K, Ambrose CS, et al. Efficacy of live attenuated influenza vaccine in children against influenza B viruses by lineage and antigenic similarity. Vaccine 2010;28(9):2149–56.

[61] Ambrose C, Levin M. The rationale for quadrivalent influenza vaccines. Hum Vaccin Immunother 2012;8(1):81–8.

[62] Domachowske JB, Pankow-Culot H, Bautista M, et al. A randomized trial of candidate inactivated quadrivalent influenza vaccine versus trivalent influenza vaccines in children aged 3-17 years. J Infect Dis 2013;207(12):1878–87.

[63] Block SL, Falloon J, Hirschfield JA, et al. Immunogenicity and safety of a quadrivalent live attenuated influenza vaccine in children. Pediatr Infect Dis J 2012;31(7):745–51.

[64] U.S. Food and Drug Administration. Pediatric labeling information database. Available at: http://www.fda.gov/ScienceResearch/SpecialTopics/PediatricTherapeuticsResearch/default.htm. Accessed December 9, 2013.

[65] Fraser IP, Han L, Han TH, et al. Pharmacokinetics and tolerability of rizatriptan in pediatric migraineurs in a randomized study. Headache 2012;52(4):625–35.

[66] Ho TW, Pearlman E, Lewis D, et al. Efficacy and tolerability of rizatriptan in pediatric migraineurs: results from a randomized, double-blind, placebo-controlled trial using a novel adaptive enrichment design. Cephalalgia 2012;32(10):750–65.

[67] U.S. Food and Drug Administration. Maxalt MLT (rizatriptan benzoate): cross discipline team leader review—addendum. Available at: http://www.fda.gov/downloads/Drugs/DevelopmentApprovalProcess/DevelopmentResources/UCM289413.pdf. Accessed December 9, 2013.

[68] Arruda M. No evidence of efficacy or evidence of no efficacy. JAMA Pediatr 2013;167(3):300–2.

[69] Sun H, Bastings E, Temeck J, et al. Migraine therapeutics in adolescents: a systematic analysis and historic perspectives of triptan trials in adolescents. JAMA Pediatr 2013;167(3):243–9.

[70] El-Chammas K, Keyes J, Thompson N, et al. Pharmacologic treatment of pediatric headaches: a meta-analysis. JAMA Pediatr 2013;167(3):250–8.

[71] Manitpisitkul P, Shalayda K, Todd M, et al. Pharmacokinetics and safety of adjunctive topiramate in infants (1–24 months) with refractory partial-onset seizures: a randomized, multicenter, open-label phase 1 study. Epilepsia 2013;54(1):156–64.

[72] Chamberlain JM, Capparelli EV, Brown KM, et al. Pharmacokinetics of intravenous lorazepam in pediatric patients with and without status epilepticus. J Pediatr 2012;160(4): 667–72.

[73] Silbergleit R, Durkalski V, Lowenstein D, et al. Intramuscular versus intravenous therapy for prehospital status epilepticus. N Engl J Med 2012;366(7):591–600.

[74] Writing Committee for the American Lung Association Asthma Clinical Research Centers, Holbrook J, Wise R, et al. Lansoprazole for children with poorly controlled asthma: a randomized controlled trial. JAMA 2012;307(4):373–81.

[75] Lima JJ, Lang JE, Mougey EB, et al. Association of CYP2C19 polymorphisms and lansoprazole-associated respiratory adverse effects in children. J Pediatr 2013;163(3): 686–91.
[76] Kelly H, Sternberg A. Effect of inhaled glucocorticoids in childhood on adult height. N Engl J Med 2012;367(10):904–12.
[77] The Childhood Asthma Management Program Research Group. Long-term effects of budesonide or nedocromil in children with asthma. N Engl J Med 2000;343(15):1054–63.
[78] Meltzer E, Jacobs R, LaForce C, et al. Safety and efficacy of once-daily treatment with beclomethasone dipropionate nasal aerosol in subjects with perennial allergic rhinitis. Allergy Asthma Proc 2012;33:249–57.
[79] Vertex Pharmaceuticals, Inc. Kalydeco™ (ivacaftor) prescribing information. Available at: http://www.accessdata.fda.gov/drugsatfda_docs/label/2012/203188lbl.pdf. Accessed December 30, 2013.
[80] Ceelie I, de Wildt S, van Dijk M, et al. Effect of intravenous paracetamol on postoperative morphine requirements in neonates and infants undergoing major noncardiac surgery: a randomized controlled trial. JAMA 2013;309(2):149–54.

Advances in Pediatrics 61 (2014) 33–74

ADVANCES IN PEDIATRICS

ELSEVIER
MOSBY

Advances in the Care of Children with Spina Bifida

Susan D. Apkon, MD[a,b,*], Richard Grady, MD[c],
Solveig Hart, PT, MSPT, PCS[d], Amy Lee, MD[e],
Thomas McNalley, MD, MA[f], Lee Niswander, PhD[g],
Juliette Petersen, MS[h], Sheridan Remley, PT, DPT[d],
Deborah Rotenstein, MD[i], Hillary Shurtleff, PhD[j,k],
Molly Warner, PhD, ABPP-CN[j,l], William O. Walker Jr, MD[m]

[a]Rehabilitation Medicine, University of Washington, Seattle, WA, USA; [b]Rehabilitation Medicine, Seattle Children's Hospital, 4800 Sand Point Way Northeast, M/S OB-8414, Seattle, WA 98105, USA; [c]Section of Pediatric Urology, Seattle Children's Hospital, University of Washington School of Medicine, 4800 Sand Point Way Northeast, Seattle, WA 98105, USA; [d]Rehabilitation Services, Seattle Children's Hospital, 4800 Sand Point Way Northeast, Seattle, WA 98105, USA; [e]Pediatric Neurosurgery, Seattle Children's Hospital, University of Washington, 4800 Sand Point Way Northeast, M/S W7729, PO Box 5371, Seattle, WA 98105, USA; [f]Rehabilitation Medicine, Seattle Children's Hospital, University of Washington, 4800 Sand Point Way Northeast, M/S OB-8404, Seattle, WA 98105, USA; [g]Department of Pediatrics, Children's Hospital Colorado, Howard Hughes Medical Institute, University of Colorado School of Medicine, Mail Stop 8133, Building RC1 South, Room L18-12106, 12801 East 17th Avenue, Aurora, CO 80045, USA; [h]Molecular Biology Program, University of Colorado Denver Anschutz Medical Campus, Mail Stop 8133, Building RC1 South, L18-12400D, 12801 East 17th Avenue, Aurora, CO 80045, USA; [i]Pediatric Endocrinology, Endocrine Division, Pediatric Alliance, 1789 South Braddock Avenue, Suite 294, Pittsburgh, PA 15218, USA; [j]Department of Neurology, University of Washington School of Medicine, Seattle, WA, USA; [k]Department of Child Psychiatry, Seattle Children's Hospital, 4800 Sand Point Way Northeast, Seattle, WA 98105, USA; [l]Neuropsychology Consult Service, Department of Psychiatry, Seattle Children's Hospital, 4800 Sand Point Way Northeast, Seattle, WA 98105, USA; [m]Division of Developmental Medicine, Seattle Children's Hospital, University of Washington School of Medicine, 4800 Sand Point Way Northeast, M/S OC.9.940, Seattle, WA 98105, USA

Keywords
• Advances • Care • Children • Spina bifida

*Corresponding author. Rehabilitation Medicine, Seattle Children's Hospital, 4800 Sand Point Way Northeast, M/S OB-8414, Seattle, WA 98105. *E-mail address*: Susan.apkon@ seattlechildrens.org

0065-3101/14/$ – see front matter
http://dx.doi.org/10.1016/j.yapd.2014.03.007
© 2014 Elsevier Inc. All rights reserved.

EPIDEMIOLOGY AND RISK FACTORS

Key points
- The risk of a mother with 1 neural tube defect (NTD)-affected pregnancy having another NTD-affected pregnancy triples.
- Adequate consumption of folic acid periconceptionally can prevent 50% to 70% of NTDs.
- Ultrasonography is a reliable method to identify NTDs by the end of the first trimester of gestation.

Introduction

Neural tube defects (NTDs) are a multifactorial disorder that results from a complex combination of genetic and environmental interactions. The worldwide incidence of NTDs ranges from 1.0 to 10.0 per 1000 births in specific geographic locations, with almost equal frequencies between 2 major categories: anencephaly and spina bifida [1,2]. The birth prevalence of NTDs in specific populations is influenced by the availability of prenatal diagnosis and elective pregnancy termination; higher frequencies occur in miscarriage material [3]. Each year, 300,000 to 400,000 infants worldwide are born with 1 of these 2 forms of NTDs.

Risk factors

Current identified risk factors for NTDs include a mother who previously had an NTD-affected pregnancy, maternal pregestational insulin-dependent diabetes, maternal pregestational obesity, hyperthermia, other environmental exposures, specific anticonvulsant drugs, including valproic acid, genetic variants, race/ethnicity, and nutrition (particularly folic acid [FA] insufficiency) [4]. The teratogenic potential of maternal pregestational diabetes is well established and includes a 2-fold to 10-fold increase in the risk of central nervous system malformations (including NTDs) among the offspring of affected women, relative to the general population. Women in the highest body mass index (BMI, calculated as weight in kilograms divided by the square of height in meters) categories (usually defined as a prepregnancy body mass index >29 kg/m^2) have a 1.5-fold to 3.5-fold higher risk than women with lower indices. There is evidence that maternal hyperthermia increases the risk of having a child with an NTD by up to 2-fold. The fungal product fumonisin caused a doubling of NTD incidence along the Texas-Mexico border in the early 1990s. Among women taking valproic acid or carbamazepine, the risk of having a pregnancy affected with spina bifida may be as high as 1% to 2%. In a few cases, anencephaly and spina bifida occur as part of malformation syndromes that result from teratogenic exposures [5]. Of particular clinical significance is valproic acid, an anticonvulsant that increases the risk of spinal NTDs by roughly 10 times when taken early in pregnancy. Although the teratogenic mechanisms are hypothesized to involve antifolate effects, particularly for carbamazepine, studies of valproic acid suggest potent histone deacetylase inhibitory activity. NTDs can also occur as part of malformation syndromes resulting from known chromosomal abnormalities (eg, trisomy 13, 18, and 21) and single gene disorders (eg, Meckel-Gruber and Waardenburg syndromes). However, the population burden of human NTDs explained by known genetic polymorphisms remains small.

Epidemiology

The prevalence estimates of spina bifida among children and adolescents varies according to region, race/ethnicity, and gender, which suggests possible variations in prevalence at birth or inequities in survival rates [6]. With the advent of antenatal diagnosis and elective termination of pregnancy (TOP), the prevalence of NTDs at birth is no longer reliable as an estimate of incidence. TOP is the most common outcome of pregnancy after prenatal diagnosis of anencephaly and spina bifida [3]. One systematic review showed an overall frequency of TOP after prenatal diagnosis to be 83% for anencephaly (range, 59%–100%) and 63% for spina bifida (range, 31%–97%). TOP for spina bifida was more common when the prenatal diagnosis occurred at less than 24 weeks' gestation (86 vs 27%), with defects of greater severity, and in Europe versus North America (66 vs 50%) [3]. The few fetuses with NTDs presenting as live births presents challenges to investigators conducting studies in which not all terminated NTD-affected pregnancies are included.

Regional differences in average gestational age at prenatal diagnosis are a possible explanation for some of the observed between-study variability in frequency of TOP. A greater frequency of TOP could be expected at earlier gestational ages because many regions have laws restricting the gestational ages at which TOP can be performed. These results suggest the importance of considering characteristics that delay prenatal diagnosis as potential sources of selection bias. Pregnancies complicated by a severe NTD or one accompanied by multiple major malformations might be more likely to end in TOP than an isolated NTD or a less severe case. Severity of the defect is more relevant for spina bifida than anencephaly, because the latter is uniformly lethal.

There are multiple challenges to and no agreement in determining accurate familial recurrence rates for NTDs [1]. Studies estimate that with each subsequent NTD-affected pregnancy after the first, the risk of another NTD-affected pregnancy triples. Risks for first-degree relatives of a mother having an NTD affected fetus (parent, sibling, child) range from 1 in 30 to 1 in 140. Risks for second-degree relatives (uncle, aunt, nephew, niece, grandparent, grandchild or half-sibling) range from 1 in 90 to 1 in 220. The recurrence rate in affected mothers having a child with an NTD is reported to range from 1 in 100 to 1 in 200. These variances in results may also be affected by low parent to child transmission rates secondary to decreased reproductive abilities in affected individuals, increased risk of spontaneous abortion in mothers with an NTD-affected pregnancy, high perinatal mortality, and the increased rate of elective terminations.

FA

Although the causes of NTDs are only now beginning to be understood, 2 significant advances have been made in their prevention and treatment. First, it is widely known that taking FA during childbearing years can significantly reduce a woman's risk of having a baby with an NTD. Second, recent studies have reported that in utero repair of spina bifida significantly improves patient outcomes (see section on prenatal surgery).

NTDs stand out as one of few birth defects for which primary prevention strategies are available. Both observational and intervention studies, including randomized, controlled trials, showed that adequate consumption of FA periconceptionally can prevent 50% to 70% of NTDs.

Fortifying foods with FA has been a highly effective intervention compared with dietary improvement or supplementation, because fortification made FA accessible to all women of childbearing age without requiring behavior change. In 1992, the US Public Health Service recommended that all women of childbearing age capable of becoming pregnant consume 400 µg of FA per day to prevent NTDs. In 1998, the United States was the first country to require mandatory FA fortification of standardized enriched cereal grain products, infant formulas, medical foods, and foods for special dietary use [7]. This public policy change resulted in a substantial increase in blood folate concentrations and a concomitant decrease in NTD prevalence. The percentage of the population with low serum folate (<3 ng/mL) levels declined from 21% in the period before fortification (1988–1994) to less than 1% of the total population in the period immediately after fortification (1999–2000). NTD prevalence decreased by 36% after fortification, from 10.8 per 10,000 population during 1995 to 1996 to 6.9 at the end of 2006. However, Hispanic women continue to be at significantly greater risk (prevalence ratio = 1.21; 95% confidence interval = 1.11–1.31) for having a baby affected by an NTD than non-Hispanic white women. Non-Hispanic black women have consistently had a lower NTD prevalence than Hispanic women and non-Hispanic white women, despite having the lowest folate levels before and after mandatory fortification.

The reasons for the disparity in declines in the prevalence of NTDs since FA fortification are unknown. Differences in FA consumption through diet and supplement use are unlikely to be the cause of the observed higher rate of NTD-affected pregnancies among Hispanic women and lower rates among non-Hispanic black women. It is likely that a combination of genetic and environmental factors is responsible. Contributing factors to this disparity could include genetic differences in folate metabolism, maternal diabetes, and obesity, which are known to vary by race and ethnicity. Other possibilities are a variable intake of nutrients other than FA, such as vitamin B_{12} [8]. This theory implies that folate deficiency is a risk factor for NTDs, but only in the presence of a predisposing genotype [2].

The fortification program seems to be preventing approximately 50% of NTDs, based on high-quality studies from Canada. Because the Canadian and US programs are almost the same, there seems to be little reason to think that the United States is not close to the target of preventing 50% of NTDs [9].

FA fortification of the food supply seems to represent the first successful, population- based strategy for the primary prevention of a common congenital malformation. Published economic evaluations have shown that FA food fortification is cost saving and cost effective in the United States and other countries: annual savings of about $300 million, or $100 for each $1 invested in fortification. Similarly, economic evaluations suggest that periconceptional supplementation of FA is a good use of health care resources and justifies further promotion of the use of FA supplementation before pregnancy. However, no European countries, including the United Kingdom, had implemented mandatory food fortification, as of June, 2013 [10].

How FA acts to prevent NTDs in some individuals and does not appear to have any prevention ability in 30% to 50% of cases remains an important but unanswered question. The answer to this question is likely complex, because folate is central to numerous cellular reactions. There is limited information to explain either FA-responsive NTD models or FA-resistant NTD models at a mechanistic level. Deficits in FA metabolism could affect cell proliferation, cell survival, transcriptional regulation, or a host of other cellular reactions. Cell multiplication has an important role in neural tube closure, encouraging the hypothesis that enhanced cell proliferation could be a key effect of FA. The variation in NTD risk depending on the length of FA exposure points toward the possibility of epigenetic changes. Methylation of genomic DNA and histone modification are increasingly being implicated in the epigenetic regulation of gene expression and could underlie the action of FA in the prevention of NTDs. Epigenetic influence has also been suggested to help explain the predominance of cranial NTDs in females versus males: X chromosome inactivation is maintained by DNA methylation, and there is more demand on the methylation cycle in female cells after every division relative to male cells [4].

Diagnosis

Screening to identify pregnant women at risk for carrying NTD-affected fetuses can be achieved by evaluation of maternal serum α-fetoprotein levels, amniocentesis, and ultrasonographic imaging. The first methods for prenatal diagnosis of open NTDs were developed in the 1970s. Initially, diagnosis was based on measurement of α-fetoprotein concentration in the maternal blood during the second trimester. If abnormal, this test was frequently followed by amniocentesis and direct measurements of α-fetoprotein and acetylcholinesterase concentrations.

Measurement of maternal serum α-fetoprotein is part of the triple test (α-fetoprotein, human chorionic gonadotropin, and estradiol) and the quad screen (α-fetoprotein, human chorionic gonadotropin, estradiol, inhibin A). α-fetoprotein levels are reported as multiples of the median (MoM); concerning results for an open NTD are greater than 2.5 MoM.

Screening for increased maternal serum α-fetoprotein levels in the second trimester of pregnancy could identify more than two-thirds of fetuses with open NTDs (defects that are not covered by skin), including almost all fetuses with anencephaly. If a neural tube abnormality occurs between the 17th and 30th day after ovulation, the defect is open; later lesions are covered by skin and are described as closed or occult. Skin-covered dysraphism represents approximately 15% of cases and is usually asymptomatic or associated with cutaneous lesions, such as lipoma, hypertrichosis, hemangioma, and telangiectasia. Occult dysraphisms are rarely diagnosed prenatally.

Technological improvements enabled ultrasonography to replace α-fetoprotein measurement as the mainstay of prenatal diagnosis. Efforts to use ultrasonography have focused on changes in intracranial structures and abnormalities along the spine itself. There have been several evaluations of the diagnostic benefit for specific ultrasonographic findings. The usefulness of specific cranial ultrasonography signs in the diagnosis of spina bifida has been well known since the 1980s. However, these markers are specific for open spinal defects and represent the consequence of the associated Chiari II malformation. The sequence of these sonographic signs has not been established; investigators disagree whether cerebellar signs precede cerebral signs or vice versa. It is believed that ultrasonography is a reliable method to identify NTDs by the end of the first trimester of gestation.

Common cranial ultrasonographic signs described in spina bifida include [11]:

1. The lemon sign (overlapping of the frontal bones)
2. Small cerebellum (transcerebellar diameter <10th percentile)
3. Effacement of the cisterna magna (width <2 mm on axial scan of posterior fossa)
4. The banana sign (small cerebellum hemispheres curling anteriorly and obliteration of the cisterna magna as a result of downward displacement of the hindbrain structures)
5. Ventriculomegaly (atrial width: severe: >14 mm; borderline: >10 mm)
6. Funneling of the posterior fossa (clivus-supraocciput angle <72°)

Posterior fossa signs are the most specific ones to detect open spinal defects. Ventriculomegaly typically appears after 22 weeks' gestation, and with its development, the lemon sign resolves. In 1 study, posterior fossa funneling in conjunction with a small cerebellum and effacement of the cisterna magna identified more than 90% of affected fetuses, whereas ventriculomegaly occurred in about 80% of cases. Several studies have found that by the end of the first trimester, the biparietal diameter (BPD) of fetuses with spina bifida was significantly smaller compared with normal fetuses. However, 1 study found that only 50% of cases with spina bifida had a BPD lower than the fifth percentile, making BPD measurement alone a poor screening tool, because it would theoretically misdiagnose half the cases of spina bifida.

The assessment of first trimester screening (11–13 weeks) for nuchal translucency (midsagittal view of the face) as a potential marker for trisomy 21 and other aneuploidies has become more commonplace. Using this same fetal ultrasonographic view, intracranial translucency can be assessed. The identified loss of intracranial translucency is believed to be the result of fourth ventricle compression between the brainstem and choroid plexus and may allow earlier detection of NTDs by ultrasonography before posterior fossa ultrasonographic signs.

Besides their contribution to facilitate early prenatal diagnosis of spina bifida, these ultrasonographic signs also confirm that NTDs affect early fetal brain development. The changes reflect the caudal displacement of infratentorial structures secondary to an early decrease of both the vermis and cerebellar tonsils and caudal portion of the brainstem through an enlarged foramen magnum into the cervical spinal canal. None of these signs has shown consistent prognostic power regarding outcome, functional level, or even the need for future ventricular shunting.

Studies using magnetic resonance imaging (MRI) have also tried to look at various findings as predictors of outcome: lesion level, interpediculate distance, vertebral segment span, and presence or absence of a covering membrane. Higher lesion level, lesion size, and lack of a covering membrane were associated with several adverse outcomes in children with spina bifida. These findings may be helpful in counseling families and informing physicians caring for the child with spina bifida in postnatal follow-up [12].

Because the brain anomalies associated with spina bifida are helpful in detecting only the open spinal defects, the screening for spina bifida should not be limited to the examination of fetal brain but should include the evaluation of the whole spine to detect closed defects. Spinal defects are usually identified during the second trimester. However, there is some disagreement on what can and cannot be said about the cystic structure and its covering (open or closed). In human and mouse embryos, the persistently open spinal cord undergoes relatively normal neuronal differentiation during the embryonic period, including development of spinal motor and sensory function below the lesion, which shows that neural tube closure is not needed for subsequent events of neuronal differentiation. However, as gestation progresses, neurons die within the exposed spinal cord, suggesting that the amniotic fluid environment is toxic for cells (the 2-hit hypothesis) [2].

GENETICS OF NTDS

Key points
- NTDs are considered to be a multifactorial disorder, arising from a complex combination of genetic and environmental factors.
- Disruption of 3 main gene pathways has been associated with NTDs.
- FA fortification in grains has led to a significant reduction in the prevalence of spina bifida.

NTDs are considered to be a multifactorial disorder, arising from a complex combination of genetic and environmental factors [2,13]. In humans there is a poor understanding of the genetic basis of NTDs. A genetic component for NTDs is suggested by the increased recurrence risk for a sibling of an affected individual (2%–5%), as well as an association of NTDs with several syndromes, including Meckel-Gruber syndrome (MKS) and Joubert syndrome [2,14,15]. Chromosomal abnormalities are also associated with NTDs, with a higher prevalence of NTDs occurring in conjunction with trisomy 13 and 18 [13]. To inform genetic studies in humans, attention has turned to knowledge gained from animal models, including mouse, in which more than 200 genes critical for neural tube closure have been identified [16]. Genetic risk factors for NTDs in humans fall into 3 main categories: noncanonical Wnt/planar cell polarity (PCP) pathway genes, cilia genes, and folate 1-carbon metabolism (FOCM) genes.

Genetic causes of NTDs

Noncanonical Wnt/PCP pathway genes

Noncanonical Wnt/PCP signaling is required for convergent extension, the process by which cells elongate and intercalate along the midline, leading to extension along the anterior-posterior axis of the body, with concomitant narrowing of the mediolateral axis [17]. Genes involved in the PCP pathway have been implicated in NTDs in both humans and mice. In humans, mutations in the core PCP gene *Celsr1* and the PCP-associated gene *Scrib* have been associated with craniorachischisis, the most severe NTD in which the entire neural tube remains open [18]. However, there is not a strict correspondence between genotype and phenotype, because mutations in *Celsr1* and *Scrib* have also been associated with milder forms of NTD and spina bifida [18,19]. Functional studies suggest that the mutations disrupt protein localization to the membrane. Several missense mutations in *Dact1*, which mediates Wnt signaling downstream of *DISHEVELLED* (*DVL*), were identified in a cohort of stillborn or miscarried fetuses with craniorachischisis, including 2 mutations that appeared to increase DVL2 degradation and alter JNK phosphorylation [18]. Several variants in core PCP genes *Vangl1* and *Vangl2* have been identified in human cases of both open (myelomeningocele [MMC]) and closed (tethered cord) spina bifida, as well as anencephaly, as have mutations in *Prickled1* [15,18,20]. The VANGL1 Val293Ile variant disrupts binding of VANGL1 with its cytoplasmic partners, *DISHEVELLED* (*DVL1*, *2* or *3*) [18]. Rare mutations in *Dvl2* have been found in NTD cohorts, as have 5 rare mutations in the Wnt receptor *Fzd6*, all of which are predicted to affect protein function [21]. Several mutations have been identified in the PCP effector *Fuz* in cases of MMC, including at least 1 substitution, Arg404Glu, which also resulted in defective ciliogenesis. Much of our understanding of the mechanisms underlying PCP function and its role in neural tube closure come from animal studies, and mutations in all of these genes as well as other members of the PCP pathway have been implicated in NTDs in mice [18]. Together, the substantial number of PCP genes implicated in human NTDs suggests that mutations in the PCP pathway represent a strong genetic risk factor in the development of NTDs.

Cilia genes

There is a link between the PCP pathway and ciliogenesis, as highlighted by the *Fuz* mutation. MKS is a ciliopathy disorder and is associated with NTDs. Several genes have been identified in patients with MKS that are linked to human NTDs, including *Mks1* and *Mks3* (*Tmem67*), *Rpgrip1l*, *Tmem216*, *Cep290* (*Mks4*), *Cc2d2a*, *B9D1*, and *B9D2* [22–24]. Multiple mutations have been identified in *Mks1* and *Mks3*, and these account for ~7% of MKS cases [25]. Functional studies of the aforementioned genes in human primary cells, mouse, zebrafish, and cell culture have shown all of these genes to be required for proper ciliogenesis and cilia function, which in turn is required for correct *SONIC HEDGEHOG* (*SHH*) signaling [26]. Moreover, analysis of MKS and Joubert syndrome fetal samples has shown impaired SHH-signaling [27]. Many genes implicated in mouse NTDs are required for ciliogenesis and PCP signaling, suggesting that cilia-related genes are excellent targets for future human studies. Recent whole-genome copy number variation analysis of NTD cases showed a strong association between cilia genes and NTDs [28].

FA metabolism genes

Although genetic factors are believed to account for up to 70% of NTDs, it is known that risk factors such as maternal diabetes, obesity, antiepileptic drugs, and maternal folate levels also play an important role in the cause of NTDs [2,14,29]. An association between folate deficiency and NTDs was first reported in 1965. Subsequent studies, culminating in a landmark study by the Medical Research Council in 1991, indicated that periconceptual FA supplementation (0.4 mg/d) could reduce the risk of recurrence of an NTD-affected pregnancy by up to 72% [14]. Since FA fortification of grains in 1998, the rate of NTDs in the United States has decreased substantially in the general population (31% decrease in spina bifida incidence and 16% decrease in anencephaly incidence) [30]. Thus, the search for genetic causes of NTDs focused on genes involved in folate metabolism. More than 40 genes involved in FOCM have been analyzed as potential risk factors for NTDs in humans. Much attention has focused on the common $677C \rightarrow T$ mutation in 5,10-methylenetetrahydrofolate reductase (*Mthfr*), which generates a protein with reduced enzyme activity and results in increased plasma homocysteine levels [31]. Data are conflicting as to whether the T allele in either the mother or patient is a risk factor for NTDs or not, suggesting a population-specific effect of the polymorphism [15]. Recent meta-analyses of the data concluded that there is an overall risk associated with the $677C \rightarrow T$ allele, and this risk can be reduced with FA supplementation [32–34]. A second polymorphism identified in *Mthfr*, $1298A \rightarrow C$, is also implicated as a risk factor for NTDs, although meta-analysis indicates that by itself, the polymorphism is not a significant risk factor [34,35]. Similarly, meta-analyses of polymorphisms in *Mtrr* ($66A \rightarrow G$) and *Mtr* ($2756A \rightarrow G$) showed no significant increase in risk, although the *Rfc-1* $80A \rightarrow G$ polymorphism may be associated with increased NTD risk. There seems to be more conclusive evidence for polymorphisms in *Mthfd1*, at least in the presence of underlying folate deficiency [36]. Studies that did not take into account maternal folate levels are less conclusive [15]. A common deletion/insertion polymorphism in the mitochondrial paralogue of *Mthfd1*, *Mthfd1l*, was recently identified as a risk factor for NTDs, and this may be through alternative splicing of MTHFD1L and microRNA regulation [37,38]. The glycine cleavage system, part of mitochondrial FOCM, is also implicated in NTDs. Several nonsynonymous mutations in *Amt* and *Gldc* were identified, and all the NTD-associated *Gldc* mutations showed reduced enzymatic activity, supporting the idea that these mutations are causative [2]. Despite the extensive studies on folate pathway genes and the importance of folate in neural tube closure established almost 50 years ago, the data remain inconclusive for most of the FOCM genes, highlighting how much is yet to be learned about the role of FA in neural tube closure.

Summary

Many gene-NTD correlation studies have failed to investigate the functional importance of the variants identified, which limits the power of the findings in showing causative mutations. The 3 pathways discussed earlier clearly do not complete our understanding of the genetic causes of human NTD, yet the large number of genes within each of these pathways indicates their importance in neural tube closure. Animal models still have much to contribute to research in this field by providing functional studies of potential risk alleles and through continued identification of genes necessary for neural tube closure. Combined efforts of developmental biologists, geneticists, epidemiologists, and clinicians will lead to a greater understanding of this complex and multifactorial birth defect.

NEUROSURGICAL ISSUES

Key points

- Neurosurgical management of the patient with spina bifida is lifelong.
- Shunt malfunction may present with signs and symptoms similar to Chiari malformation, tethered cord, or syringohydromyelia.
- Any neurologic deterioration should begin with an evaluation of shunt function.
- Surgical treatment of hydrocephalus, Chiari malformation, tethered cord, or syringohydromyelia may result in stabilization of, and often improvement in, neurologic function.

Introduction

Neurosurgical management of the child with spina bifida is a lifelong commitment that involves:

1. Closure of the MMC
2. Assessment and treatment of hydrocephalus
3. Management of shunt malfunctions, symptomatic Chiari malformations, tethered spinal cord, and syringohydromyelia

Prenatal detection allows parents to have sufficient time to understand the potential problems associated with the diagnosis. The unanticipated MMC at birth requires a multidisciplinary approach to help parents arrive at optimal and surgical treatments for their child.

Neonatal assessment and surgical treatment

On delivery, the infant's MMC should be kept clean, promptly covered with gauze dressing soaked in sterile saline, followed by plastic wrap over the gauze to keep the dressing moist. Substances containing neurotoxic iodine should be avoided. Prophylactic intravenous antibiotics, such as ampicillin and gentamicin, are administered.

Neurosurgical evaluation includes:

1. Size and shape of the defect determines proper surgical planning
   a. Kyphotic deformity may require kyphectomy at time of closure
2. Sensorimotor function
   a. See Table 1
3. Hydrocephalus
   a. Examine fontanelle for fullness
   b. Look for splaying sutures
   c. Enlarging head circumference over time
4. Symptomatic Chiari malformation, as shown by:
   a. Apneic spells
   b. Dysfunctional swallowing
   c. Lower cranial palsies
   d. Hypotonia

MMC repair

The MMC can be repaired within the first 48 to 72 hours after birth without significant neurologic morbidity or infectious complications [39]. The operative technique for closure involves [40–42]:

1. Entering the sac in an area with no visible neural tissue
2. Dissecting the margin of the exposed neural placode from the surrounding skin (Fig. 1A)
3. The neural tube is recreated by reapproximating the margins of the placode in the midline

Table 1
Motor and sensory function by neurologic level

Neurologic level	Motor	Sensory
L2	Hip flexion	Anteromedial thigh
L3	Knee extension	Anterior shin
L4	Ankle dorsiflexion	Dorsum of foot
L5	Long toe extension	First–second interspace
S1	Ankle plantar flexion	Plantar aspect of foot

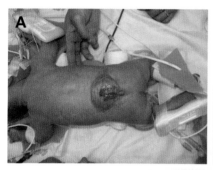
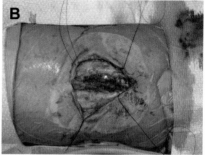
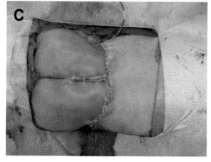

Fig. 1. Closure of the MMC. (A) Lumbosacral MMC with placode in the center and attached to the surrounding skin. (B) Dural dissection has been completed and closed over newly closed neural tube. (C) Muscle and fascial layers have been mobilized to close the defect. (*Courtesy of* Dr Craig Birgfeld, Seattle Children's Hospital, Seattle, WA.)

4. The dura is dissected at the junctional zone where it meets the skin; a dural sac is created and subsequently closed over the newly closed neural tube (see Fig. 1B)
5. The subcutaneous tissue and skin are mobilized to close the defect (see Fig. 1C)

Management of hydrocephalus

Approximately 80% to 90% of children with spina bifida undergo shunt placement for hydrocephalus [43,44]. The signs and symptoms of a shunt malfunction are closely monitored throughout the patient's lifetime. Shunt malfunction may present with the classic symptoms such as headache, nausea/vomiting, lethargy, or sunsetting eyes. It may also present with signs and symptoms of a tethered cord, such as syringomyelia or brainstem compression from Chiari malformation. Initial evaluation of any neurologic deterioration in these patients should first begin with investigation of the shunt. A computed tomography scan may show enlargement of the ventricles compared with baseline scans. However, some patients have ventricles that remain unchanged despite symptoms. For these patients, a shunt tap to determine opening pressure may be necessary. Alternatively, a nuclear medicine study with injection of radionuclide tracer into the shunt reservoir may ascertain system patency. As with all shunt failures, the clinical status of the child is paramount in the diagnosis.

Endoscopic third ventriculostomy (ETV) has emerged as an alternative to shunt placement in this population, with reported overall success rates of up to 72% [45]. Candidates for ETV should have radiographic evidence of noncommunicating hydrocephalus. Because of the high incidence of abnormal third ventricular anatomy in this population, patients must have careful examination of imaging before ETV to avoid surgical complications.

Management of Chiari malformation

Virtually all children with MMCs have Chiari II malformations. Chiari II malformations are best evaluated on sagittal T1-weighted or T2-weighted MRI. They present as displacement of the cerebellar tonsils, vermis, and caudal medulla below the foramen magnum, a beaked tectum, dysgenesis of the corpus callosum, and enlarged massa intermedia. Many have no clinical symptoms, but clinical manifestations may include dysphagia, apneic spells, stridor, hoarse or high-pitched cry, weakness or spasticity or the upper extremities, oculomotor dysfunction, and scoliosis.

Symptomatic Chiari malformation can be treated surgically with cervical laminectomy with or without duraplasty. Foramen magnum or occipital bony decompression is rarely necessary. Opening the posterior fossa carries greater bleeding risk, because of anatomically low venous sinuses.

Management of tethered spinal cord

Overall, one-third of children with spina bifida require surgery for a tethered spinal cord [46]. Signs and symptoms of tethered cord include:

- Pain in the back or legs
- Deterioration in motor function or gait
- Sensory changes
- Deterioration in bowel or bladder function
- Progressive orthopedic deformities of the lower extremities or spine

If shunt malfunction is ruled out, and there is clinical suspicion of cord tethering, objective measures such as manual testing of muscle strength and urodynamics can be obtained to confirm the diagnosis.

Detethering the spinal cord requires opening the original surgical closure site, extending it cranially, and identifying the last level of formed posterior elements, which are removed to expose normal dura. The dura is then opened to identify normal spinal cord. The incision is then extended caudally to facilitate dissection of the scarred placode and associated nerve roots off the dura. Adhesions are transected until the placode is released circumferentially. The dura is then reapproximated and closed. The wound is subsequently closed in layers to minimize leakage of cerebrospinal fluid (CSF).

Surgical outcome is excellent. Preoperative motor deficit improvement can be seen in 72% of patients after surgery, stabilization of deficit in 25%, and deterioration in 3%.

Management of syringohydromyelia

The syringomyelia is a cavity in communication with the central canal that develops within the spinal cord. Hydromyelia is dilatation of the central canal. Because it is often difficult to differentiate between the 2, the term syringohydromyelia is used. It is present in 50% to 80% of patients with spina bifida, but becomes symptomatic in less than 5% [47,48]. Symptomatic syringohydromyelia may be a result of shunt failure, and symptoms may resolve after revision. Because syringohydromyelia, Chiari malformation, and spinal cord tethering have similar clinical presentations, surgical options depend on specific symptomatology. There is little strong evidence to support firm recommendations for Chiari decompression, spinal cord detethering, or shunting of syringes.

Summary

Neurosurgical management of the patient with spina bifida is lifelong. Shunt malfunction may present with signs and symptoms similar to Chiari malformation, tethered cord, or syringohydromyelia. Any neurologic deterioration should begin with an evaluation of shunt function. Surgical treatment of hydrocephalus, Chiari malformation, tethered cord, or syringohydromyelia may result in stabilization of, and often improvement in, neurologic function.

BOWEL AND BLADDER MANAGEMENT

Key points

- Options to optimize bladder storage pressures now include overnight bladder drainage and the use of intravesical botulinum toxin injection in addition to clean intermittent catheterization and anticholinergic medication.
- Antegrade continence enema (ACE) irrigation times can be frustratingly long for some patients. The use of a left-sided ACE addresses the concern.
- The TOMAX procedure (to maximize sensation, sexuality, and quality of life) is a new and underused procedure for the adult male patient with poor or no sensation in the glans penis.

Management of the neurogenic bladder

Introduction

Eighty-five percent of patients with spina bifida have an underlying neurogenic bladder [49]. Bladder management includes the use of clean intermittent catheterization, anticholinergic medications, and α-blockade medication. Botulinum toxin A is a relatively new addition to the therapeutic armamentarium for these patients, and onabotulinumtoxinA (Botox) has recently received US Food and Drug Administration approval for use in patients with neurogenic bladder conditions. Overnight catheter drainage has also been effectively used in a select group of patients with small poorly compliant neurogenic bladders to decrease the risk of upper urinary tract deterioration.

Evaluation

Patients should be evaluated with renal ultrasonography and urodynamic studies every 6 to 12 months to detect evidence of hydronephrosis. If the urodynamic study does not have a fluoroscopic component included with it, voiding cystourethrography is a useful radiographic modality to assess for the presence of vesicoureteral reflux. Based on these studies, an optimal bladder management strategy may be proposed to keep bladder storage pressures within safe limits and to optimize urinary control.

Nonpharmacologic treatment options

Clean intermittent catheterization remains a mainstay of treatment of most patients with neurogenic bladder conditions like spina bifida, with the goal of maximizing bladder emptying and preserving upper urinary tract function in the setting of a poorly compliant neurogenic bladder. Children with spina bifida can be taught to independently catheterize themselves between 5 and 10 years in girls in boys. Overnight urinary catheterization can be introduced to decrease bladder pressures for prolonged periods in patients with functionally small, poorly compliant bladders before the implementation of surgical urinary diversion. Overnight catheter drainage preserves bladder capacity, which facilitates later urinary reconstruction. Patients and their families are instructed to insert a urinary retention catheter in the evening before sleeping and remove it in the morning.

Pharmacologic treatment options for the neurogenic bladder

The use of medications via the oral route, transdermally, and via intravesicular injection is frequently recommended to decrease bladder storage pressure and improve urinary continence (Table 2). Several small case series studies have reported increased bladder compliance and improved urinary continence [50]. OnabotulinumtoxinA is reconstituted and diluted to a concentration of 10 to 20 units/mL for a bladder injection or 50 to 100 units/mL for a bladder neck

Table 2
Common medications for management of the neurogenic bladder

Medication	Mechanism of action	Route	Dosage	Timing
Oxybutynin	Anticholinergic	By mouth/ intravesical	Immediate 5 mg in >5 y	2–3×/d
			Extended release 5 mg in >6 y with maximum of 20 mg	1×/d
Oxytrol R	Anticholinergic	Transdermal	1 patch	2× wk
Tolterodine	Anticholinergic	By mouth	1–2 mg	1–2×/d
Tamsulosin	α Blockade	By mouth	0.2–0.4 mg	Every day
Botulinum toxin A (Botox)	Neuroparalytic	Intravesical or intraurethral	100–200 units	Every 6–12 mo

injection. The injection is performed transurethrally in a series of 0.5-mL to 1.0-mL injections along the posterior lateral aspect of the bladder using up to 200 units of onabotulinumtoxinA or up to 100 units of onabotulinumtoxinA diluted in 1 to 4 mL normal saline injected into the bladder neck and external urethral sphincter. Methylene blue may be added to the diluent to assist in visualizing the injection sites. Table 2 highlights the most common pharmacologic treatments for bladder management in patients with spina bifida. Most have not been approved for treatment in children.

Combination therapies
Pharmacologic and nonpharmacologic therapies may be combined in any combination that achieves the desired outcome.

Surgical treatment options
Surgical interventions for children with spina bifida are used frequently to preserve upper tract function, increase continence, and enhance independence in care. A vesicostomy is useful when safe urine storage pressures cannot be achieved with nonsurgical options. This surgical procedure is typically performed in the infant. Refluxing ureterostomy is useful when safe urine storage pressures cannot be achieved with nonsurgical options and the patient has a refluxing ureter. The anterior wall of the distal ureter is mobilized and anastomosed to the skin to allow free efflux of urine. It has the advantage of being technically easier to perform than a vesicostomy and preserves bladder capacity. The Mitrofanoff procedure is used to create a nonorthotopic catheterizable channel to the bladder. It can be constructed from appendix, ureter, small intestine, or any other luminal structure in the body. It allows the patient or caregiver access to catheterize the bladder without using the urethra.

Management of the neurogenic bowel
Introduction
Ninety percent of patients with spina bifida have an underlying neurogenic bowel, which prevents normal toilet training and frequently results in fecal incontinence when unmanaged. Advances in bowel management through dietary modification and the use of stool softeners and laxatives have improved bowel control [51]. Surgical alternatives such as the Chait tube and the ACE or Malone ACE (MACE) procedure have also been useful additions for patients who want independence in their bowel management programs and who have responded well to retrograde bowel management. Social continence with controlled defecation occurring in a socially appropriate location and time remain the goal of bowel management, in conjunction with the minimization of clinically significant constipation and obstipation.

Surgical treatment options
The original description of the MACE involves placement of the stoma on the right side of the colon, with the intention to evacuate the entire colon with enema administration. Recent modifications to the location of the MACE include placement on the left side of the colon. Shorter flush times were found

when patients used the MACE in a left-sided location. Stomal complications were slightly less common as well in this location [52].

Management of sexual dysfunction in men with spina bifida
Introduction
Many male patients with spina bifida have decreased or no penile sensation, despite the ability to achieve erections, ejaculation, and orgasm. Approximately 70% of male patients can achieve erections, dripping ejaculation in 54%, and orgasm occurring in 20%. Normally, penile sensory impulses transmit via the 2 dorsal nerves of the penis and pudendal nerves to the penis to the S2-S4 sacral nerve roots, but this is disrupted in men with spina bifida. The TOMAX procedure (to maximize sensation, sexuality, and quality of life) represents a microneurorraphy procedure that joins the ileoinguinal nerve to the dorsal nerve. In the 1 reported case series, all 3 patients achieved increased sensation in the glans penis after the operation and reported improved quality of life [53]. Larger-scale studies are needed to gain a deeper understanding of the success and applications of this procedure. This operation remains underused, likely because of lack of awareness of the operation or lack of familiarity with neurorraphy procedures among urologists.

ENDOCRINE ISSUES

Key points
- The hypothalamic-pituitary axis can be disrupted by hydrocephalus seen commonly in children with spina bifida.
- Leptin secretion may be dysregulated and related to obesity in children with spina bifida.

MMC remains a complex disease that affects the central nervous system and therefore the endocrine system. Anatomically, the floor of the third ventricle is just above the hypothalamus, which communicates via the portal system to the anterior pituitary. Alteration in cerebral spinal fluid flow, as observed with hydrocephalus, can change the physical environment of the maturing hypothalamic pituitary axis, potentially altering stimulatory and inhibitory input. In recent years, endocrine issues, including leptin secretion, precocious puberty, and growth hormone (GH) deficiency, have been studied in patients with MMC, some of which have a therapeutic benefit:

Leptin
Leptin, derived from adipose tissue, is a satiety signal (anorexigenic) involved in long-term regulation of weight. It activates the proopiomelanocortin gene in the hypothalamus. Leptin receptor mutations have been associated with early onset obesity and failure of sexual maturation. Treatment with leptin results in reduction in weight and resumption of puberty. Transport of leptin across the

blood-brain barrier is important in leptin regulation, and thus, shunt-dependent hydrocephalus with intermittent change in intracranial pressure may influence leptin secretion of patients with MMC. Trollmann and colleagues [54] studied 10 prepubertal children with MMC, all of whom had GH deficiency and shunt-dependent hydrocephalus. Motor level of lesion was lower than L2 for 4, higher than L2 for 3, and L3-4 for 3 children. They had normal BMI for age and sex. Leptin levels of patients with MMC were compared with 10 prepubertal children with GH deficiency as well as 12 healthy prepubertal short children who were GH sufficient. GH-deficient children with MMC had abnormal nocturnal leptin secretion compared with both control groups. The MMC group did not show the expected decline in leptin in the morning hours nor did their leptin levels correlate with BMI, as observed among the control groups. The investigators concluded that the pattern of leptin secretion of these patients with MMC and GH deficiency may reflect hypothalamic dysregulation.

Precocious puberty

Hydrocephalus, with or without MMC, has been associated with early puberty. Proos and colleagues [55] found that perinatally increased intracranial pressure in girls with MMC predicts early and precocious puberty. These investigators observed the same association with boys who have MMC [56]. Of the 38 (37 with hydrocephalus) boys whom they evaluated retrospectively, 21% had pubertal changes before the age of 9 years. Early brainstem dysfunction has the highest explanatory value in predicting early puberty. Central precocious puberty is treated with gonadotropin-releasing hormone analogues, which reduce the pulsatile secretion of luteinizing hormone and follicle-stimulating hormone to a flat profile and stops the progression of puberty.

GH deficiency

Since the first description by Rotenstein and colleagues [57] in 1989 of increased growth velocity of GH-deficient children with MMC treated with GH, data have accumulated with respect to efficacy and attainment of near adult stature. From various estimates, 30% to 70% of children with MMC have GH deficiency, possibly related to hydrocephalus in utero and alterations of their hypothalamic pituitary axis, as discussed earlier. Trollmann and colleagues [58] evaluated growth of children with MMC on GH treatment within KIGS (Pfizer International Growth Database). Of 52 patients with documented GH deficiency, 21 were prepubertal at the start and during GH treatment. With 3 years of longitudinal growth analyzed, the patients showed a significant increase in growth velocity standard deviation score (SDS) and an improvement in height SDS from −3.25 at the start to −1.87 at 36 months. The BMI SDS remained unchanged during GH treatment, with no major side effects observed. The data from the KIGS study reflect the overall height increase observed by Rotenstein and Breen [59], who analyzed data from the Genentech database in the United States as well as data on fewer patients in other reports. Although there are weaknesses in registry data and a lack of controls and MMC-specific factors, such as motor level of lesion, the investigators concluded that GH treatment of MMC children is a means to achieve improved stature. Rotenstein and Bass reported retrospective evaluation of 20 GH-deficient patients with MMC (12 males) treated with GH for a mean of 8.7 years [60]. GH treatment significantly improved the SDS for stature of the patients with MMC compared with both untreated adult patients with MMC and with normal adults. Fifteen of 20 patients achieved stature between the third and 10th percentile of the normal population. Scoliosis did not progress and BMI was less than untreated adult patients with MMC.

Summary
In view of the multiple problems that face patients with MMC, such as obesity, short stature, and decreased muscle strength and ambulation, treatment with GH may offer the possibility of normalization of stature and increase in muscle strength, which may improve ambulation. Clearly, GH has major advantageous metabolic effects, which need further study and evaluation to improve the functional lives of patients with MMC beyond stature.

ORTHOPEDICS AND BONE HEALTH ISSUES

Key points
- Both congenital and acquired orthopedic deformities are commonly seen in children with spina bifida.
- Surgical intervention may be indicated to improve ambulation, function in sitting and transfers, and alignment to protect the insensate skin.
- Fractures unrelated to significant trauma are common and related to limited weight bearing.

Introduction
Congenital and acquired orthopedic deformities are commonly seen in children with spina bifida. These deformities are seen at the spine, hip, knee, and foot and ankle and result from positioning, muscle imbalance, and paralysis [61]. To assist in the evaluation and treatment, a pediatric orthopedic surgeon is an integral team member in the care of children with spina bifida.

Spine
Spinal deformities are commonly observed in children with spina bifida and include scoliosis, kyphosis, and lordosis. Congenital vertebral anomalies, including hemivertebra, unsegmented vertebra, butterfly vertebra, and the condition defining failure of fusion of the posterior arch, lead to the high prevalence of these deformities. Scoliosis is present in approximately 50% of children with spina bifida, with those having a thoracic level at a 90% prevalence rate, midlumbar 40%, and low lumbar 10% [62].

Acquired scoliosis is considered neuromuscular in nature and related to spinal muscle weakness and it increases with the age of the child. The presence of a tethered cord or syringomyelia should be considered when the scoliosis curve increases at a higher than normal velocity. Nonsurgical treatment options are generally ineffective and include bracing and use of supportive seating systems. Surgical interventions are warranted when the curve progresses beyond 30°, because progression of the curve beyond that point is expected. A spinal fusion is the definitive treatment but is traditionally limited to children who have completed most of their growth. With the introduction of growing constructs such as the vertically expanding prosthetic titanium rib systems and growing rods, children with severe scoliosis at younger ages can undergo a spine stabilization procedure without sacrificing the final truncal height [63].

Hips

Hip deformities in children with spina bifida include contractures, subluxation, and dislocation and are more common in those with higher-level neurologic involvement [64]. Muscle imbalance with weakness is responsible for the high incidence of dislocated hips. Historically, attempts were made to relocate the dislocated hip but were not successful. The dislocated hip remains relatively pain free in the child with spina bifida, because of decreased sensation. In the ambulatory child, a unilateral or bilateral dislocated hip did not affect the symmetry of gait, and in the case of an asymmetric dislocation, did not affect the walking speed compared with those without a dislocated hip. Treatment goals are focused on maintaining range of motion with contracture release procedures to allow for a level pelvis and symmetry, without a focus on the dislocation.

Knees

Knee flexion and extension contractures are observed in children with spina bifida, with those having a higher-level lesion experiencing it more frequently [64]. Knee flexion contractures are seen more often when nonambulatory and are related to prolonged periods of sitting with knees in the flexed position and quadriceps weakness. Knee flexion contractures in the ambulatory child are less common and interfere with gait efficiency when the contractures are greater than 20°. Surgical intervention is indicated when the contractures are significant enough to interfere with sitting balance or gait. Knee extension contractures are less common and observed in the child with a midlumbar level spina bifida with unopposed quadriceps activity. For those who are wheelchair dependent, persistent knee extension can make transfers challenging, as well as positioning in a wheelchair, prompting a surgical intervention.

Foot and ankle

Foot and ankle problems are almost universal in children with spina bifida. Congenital clubfoot and vertical talus are the most common, with a clubfoot presenting in up to 50% of infants. Both clubfoot and vertical talus can affect ambulation, tolerance of orthoses, or positioning of the feet on a wheelchair footplate. Foot deformities also lead to issues with skin breakdown. The goal of any intervention is for the child to have a plantargrade foot. Management of the clubfoot is primarily surgical in nature, although manual manipulation and serial casting using the Ponseti method has shown some benefit [65,66].

Acquired foot and ankle deformities are typically caused by muscle weakness and subsequent imbalance of forces. A calcaneus foot (ankle is in extreme dorsiflexion) is caused by an unopposed anterior tibialis muscle seen in someone with an L4 or L5 level lesion. At this level, the child is frequently ambulatory, so surgical intervention is warranted if the deformity is interfering with gait. The presence of a tethered cord or syrinx should be considered when a progressive deformity of the foot is seen, such as development of a cavus foot. Inspection of the feet with a special focus on the skin and the structure of the foot should be an integral part of every clinical examination.

Fractures

The incidence of fractures is reported to be 11% to 30% in children with spina bifida [67–69]. The high rate is believed secondary to reduced bone mineral density in the setting of limited ambulation and muscle weakness [70]. Fractures frequently occur without a history of significant trauma, and there is frequently no report of any type of trauma that preceded the fracture. In the setting of a child with reduced sensation, the fracture is identified by radiograph in the setting of a swollen and warm limb. Full-time ambulators had better bone density compared with those children who were wheelchair dependent or part-time ambulators and had a higher neurologic level [71]. Use of bisphosphonates has not been universally accepted in children with spina bifida, although consideration should be given when a child has had a fracture of a long bone unrelated to trauma [72].

Summary

Congenital and acquired orthopedic issues are common in children with spina bifida and are seen in the spine, hips, knees, and ankles. Participation in the interdisciplinary spina bifida clinic by an orthopedic surgeon is critical to assure a proactive approach to management of the deformities. The focus of the nonsurgical and surgical approaches should be on improving or maintaining ambulatory function, sitting posture in a wheelchair, and orthosis and shoe wear, and skin integrity.

REHABILITATION CARE

Key points

- The functional level of a child with MMC is determined primarily by their motor level.
- Use of orthoses and adaptive equipment such as crutches or walkers is typical in children with midlumbar and low lumbar MMC.
- Children at or lower than the L5 level are likely to be community ambulators.

Introduction

The comprehensive management of functional issues in children with spina bifida is dependent on a thorough clinical examination. It is important to identify
the individual's neurologic level, which can help determine functional prognosis and guide care over time. The neurologic level is determined by evaluating patterns of muscle function [73] and cutaneous sensation [74]. The
motor level can be established based on active isolated movement, which is
observed or determined through resisted manual muscle testing, which is typically reliable after age 5 years. Existing strength greatly affects the individual's
functional mobility and ambulation status [75].

Independent mobility for people with spina bifida is influenced by muscle
function level and the presence of secondary impairments such as contractures
and orthopedic as a result of changes associated with growth and muscle imbalance [76]. Table 3 highlights the functional, equipment, and orthotic expectations by neurologic level. Other factors that affect independence and
participation in daily life include cognitive abilities and the presence of a shunt
[75], familial support [77], and access to resources, including equipment and education regarding health and maintenance.

Table 3
Rehabilitation needs by functional motor level

Functional motor level	Expected muscle function	Functional mobility	Equipment use	Orthotic use
Thoracic	Abdominals, paraspinals, quadratus lumborum	Nonfunctional ambulation/ standing during therapy, school or at home, wheelchair for mobility	Standing frame, wheelchair, parapodium	Trunk-hip-knee-ankle-foot orthosis
High lumbar L1-L3	Hip flexion, hip adduction	Limited household ambulation, wheelchair for mobility	Wheelchair, walker, forearm crutches	Reciprocating gait orthosis, hip-knee-ankle-foot orthosis
Midlumbar L3-L4	Knee extension	Household, limited community ambulation	Wheelchair, walker, forearm crutches	Knee-ankle-foot orthosis
Low lumbar L4-L5	Hip abduction, knee flexion, ankle dorsiflexion, ankle inversion, toe extension	Household, community ambulation, wheelchair for long distances	Wheelchair, forearm crutches	Ankle-foot orthosis
Sacral S1S2	Hip extension, ankle plantar flexion, ankle eversion, toe flexion	Community ambulation	—	Supramalleolar-foot orthosis, foot orthotic

Functional expectations by motor levels

Thoracic level

At the thoracic level of muscle function, children have intact upper extremity function but lack volitional control of muscles in the lower extremities. There is active shoulder and neck muscle function, as well as trunk (abdominal and paraspinal) muscle function, depending on the level of spinal defect. Children with function lower than T11 (T12–L1) most likely have good trunk strength, resulting in fair to good sitting balance, and varying ability to assist with bed mobility and transfers. Quadratus lumborum may be present to allow hip hiking, which makes the use of a parapodium possible. Otherwise, at this level, ambulation is not functional. Standers are often used for upright positioning, and children typically use a wheelchair for primary locomotion in the household and out in the community. Use of a manual wheelchair is common in children at this level, unless they have poor trunk control and weak upper extremities. In this case, use of a power wheelchair provides independent mobility.

High lumbar level

At the high lumbar level of muscle function, there is hip flexion, hip adduction, and internal and external hip rotation. At the L1 level, there is weak hip flexion, and at L2, there is functional hip flexion plus hip adduction and rotation. It is possible for smaller children to perform short distance household ambulation with a reciprocating gait orthosis (RGO). Generally, a manual wheelchair is required for home and community mobility in older children, and most are independent for transfers.

Midlumbar and low lumbar levels

Five muscle groups have been shown to significantly determine ambulatory status: iliopsoas, quadriceps, gluteus medius, gluteus maximus, and anterior tibialis [73]. At the L3 level, children show strong hip flexion and adduction, with functional knee extension. Household ambulation is possible with use of knee-ankle-foot orthoses (KAFO), ankle-foot ortheses (AFOs), or ground reaction AFOs and Lofstrand forearm crutches or a walker. These children primarily use a wheelchair for community mobility. At L4, knee flexion is available via the medial hamstrings, and ankle dorsiflexion is functional. Although a wheelchair is usually used for longer distances, community ambulation is possible with KAFOs or AFOs, and forearm crutches or a walker. At the L5 level, there is functional knee flexion, ankle dorsiflexion, and inversion, but weak hip abduction and extension. Typically, children at the L5 level are community ambulators, but often with the assistance of AFOs, and sometimes, forearm crutches or a walker.

Sacral level

The sacral level is consistent with the presence of plantar flexors and hip abduction and extension. Children at the S1 level can ambulate in the community without orthoses or assistive devices. Bracing at the foot and ankle may be required as a result of biomechanical malalignment from muscle imbalance and orthopedic changes and to improve stability. At the S2 and S3 levels, near normal or normal strength is present throughout the lower extremity muscles. These children may require a foot orthosis or shoe inserts to provide stability and maintain optimal ankle and foot alignment. The gait pattern is typical, with the possible exception of mildly decreased force of push-off.

Cutaneous sensation

Cutaneous sensation of pain, light touch, temperature, and pressure usually corresponds with muscle function level. Testing sensation can be preferable to muscle testing because it remains stable and is not affected by surgery, disuse, or contractures [74]. A dermatome map is used to identify areas of sensory deficit. A sensory level is generally assigned as the lowest level of intact sensation for both the right and left lower extremities. Lack of cutaneous sensation places the individual at risk for injury, skin breakdown, and pressure sores, which may go undetected.

Orthotic management

For children with high lumbar and thoracic motor levels, a standing frame, swivel walker, or parapodium can be used to promote upright positioning. Weight bearing in an upright position may maintain lower extremity range of motion and provide positioning for social interaction. In other populations, passive weight bearing has been associated with improved bone mineral density and reduced urinary tract infections by more complete emptying of the bladder [78,79]. Upright mobility is possible using an RGO in conjunction with a walker. For children with midlumbar to low lumbar spina bifida, the use of a solid AFO has been shown to increase stability during walking, with increased stride length, increased speed, decreased double stance time, decreased oxygen consumption, and increased power at terminal stance [80]. A floor reaction style that limits anterior movement of the tibia during stance phase can be used in the presence of weak quadricep and gastrocnemius soleus muscles. For children requiring only medial-lateral stability or the correction of varus or valgus deformities in the foot, a supramalleolar foot orthosis or foot orthosis may be used. Orthoses are typically custom molded for a child by an orthotist or some physical therapists, and adjustments are needed every few months, with replacements every 12 months for growth.

Therapeutic intervention

A comprehensive team of providers is optimal in the functional management of children with MMC and consists of specialists in orthopedics, developmental pediatrics, rehabilitation medicine, orthotic management, and therapies, including physical, occupational, and sometimes, speech therapy [81].

The physical therapist can play in integral role in the care of individuals with spina bifida. The focus of therapy changes throughout the individual's life span but always emphasizes function, independence, and self-esteem [81]. Independence with mobility, regardless of means, has been found to strongly correlate with quality of life [75].

Therapeutic intervention is based on maximizing independence and efficiency with regard to the person's motor level in conjunction with their specific concerns and goals. Interventions generally emphasize patient and family education regarding functional skills, mobility, information on skin care and pressure relief, and instruction on a home maintenance program. The therapist also addresses appropriate equipment and orthotic support, as well as resources for community-based recreational and physical opportunities for people with special needs. Home programs target active and passive range of motion, stretching, functional strengthening, supported standing programs for weight-bearing benefits, and positioning to maintain neutral alignment through appropriate equipment and orthotic prescription.

Treatment of individuals with thoracic level lesions emphasizes modified independence, with bed mobility, assisted transfers from supine to sitting, static sitting balance, and wheelchair mobility. At the high lumbar level, therapy focuses on dynamic sitting balance, wheelchair transfers, wheelchair mobility, and possibly, household ambulation, using an RGO for exercise. The therapeutic focus for midlumbar and lower lumbar levels is balance, postural control, biomechanical alignment in standing and assisted walking, gait training using Lofstrand forearm crutches or a walker, and independence with accessing the home and community environments. Sacral level therapeutic intervention targets higher-level balance activities, bilateral coordination, support for participation in sports, and fine tuning gait if affected by muscle imbalance, such as decreased push-off.

Occupational therapists play an integral part in the care of children with spina bifida. Similar to their physical therapy counterparts, they evaluate and treat children in the hospital, birth to age 3 year settings, outpatient clinics, and schools. Functional mobility is a focus for occupational therapy as well as physical therapy in the promotion of developmental skills. Positioning for play and optimal upper extremity use is essential for fine motor skills, activities of daily living, and independent mobility. Occupational therapists also address play skills, visual motor integration, sensory processing, social skills, equipment acquisition, and prevocational training. In the setting of upper extremity weakness, they focus on functional strengthening, bracing to maintain range of motion, and use of adaptive equipment to maximize function [82].

NEUROPSYCHOLOGICAL FUNCTION

Key points
- Structural brain abnormalities in spina bifida are important determinants of the neuropsychological profile.
- The impairments in language, mathematics, and executive functioning are not delayed but persist throughout life.
- Neuropsychological profiles can delineate individual phenotypes and assist in improving functioning and outcomes.

Introduction
The neuropsychological model of children with spina bifida has evolved over the past 50 years. It has emphasized IQ, spinal lesion level, perceptual motor

issues, cocktail chatter, reading issues, language deficits, nonverbal learning disabilities, executive functioning problems, and mathematic deficits. The current focus is on a spina bifida phenotype, the product of multiple complex processes, as opposed to a dichotomy such as visual versus auditory perception or verbal versus nonverbal learning disability. The current evolving neuropsychological model involves a complex cognitive pattern, with a naturally occurring variability in neural phenotype and environmental factors, leading to the variability of the cognitive phenotype.

Structure versus function

An increasing body of work supports the concept that specific intellectual deficiencies in individuals with spina bifida can be attributed to structural brain defects. Historically, patients with spina bifida who had associated hydrocephalus and episodes of shunt malfunction (blockage and infection) were believed to have lower intelligence than those who did not have hydrocephalus. More recently, improved imaging techniques and neuroanatomic studies (such as of the cerebellum) have identified additional inherent structural brain abnormalities; the Chiari II malformation and tectal beaking may be more important determinants of cognitive outcome than the number of shunt malfunctions or shunt revisions [83,84]. Three core deficits are described in spina bifida: timing, attention, and movement.

- Deficits in timing are related to the volume of the cerebellum.
- Deficits in attention are related to the status of the midbrain, posterior cortex, and corpus callosum.
- Deficits in movement are related to spinal cord dysfunction and cerebellar dysmorphologies that affect sensory motor timing and motor regulation.

Level of lesion

Children with upper versus lower level spinal lesions differ in terms of their anomalous brain development and behavioral outcomes. A higher level of spinal lesion has been used as a marker for more severe anomalous brain development. MRI obtained in children with upper-level spinal lesions (T12 and above) show more qualitative abnormalities in the midbrain and tectum, pons, and splenium compared with images obtained in children with lower-level spinal lesions [85]. Cerebellar anomalies were frequent in both groups and did not occur at a different rate in higher-level or lower-level lesions. However, upper-level lesions were associated with reductions in overall and regional cerebrum and cerebellum volumes. The smaller brain volumes are a result of a loss of gray and white matter.

Studies comparing lesion level and measures of intelligence, academic skills, and adaptive behavior are not consistent. Some studies report no relationship between IQ and lesion level, whereas some report that only thoracic lesions are associated with lower IQ. Others report that only lesions above L2 are related to poorer neurobehavioral outcomes; these outcomes may affect future levels of independent functioning. These differences do not seem to represent the effects of hydrocephalus.

Assembled versus associative processing

The neuropsychological model in children with spina bifida involves several factors that determine functional assets and weaknesses. Particularly important are deficits in assembled processing (the ability to assemble, construct, and integrate information) and relatively intact associative processing (the ability to activate or categorize information) [86]. Assembled processing is based on dissociation, suppression, disengagement, and contingent relations. It requires the assembly of input across various content domains. Weaknesses in assembled processing disrupt exogenous attention, predictive movement, coordination of visual perception, spatial construction, constructed language (reading comprehension), text-level literacy, most types of mathematical problem solving/computation, and aspects of memory and executive function. Associative processing is data driven and is the basis for relative strengths in endogenous attention, categorical perception, retrieved language, word-level literacy (word reading, vocabulary), and numeration and calculation procedures.

Children with spina bifida learn, remember, and activate old knowledge better than they assemble meaning using old and new knowledge. The combination of intact associative processing and impaired assembled processing results in variability in functioning, which can be confusing and frustrating to individuals with spina bifida and those working with them.

Secondary phenotype moderators

There are 2 additional phenotype moderators: secondary central nervous system insults (hydrocephalus) of the neural phenotype, which impair assembled processing, and environmental factors (poverty, parenting, and education), which impair associative processing. The distinctive cognitive phenotype seen in people with spina bifida is expressed as variations across content domains (eg, higher verbal IQ, better reading than mathematics) as well as variations within content domains (eg, facility with grammar and vocabulary, but poor pragmatic language).

To maximize functioning and outcome, it is crucial for adults working with children with spina bifida to see beyond the physical disabilities and toileting issues and to really understand the hidden issues and complexities along with the underlying strengths and weaknesses of each individual's phenotype.

Timing and rhythm

Children with spina bifida have difficulties in the perception and production of timing and rhythm, which are essential components of movement and cognition [87]. For example, those individuals with a characteristic brain abnormality, beaking of the midbrain tectum, show attenuated inhibition of return, expressed as a longer time to return to a previously attended cue location compared with a new cue location. Many eye-hand tasks require the constant modulation of motor timing, and many cognitive tasks require attention, particularly the return of attentional focus to prior cues.

Reading

Children with spina bifida can decode words better than they can understand texts. They show appropriate development in the areas of basic language skills (vocabulary and syntax) and language-related academic skills (reading decoding, reading fluency, spelling). They show weaknesses in reading comprehension (integration and inferencing). Reading decoding requires the activation of previously formed associations; in contrast, reading comprehension requires assembled processing, because it combines world knowledge with text to construct meaning. Reading comprehension, but not reading decoding, is related to general cognitive ability. Reading comprehension is poorer in children with spina bifida than in controls, even when reading decoding is precisely matched. With increasing age, reading profiles tend to stay relatively constant.

Mathematics

About 25% of school-aged children with spina bifida have a mathematical learning disability; the neural correlates of these deficits have not been fully examined. Preschoolers have weaknesses in early number sense (one-to-one correspondence/cardinality, rote counting/counting errors, matching quantities/number constancy). School-aged children show weaknesses in mathematical fact retrieval (slower and less accurate), use of immature strategies, and in arithmetical procedures (carrying and borrowing) [88]. These weaknesses are not delays, because these mathematical difficulties, including difficulties with computation accuracy and speed, problem solving and functional numeracy, persist into adulthood. Functional numeracy (the numbers you need to get you through the day) is a better predictor of functional, social, personal, financial, and community independence than functional literacy.

Executive functioning

Executive functioning typically describes a group of abilities associated with controlling goal-directed cognitive, behavioral, and emotional functioning. Deficits in executive functioning are often first observed in the classroom environment. Executive functioning is generally associated with the frontal lobes, yet it can be affected by other brain structures, including systems often affected in spina bifida, such as the cerebellar-subcortical-cortical systems. Further, executive functioning is not an all or nothing phenomenon, and a more accurate perspective is that children with spina bifida have difficulties with specific aspects of executive functioning: problem solving, planning and goal-directed behavior, focused attention, ability to shift attention, response inhibition, and working memory [89]. Further, expected developmental improvements in executive functioning skills over time do not typically occur in individuals with spina bifida. As a result, children may require targeted interventions and modifications to address specific aspects of executive dysfunction into young adulthood to promote functional independence and autonomy. From a practical point of view, these persistent deficits have implications in areas such as medical adherence and quality of life [90].

Attention

Children with spina bifida show greater impairments on objective and subjective measures of attention, even when controlling for differences in intellectual functioning. However, assessment of attention functions by traditional tests may be misleading, because of complex cerebral malformations, such as tectal beaking and resultant difficulties with cognitive and visual-motor functions. Children with spina bifida have a higher incidence of attention-deficit/hyperactivity disorder (ADHD) than the general population and typically show problems with inattention rather than with impulsivity and hyperactivity. Children with ADHD have more difficulty on tasks that draw on anterior attention systems (eg, sustained attention), whereas children with spina bifida show more difficulty on tasks that place greater demands on the posterior attention networks of the brain (eg, focus and shifting). Children with spina bifida take longer to disengage from what has captured their attention, but do not show deficits in orienting to cognitively interesting stimuli, which is more goal directed. This difference in the neurocognitive ability of children with spina bifida may seem solely volitional to adults working with children with spina bifida, causing inaccurate blaming; clear identification of this difference is crucial for effective intervention.

Memory

Fiber tract anomalies in the limbic system are correlated with memory deficits. Children with spina bifida have relatively intact implicit memory, which is a function of associative processing. Implicit memory is the learning or facilitation of performance by exposure without the intention to remember. Implicit memory is in contrast to explicit memory, which is the conscious effort to recognize or recall, and is a function of assembled processing.

In addition, memory can be affected by other aspects of cognition such as attention, language, and executive function, which, if addressed, assist memory functioning. For example, children with spina bifida often focus on extraneous details and may seem to have difficulty remembering underlying messages, but using relative strengths in metacognitive abilities may moderate deficits in specific memory-related tasks such as reading comprehension [91].

Language

Although language was once viewed as an asset for children with spina bifida, recent psycholinguistic and experimental studies of language have shown a profile of intact and impaired language skills. Their strengths are in the formal, fixed structures of grammar, and single words or phrases (vocabulary) and meanings that represent stored associations (semantically retrieved meaning). They generally have intact syntax, morphology, and phonology. Interpersonal rhetoric is preserved in children with spina bifida; they are polite and friendly, sociable, cooperative, and interested in talking. In conversations, they initiate appropriate conversational turns and exchanges. Their weaknesses are in assembling online (dynamically constructed) meaning by integrating words, world knowledge, and context. They have particular difficulties with supralinguistic and pragmatic tasks. Their textual rhetoric is impaired, and their communication is difficult to process, uneconomic, and unclear. These language weaknesses adversely affect their success in social discourse settings.

Social skills

Although children with spina bifida are often described as sociable, particularly for reasons described in the preceding section, they often have difficulties with behavioral regulation and perform at a lower level of social cognitive functioning than typically developing peers. Difficulties include identifying the rules, maintaining goal-directed activities during play, performance in unstructured social situations, showing inappropriate social distance, hyperverbosity, inappropriate use of language, tangential speech, and a failure to benefit from feedback or instruction about their behavior. There are limited studies of neural correlates of these behavioral difficulties, with no specific correlations identified.

Outcomes

The pattern of relative strengths and weaknesses present in individuals with spina bifida is often confusing to parents, educators, peers, and employers. Children with spina bifida are typically articulate, grammatically correct, and look like they have only physical issues. However, inherit and often hidden difficulties with inattention, mathematical computational and fact retrieval skills, and reading comprehension (in contrast to their good reading decoding skills) as well as other issues outlined earlier are likely hard wired and directly related to specific neuroanatomic differences, which can combine with the effects of other secondary medical conditions (hydrocephalus, shunt malfunction) and environmental factors. Further, there is not a linear correlation between the degree of physical and intellectual disability. As a result, individuals with lesser degrees of physical impairment may still have significant neurocognitive difficulties and thus may require additional supports that go beyond a school being barrier free and accommodations for appropriate bathroom access.

What is even clearer is that these differences do not resolve with time; the skills are not simply delayed. Instead, these differences can affect not only individual adult skills, such as functional literacy and functional numeracy, but can determine functional independence and quality of life. To help mediate these problems, neuropsychological evaluations can provide important information in the assessment of and planning for individuals with spina bifida, particularly in the early childhood years, and can assist with optimizing not only school success and issues of medical adherence, but also with improving adult outcomes such as independent living and financial independence [92].

FETAL REPAIR OF MMC

Key points
- Infants undergoing fetal repair of the spinal defect had a decreased need for postnatal ventriculoperitoneal shunt placement.
- There is an increased risk of premature delivery of the infant undergoing fetal repair.
- Fetal repair is predicted to be cost-effective over the course of a child's life.

Introduction

The optimal management of the child with an MMC begins before birth. Because prenatal diagnosis can now occur during the first trimester of pregnancy, there is the opportunity to prepare the family by presenting the full range of treatment options and developing an appropriate management plan: pregnancy termination, fetal repair, delivery method, postnatal repair. Any discussion of fetal intervention should follow the recommendations of the 2011 American College of Obstetricians and Gynecologists and American Academy of Pediatrics joint report *Maternal-Fetal Intervention and Fetal Care Centers*:

1. Explicit informed consent by the mother
2. The evidence base for any proposed intervention
3. A discussion of all risks and benefits to the fetus and the mother
4. The range of treatment options available
5. Procedural safeguards
6. Appropriate social supports and medical professionals in place

Fetal MMC (fMMC) repair represented a significant shift in the application of in utero therapies. Although the goal of previous fetal interventions was to prevent fetal/neonatal demise, the goal of fMMC repair was to improve long-term outcome in a condition that already had an effective postnatal treatment. The presumption is that in utero surgery provides superior outcomes for the offspring than postnatal surgery.

Animal models

The theoretic reasoning behind fetal repair evolved from animal experimental work, which suggested that early fetal repair might ameliorate the adverse effects believed to be a result of a 2-hit mechanism [93]:

1. Hit one: a primary congenital abnormality in anatomic development (an incompletely formed neural tube) occurs during the fourth week of gestation.
2. Hit two: a relatively normal spinal cord is further damaged by amniotic fluid exposure, direct trauma, hydrodynamic pressure, or a combination of these intrauterine milieu factors throughout the remainder of the pregnancy.

Repair between 19 and 25 weeks of gestation was believed to minimize the length of time during which neuronal damage to the exposed cord could occur, still taking into account the technical difficulty of surgery on fetal tissues before this age. Reversal of hindbrain herniation after fMMC surgery in these animals also supported the hypothesis that excessive drainage of CSF through the open MMC defect led to loss of hydrostatic pressure and subsequent downward herniation and caudal displacement of the cerebellar vermis and brainstem into the cervical spinal canal. Hydrostatic backpressure could be reestablished in the posterior fossa with fMMC repair that disimpacts the brain from the spinal canal and reestablishes a more normal CSF drainage. It was also believed that early repair might limit the progression of hydrocephalus, because increasing ventricular size over the course of gestation is characteristic of fMMC.

Human studies

The earliest fMMC repair method (1997) used fetal endoscopy and a maternal split-thickness skin graft over the fetal neural placode. Poor results, including fetal demise, led to this method being abandoned and replaced with an open fetal surgery approach (1998). However, differences in selection criteria and the lack of comparison populations undergoing postnatal repair led the National Institute of Child Health and Human Development to initiate the Management of Myelomeningocele Study (MoMS) (2003–2010). MoMS showed the efficacy of fMMC in a specific homogeneous population under ideal circumstances. These results may not be generalizable outside the eligibility criteria set forth in MoMS. As a result, it is not clear that fMMC is effective in real patients in typical settings.

MoMS results

The initial MoMS results were published in 2011 [94]. They reported important benefits in children who underwent prenatal closure/repair compared with infants repaired postnatally:

1. Decreased need for postnatal ventriculoperitoneal shunt placement (40% vs 82%, $P<.001$)
2. Significant reversal of severe hindbrain herniation (22% vs 6%, $P<.001$)
3. Greater likelihood to walk without devices (42% vs 21%, $P = .01$)
4. Motor function 2 or more levels better than expected by anatomic level (32% vs 12%, $P = .005$).

MoMS also showed that fMMC surgery increased several risks in children who underwent prenatal closure/repair compared with infants repaired postnatally:

1. Increased risk of spontaneous rupture of membranes (46% vs 8%, $P<.001$)
2. Increased risk of oligohydramnios (21% vs 4%, $P = .001$)
3. Increased risk of preterm delivery (79% vs 15%, $P<.001$); 13% of the fetal surgery group were born before 30 weeks of gestation

Prematurity risks

The average gestational age at delivery in the fetal surgery group was 34.1 weeks of gestation compared with 37.3 weeks in the postnatal surgery group. This finding results in an increased number of late preterm infants (LPIs) (34–36 weeks' gestation). Although LPIs were previously considered similar to term infants, emerging evidence suggests that significant adverse developmental outcomes exist among LPIs [95]. LPIs have increased morbidity (neurodevelopmental disabilities, educational difficulties, early intervention needs) and mortality risks compared with term infants. LPIs should be carefully monitored for being an at-risk and not a low-risk population. Significant development of the infant brain takes place during the last 4 to 6 weeks of pregnancy.

1. There is a 4-fold increase in cortical volume during the third trimester.
2. There is an accrual of 35% of brain weight during the last 6 weeks of gestation.

Urologic outcomes

Urologic outcomes are a particular area in which the benefits of fMMC repair are unclear. Results from the MoMS population have not been published. Several other studies have compared children who underwent fMMC with those treated with postnatal repair [96]. There were no differences between the groups in their need for clean intermittent catheterization, incontinence between catheterizations, anticholinergic/antibiotic use, and urodynamic parameters.

Cost-effectiveness

MoMS showed that prenatal MMC repair is efficacious with regards to the affected neonate. At least 1 analysis has suggested that it is also cost-effective compared with postnatal MMC repair [97]. Using decision analysis models and assumptions based on the literature as well as data from MoMS, the investigators found the interests of the affected fetus compared with the mother and future offspring to be discordant:

1. Prenatal MMC repair saved $2,066,778 per 100 cases repaired
2. Prenatal MMC repair resulted in 97 quality of life years (QALYs) gained per 100 repairs.
   a. 42 fewer neonates required shunts per 100 repairs
   b. 21 fewer neonates requiring long-term medical care per 100 repairs
3. Prenatal MMC repair led to reduced maternal QALYs (23 fewer QALYs per 100 maternal-fetal surgeries)
4. Prenatal MMC repair led to reduced future sibling QALYs (9 fewer QALYs per 100 future offspring).

The future

Since the end of MoMS, multiple sites in the United States and around the world are again providing fMMC repair. This situation further complicates the questions of who receives the surgery, who should be performing the surgery, and how the surgery can be improved. The long-term durability of the benefits from this intervention will continue, ideally, to be studied in MoMS participants. The MoMS II study is ongoing at the 3 treatment sites: Children's

Hospital of Philadelphia, University of California San Francisco, and Vanderbilt University. Its primary outcome measure is to determine whether prenatal MMC repair affects adaptive behavior at 6 to 9 years of age, compared with postnatal repair using the Vineland Adaptive Behavior Scales II. Other secondary outcomes studied in MoMS II will include:

1. Motor function: does the improvement in motor function continue or is it lost over time?
2. Cognitive function: what is the natural history of their developmental milestones and measures of intelligence?
3. Brain morphology and function: does the decrease in anatomic Chiari malformations lead to better clinical outcome? Does the decreased need for shunting continue? Will the increased rate of earlier cord tethering continue?
4. Bowel and bladder function: is there any benefit?
5. Medical outcomes: is the number of procedures that these children are subjected to through the course of their life reduced? What are the long-term health outcomes?
6. Late premature outcomes
7. Quality of life: whose quality of life must be considered?
8. Maternal reproductive function: what are the future reproductive options for mothers after uterine surgery?

CARE OF THE ADULT WITH SPINA BIFIDA

Key points
- Adults with spina bifida continue to be at risk for issues that they might have faced as children (hydrocephalus, tethered cord, orthopedic complications, bowel and bladder dysfunction).
- Practitioners can help ease the transition to adult care and direct their patients to improve participation in meaningful and enjoyable activities, with the goal of improving outcomes as adults.

Introduction
As adults, persons with spina bifida face continued challenges in both remaining healthy and maintaining function [98]. The safety net (consisting primarily of family, the pediatric clinic and hospital, and school, with both academic and therapeutic supports) changes with the replacement of the pediatric hospital by adult facilities, and by the completion of school, either K-12 or graduate and postgraduate. Adult providers frequently have less experience caring for persons with childhood onset disabilities and may not have the same level of confidence caring for this population as for those with acquired disability.

Transition
In the ideal scenario, pediatric patients would begin planning for transition at age 14 years, with clear lines of communication between medical providers,

therapists, vocational and educational counselors, and community partners. Many persons with spina bifida do not have access to such coordinated transition, and so providers may need to help bridge the gap from pediatric to adult care [99]. Inherent to successful transition is the patient's assumption of greater autonomy and engagement in medical decision making, a process that can begin in teenage years.

Urologic issues

The wide prevalence of bladder dysfunction among those with spina bifida (estimates vary, up to 90% and higher) raises concern for the chronic development of renal dysfunction as well as the acute risk of urinary tract infection and possible sepsis [100]. Renal failure is likely the most common cause of death among adults with spina bifida [101]. Practitioners should have a low threshold of suspicion for infection, monitor kidney function with yearly renal ultrasonography, and involve urologic consultation as necessary. Persons with indwelling Foley catheters are at higher risk for bladder cancer and require yearly cystoscopy after 10 years of Foley catheter use [102]. More than 80% of adults do attain social bladder continence [43].

Neurologic issues

Neurologic issues can cause significant morbidity and disability, even into adulthood. Most commonly associated with adolescent growth spurts, a tethered cord can present in adulthood as well, particularly in those with history of previous surgery [103–105]. A tethered spinal cord can lead to pain, weakness, bowel and bladder changes, sensory changes, and increased spasticity. MRI remains the gold standard for evaluation, along with urgent neurosurgical referral for those with troubling or rapidly progressive symptoms. Tethered cord syndrome can be managed nonsurgically, but this must be performed in conjunction with neurosurgery.

Other neurologic concerns for adults include Chiari malformation, syringomyelia, seizures, and chronic headaches. Chiari malformation is generally type 2 and presents with bilateral upper limb weakness, sensory changes, dysphagia, headaches, and ataxia. Chiari malformations are also often associated with syringomyelia, suggesting that MRI evaluation of the entire neuraxis may be indicated. Cervical syringomyelia may present with Chiari malformations, whereas tethered cord syndrome may occur with the lower third of the cord [106,107].

Musculoskeletal

For reasons of abnormal anatomy as well as prolonged unconventional biomechanical forces, musculoskeletal problems are common among adults with spina bifida. Virtually any joint or muscle group could be at risk, especially based on level of neurologic function.

Scoliosis is most often addressed in childhood or adolescence but can progress in adulthood [108]. Pain, respiratory compromise, or positioning issues can be a cause for trial of bracing or wheelchair modifications. An orthopedic referral can also be indicated, but frequently pediatric rather than adult sur-geons are more likely to perform the surgery.

The likelihood of shoulder injury, especially in manual wheelchair users, in-creases over time, although it may be less in those who start using a wheelchair during childhood [109]. Hips are at risk for both contracture and dislocation, although the latter is less associated with functional loss than is neurologic level [110]. Knee problems include contracture but also early development of degen-erative conditions associated with abnormal biomechanics. Knee flexion contracture is more likely with higher-level neurologic impairment [111]. An-kles and feet continue to be at risk for contracture, progressive deformity requiring bracing or surgery, and Charcot arthropathy [112].

Practitioners should also be alert for signs and symptoms of osteopenia and osteoporosis [113]. Supplementation with vitamin D and calcium is important, because nonambulatory individuals are at risk for pathologic fracture. Those at risk for nephrolithiasis may need to limit calcium intake.

Obesity and metabolic syndrome

Reduced physical activity, poor diet, and increase of adipose tissue with age all contribute to the risk of obesity and its attendant morbidity, as well as meta-bolic syndrome. With loss of the pediatric safety net, persons with spina bifida may reduce activity significantly, so identifying and encouraging participation in adaptive sports is incumbent on the practitioner [114,115].

Participation

Participation is the goal of interventions based on the schema offered in the In-ternational Classification of Function. Education, work, sports, other recrea-tion, and community engagement fulfill basic human needs for connection with others. Providers caring for adults with spina bifida can encourage these activities by asking about them, having information on community resources available in clinic, and, of course, by addressing medical and psychosocial needs. Individualizing a plan to support maximum meaningful engagement in activities should be a primary goal of a long-term therapeutic alliance be-tween practitioner and patient.

Outcomes

Many adults with spina bifida face overwhelming challenges in terms of living independently, completing education, engaging socially and forming meaning-ful long-term relationships [116]. Perhaps related, young adults with spina bi-fida are more likely to report depression, low sense of self-worth, and increased suicidal thoughts. Providers may ameliorate this situation by encour-aging participation in activities and by using neuropsychological evaluation and vocational counseling to support training and work. Persons with spina bifida may have sexual dysfunction, which is not addressed by providers. Support in this domain (including discussion of relationship status, birth control, sexually transmitted disease prevention, and genetic implications of pregnancy for male and female parents) may be invaluable in improving quality of life [117,118].

Pediatricians can assist in this process by initiating discussions in adolescence and by modeling open and frank discussion of sexuality in the clinic.

References

[1] Atu K, Ashley-Koch A, Northrup H. Epidemiologic and genetic aspects of spina bifida and other neural tube defects. Dev Disabil Res Rev 2010;16:6–15.

[2] Copp AJ, Stanier P, Greene ND. Neural tube defects: recent advances, unsolved questions, and controversies. Lancet Neurol 2013;12(8):799–810.

[3] Johnson C, Honein MA, Dana Flanders W, et al. Pregnancy termination following prenatal diagnosis of anencephaly or spina bifida: a systematic review of the literature. Birth Defects Res A Clin Mol Teratol 2012;94:857–63.

[4] Wallingford J, Niswander LA, Shaw GM, et al. The continuing challenge of understanding preventing and treating neural tube defects. Science 2013;339(6123):1222002.

[5] Mitchell L. Epidemiology of neural tube defects. Am J Med Genet C Semin Med Genet 2005;135C:88–94.

[6] Shin M, Besser LM, Siffel C, et al. Prevalence of spina bifida among children and adolescents in 10 regions in the United States. Pediatrics 2010;126:274–9.

[7] Centers for Disease Control and Prevention (CDC). CDC grand rounds: additional opportunities to prevent neural tube defects with folic acid fortification. MMWR Morb Mortal Wkly Rep 2010;59:780–4.

[8] Williams L, Rasmussen SA, Flores A, et al. Decline in the prevalence of spina bifida and anencephaly by race/ethnicity: 1995-2002. Pediatrics 2005;116:580–6.

[9] Mills J, Signore C. Neural tube defect rates before and after food fortification with folic acid. Birth Defects Res A Clin Mol Teratol 2004;70:844–5.

[10] Yi Y, Lindemann M, Colligs A, et al. Economic burden of neural tube defects and impact of prevention with folic acid: a literature review. Eur J Pediatr 2011;170(11):1391–400.

[11] D'Addario V, Rossi AC, Pinto V, et al. Comparison of six sonographic signs in the prenatal diagnosis of spina bifida. J Perinat Med 2008;36(4):330–4.

[12] Chao TT, Dashe JS, Adams RC, et al. Fetal spine findings on MRI and associated outcomes in children with open neural tube defects. AJR Am J Roentgenol 2011;197(5): W956–61.

[13] Goetzinger KR, Stamilio DM, Dicke JM, et al. Evaluating the incidence and likelihood ratios for chromosomal abnormalities in fetuses with common central nervous system malformations. Am J Obstet Gynecol 2008;199(3):285.e1–6.

[14] Prevention of neural tube defects: results of the Medical Research Council Vitamin Study. MRC Vitamin Study Research Group. Lancet 1991;338(8760):131–7.

[15] Greene ND, Stanier P, Copp AJ. Genetics of human neural tube defects. Hum Mol Genet 2009;18(R2):R113–29.

[16] Harris MJ, Juriloff DM. An update to the list of mouse mutants with neural tube closure defects and advances toward a complete genetic perspective of neural tube closure. Birth Defects Res A Clin Mol Teratol 2010;88(8):653–69.

[17] Ybot-Gonzalez P, Savery D, Gerrelli D, et al. Convergent extension, planar-cell-polarity signalling and initiation of mouse neural tube closure. Development 2007;134(4): 789–99.

[18] Juriloff DM, Harris MJ. A consideration of the evidence that genetic defects in planar cell polarity contribute to the etiology of human neural tube defects. Birth Defects Res A Clin Mol Teratol 2012;94(10):824–40.

[19] Lei Y, Zhu H, Duhon C, et al. Mutations in planar cell polarity gene SCRIB are associated with spina bifida. PLoS One 2013;8(7):e69262.

[20] Bartsch O, Kirmes I, Thiede A, et al. Novel VANGL1 gene mutations in 144 Slovakian, Romanian and German patients with neural tube defects. Mol Syndromol 2012;3(2):76–81.

[21] De Marco P, Merello E, Consales A, et al. Genetic analysis of disheveled 2 and disheveled 3 in human neural tube defects. J Mol Neurosci 2013;49(3):582–8.

[22] Dowdle WE, Robinson JF, Kneist A, et al. Disruption of a ciliary B9 protein complex causes Meckel syndrome. Am J Hum Genet 2011;89(1):94–110.

[23] Hopp K, Heyer CM, Hommerding CJ, et al. B9D1 is revealed as a novel Meckel syndrome (MKS) gene by targeted exon-enriched next-generation sequencing and deletion analysis. Hum Mol Genet 2011;20(13):2524–34.

[24] Logan CV, Abdel-Hamed Z, Johnson CA. Molecular genetics and pathogenic mechanisms for the severe ciliopathies: insights into neurodevelopment and pathogenesis of neural tube defects. Mol Neurobiol 2011;43(1):12–26.

[25] Khaddour R, Smith U, Baala L, et al. Spectrum of MKS1 and MKS3 mutations in Meckel syndrome: a genotype-phenotype correlation. Mutation in brief #960. Online. Hum Mutat 2007;28(5):523–4.

[26] Ruat M, Roudaut H, Ferent J, et al. Hedgehog trafficking, cilia and brain functions. Differentiation 2012;83(2):S97–104.

[27] Aguilar A, Meunier A, Strehl L, et al. Analysis of human samples reveals impaired SHH-dependent cerebellar development in Joubert syndrome/Meckel syndrome. Proc Natl Acad Sci U S A 2012;109(42):16951–6.

[28] Chen X, Shen Y, Gao Y, et al. Detection of copy number variants reveals association of cilia genes with neural tube defects. PLoS One 2013;8(1):e54492.

[29] Imbard A, Benoist JF, Blom HJ. Neural tube defects, folic acid and methylation. Int J Environ Res Public Health 2013;10(9):4352–89.

[30] Obican SG, Finnell RH, Mills JL, et al. Folic acid in early pregnancy: a public health success story. FASEB J 2010;24(11):4167–74.

[31] Frosst P, Blom HJ, Milos R, et al. A candidate genetic risk factor for vascular disease: a common mutation in methylenetetrahydrofolate reductase. Nat Genet 1995;10(1):111–3.

[32] Lacasana M, Blanco-Munoz J, Borja-Aburto VH, et al. Effect on risk of anencephaly of gene-nutrient interactions between methylenetetrahydrofolate reductase C677T polymorphism and maternal folate, vitamin B12 and homocysteine profile. Public Health Nutr 2012;15(8):1419–28.

[33] Yan L, Zhao L, Long Y, et al. Association of the maternal MTHFR C677T polymorphism with susceptibility to neural tube defects in offsprings: evidence from 25 case-control studies. PLoS One 2012;7(10):e41689.

[34] Zhang T, Lou J, Zhong R, et al. Genetic variants in the folate pathway and the risk of neural tube defects: a meta-analysis of the published literature. PLoS One 2013;8(4):e59570.

[35] Wang XW, Luo YL, Wang W, et al. Association between MTHFR A1298C polymorphism and neural tube defect susceptibility: a metaanalysis. Am J Obstet Gynecol 2012;206(3):251.e1–7.

[36] Etheredge AJ, Finnell RH, Carmichael SL, et al. Maternal and infant gene-folate interactions and the risk of neural tube defects. Am J Med Genet A 2012;158A(10):2439–46.

[37] Minguzzi S, Selcuklu SD, Spillane C, et al. An NTD-associated polymorphism in the 3′ UTR of MTHFD1L can affect disease risk by altering miRNA binding. Hum Mutat 2014;35(1):96–104.

[38] Parle-McDermott A, Pangilinan F, O'Brien KK, et al. A common variant in MTHFD1L is associated with neural tube defects and mRNA splicing efficiency. Hum Mutat 2009;30(12):1650–6.

[39] Charney EB, Weller SC, Sutton LN, et al. Management of the newborn with myelomeningocele: time for a decision-making process. Pediatrics 1985;75(1):58–64.

[40] Cheek WR, Laurent JP, Cech DA. Operative repair of lumbosacral myelomeningocele. Technical note. J Neurosurg 1983;59(4):718–22.

[41] Macias R, Tena L. Myelomeningocele: new technique for skin repair. Childs Brain 1983;10(2):73–8.

[42] McLone DG. Technique for closure of myelomeningocele. Childs Brain 1980;6(2):65–73.

[43] Bowman RM, McLone DG, Grant JA, et al. Spina bifida outcome: a 25-year prospective. Pediatr Neurosurg 2001;34(3):114–20.

[44] Rintoul NE, Sutton LN, Hubbard AM, et al. A new look at myelomeningoceles: functional level, vertebral level, shunting, and the implications for fetal intervention. Pediatrics 2002;109(3):409–13.
[45] Teo C, Jones R. Management of hydrocephalus by endoscopic third ventriculostomy in patients with myelomeningocele. Pediatr Neurosurg 1996;25(2):57–63 [discussion: 63].
[46] Vernet O, Farmer JP, Houle AM, et al. Impact of urodynamic studies on the surgical management of spinal cord tethering. J Neurosurg 1996;85(4):555–9.
[47] Cruz NI, Ariyan S, Duncan CC, et al. Repair of lumbosacral myelomeningoceles with double Z-rhomboid flaps. Technical note. J Neurosurg 1983;59(4):714–7.
[48] Fletcher JM, Francis DJ, Thompson NM, et al. Verbal and nonverbal skill discrepancies in hydrocephalic children. J Clin Exp Neuropsychol 1992;14(4):593–609.
[49] Anderson PA, Travers AH. Development of hydronephrosis in spina bifida patients: predictive factors and management. Br J Urol 1993;72(6):958–61.
[50] Deshpande AV, Sampang R, Smith GH. Study of botulinum toxin A in neurogenic bladder due to spina bifida in children. ANZ J Surg 2010;80(4):250–3.
[51] Leibold SR. Achieving continence with a neurogenic bowel. Pediatr Clin North Am 2010;57(4):1013–25.
[52] Ellison JS, Haraway AN, Park JM. The distal left Malone antegrade continence enema–is it better? J Urol 2013;190(Suppl 4):1529–33.
[53] Overgoor ML, de Jong TP, Cohen-Kettenis PT, et al. Increased sexual health after restored genital sensation in male patients with spina bifida or a spinal cord injury: the TOMAX procedure. J Urol 2013;189(2):626–32.
[54] Trollmann R, Dorr HG, Groschl M, et al. Spontaneous nocturnal leptin secretion in children with myelomeningocele and growth hormone deficiency. Horm Res 2002;58(3):115–9.
[55] Proos LA, Dahl M, Ahlsten G, et al. Increased perinatal intracranial pressure and prediction of early puberty in girls with myelomeningocele. Arch Dis Child 1996;75(1):42–5.
[56] Proos LA, Tuvemo T, Ahlsten G, et al. Increased perinatal intracranial pressure and brainstem dysfunction predict early puberty in boys with myelomeningocele. Acta Paediatr 2011;100(10):1368–72.
[57] Rotenstein D, Reigel DH, Flom LL. Growth hormone treatment accelerates growth of short children with neural tube defects. J Pediatr 1989;115(3):417–20.
[58] Trollmann R, Bakker B, Lundberg M, et al. Growth in pre-pubertal children with myelomeningocele (MMC) on growth hormone (GH): the KIGS experience. Pediatr Rehabil 2006;9(2):144–8.
[59] Rotenstein D, Breen TJ. Growth hormone treatment of children with myelomeningocele. J Pediatr 1996;128(5 Pt 2):S28–31.
[60] Rotenstein D, Bass AN. Treatment to near adult stature of patients with myelomeningocele with recombinant human growth hormone. J Pediatr Endocrinol Metab 2004;17(9):1195–200.
[61] Westcott MA, Dynes MC, Remer EM, et al. Congenital and acquired orthopedic abnormalities in patients with myelomeningocele. Radiographics 1992;12(6):1155–73.
[62] Akbar M, Bresch B, Seyler TM, et al. Management of orthopaedic sequelae of congenital spinal disorders. J Bone Joint Surg Am 2009;91(Suppl 6):87–100.
[63] Ramirez N, Flynn JM, Emans JB, et al. Vertical expandable prosthetic titanium rib as treatment of thoracic insufficiency syndrome in spondylocostal dysplasia. J Pediatr Orthop 2010;30(6):521–6.
[64] Swaroop VT, Dias L. Orthopedic management of spina bifida. Part I: hip, knee, and rotational deformities. J Child Orthop 2009;3(6):441–9.
[65] Swaroop VT, Dias L. Orthopaedic management of spina bifida–part II: foot and ankle deformities. J Child Orthop 2011;5(6):403–14.
[66] Flynn JM, Herrera-Soto JA, Ramirez NF, et al. Clubfoot release in myelodysplasia. J Pediatr Orthop B 2004;13(4):259–62.
[67] Szalay EA, Cheema A. Children with spina bifida are at risk for low bone density. Clin Orthop Relat Res 2011;469(5):1253–7.

[68] Dosa NP, Eckrich M, Katz DA, et al. Incidence, prevalence, and characteristics of fractures in children, adolescents, and adults with spina bifida. J Spinal Cord Med 2007;30(Suppl 1):S5–9.

[69] Marreiros H, Monteiro L, Loff C, et al. Fractures in children and adolescents with spina bifida: the experience of a Portuguese tertiary-care hospital. Dev Med Child Neurol 2010;52(8):754–9.

[70] Marreiros H, Loff C, Calado E. Osteoporosis in paediatric patients with spina bifida. J Spinal Cord Med 2012;35(1):9–21.

[71] Apkon SD, Fenton L, Coll JR. Bone mineral density in children with myelomeningocele. Dev Med Child Neurol 2009;51(1):63–7.

[72] Sholas MG, Tann B, Gaebler-Spira D. Oral bisphosphonates to treat disuse osteopenia in children with disabilities: a case series. J Pediatr Orthop 2005;25(3):326–31.

[73] McDonald CM, Jaffe KM, Mosca VS, et al. Ambulatory outcome of children with myelomeningocele: effect of lower-extremity muscle strength. Dev Med Child Neurol 1991;33(6):482–90.

[74] Hunt G, Lewin W, Gleave J, et al. Predictive factors in open myelomeningocele with special reference to sensory level. Br Med J 1973;4(5886):197–201.

[75] Schoenmakers MA, Uiterwaal CS, Gulmans VA, et al. Determinants of functional independence and quality of life in children with spina bifida. Clin Rehabil 2005;19(6):677–85.

[76] Bartonek A. Motor development toward ambulation in preschool children with myelomeningocele–a prospective study. Pediatr Phys Ther 2010;22(1):52–60.

[77] Kirpalani HM, Parkin PC, Willan AR, et al. Quality of life in spina bifida: importance of parental hope. Arch Dis Child 2000;83(4):293–7.

[78] Dunn RB, Walter JS, Lucero Y, et al. Follow-up assessment of standing mobility device users. Assist Technol 1998;10(2):84–93.

[79] Pin TW. Effectiveness of static weight-bearing exercises in children with cerebral palsy. Pediatr Phys Ther 2007;19(1):62–73.

[80] Duffy CM, Graham HK, Cosgrove AP. The influence of ankle-foot orthoses on gait and energy expenditure in spina bifida. J Pediatr Orthop 2000;20(3):356–61.

[81] Ryan KD, Ploski C, Emans JB. Myelodysplasia–the musculoskeletal problem: habilitation from infancy to adulthood. Phys Ther 1991;71(12):935–46.

[82] Watson D. Occupational therapy intervention guidelines for children and adolescents with spina bifida. Child Care Health Dev 1991;17(6):367–80.

[83] Jenkinson MD, Campbell S, Hayhurst C, et al. Cognitive and functional outcome in spina bifida–Chiari II malformation. Childs Nerv Syst 2011;27(6):967–74.

[84] Hampton LE, Fletcher JM, Cirino PT, et al. Hydrocephalus status in spina bifida: an evaluation of variations in neuropsychological outcomes. J Neurosurg Pediatr 2011;8(3):289–98.

[85] Fletcher JM, Copeland K, Frederick JA, et al. Spinal lesion level in spina bifida: a source of neural and cognitive heterogeneity. J Neurosurg 2005;102(Suppl 3):268–79.

[86] Dennis M, Barnes MA. The cognitive phenotype of spina bifida meningomyelocele. Dev Disabil Res Rev 2010;16(1):31–9.

[87] Dennis M, Edelstein K, Hetherington R, et al. Neurobiology of perceptual and motor timing in children with spina bifida in relation to cerebellar volume. Brain 2004;127(Pt 6):1292–301.

[88] Barnes MA, Wilkinson M, Khemani E, et al. Arithmetic processing in children with spina bifida: calculation accuracy, strategy use, and fact retrieval fluency. J Learn Disabil 2006;39(2):174–87.

[89] Kelly NC, Ammerman RT, Rausch JR, et al. Executive functioning and psychological adjustment in children and youth with spina bifida. Child Neuropsychol 2012;18(5):417–31.

[90] O'Hara LK, Holmbeck GN. Executive functions and parenting behaviors in association with medical adherence and autonomy among youth with spina bifida. J Pediatr Psychol 2013;38(6):675–87.

[91] English L, Barnes MA, Fletcher JM, et al. Effects of reading goals on reading comprehension, reading rate, and allocation of working memory in children and adolescents with spina bifida meningomyelocele. J Int Neuropsychol Soc 2010;16(3):517–25.

[92] Dennis M, Landry SH, Barnes M, et al. A model of neurocognitive function in spina bifida over the life span. J Int Neuropsychol Soc 2006;12(2):285–96.

[93] Adzick N, Thom EA, Spong CY, et al. A randomized trial of prenatal versus postnatal repair of myelomeningocele. N Engl J Med 2011;364:993–1004.

[94] Adzick N. Fetal surgery for spina bifida: past, present, future. Semin Pediatr Surg 2013;22:10–7.

[95] McGowan J, Alderdice FA, Holmes VA, et al. Early childhood development of late-preterm infants: a systematic review. Pediatrics 2011;127:1111–22.

[96] Cuppen I, Eggink AJ, Lotgering FK, et al. Influence of birth mode on early neurological outcome in infants with myelomeningocele. Eur J Obstet Gynecol Reprod Biol 2011;156:18–22.

[97] Werner E, Han CS, Burd I, et al. Evaluating the cost-effectiveness of prenatal surgery for myelomeningocele: a decision analysis. Ultrasound Obstet Gynecol 2012;40:158–64.

[98] Cox A, Breau L, Connor L, et al. Transition of care to an adult spina bifida clinic: patient perspectives and medical outcomes. J Urol 2011;186(Suppl 4):1590–4.

[99] Thibadeau JK, Alriksson-Schmidt AI, Zabel TA. The National Spina Bifida Program transition initiative: the people, the plan, and the process. Pediatr Clin North Am 2010;57(4): 903–10.

[100] Verhoef M, Barf HA, Post MW, et al. Secondary impairments in young adults with spina bifida. Dev Med Child Neurol 2004;46(6):420–7.

[101] Singhal B, Mathew KM. Factors affecting mortality and morbidity in adult spina bifida. Eur J Pediatr Surg 1999;9(Suppl 1):31–2.

[102] West DA, Cummings JM, Longo WE, et al. Role of chronic catheterization in the development of bladder cancer in patients with spinal cord injury. Urology 1999;53(2): 292–7.

[103] Filler AG, Britton JA, Uttley D, et al. Adult postrepair myelomeningocoele and tethered cord syndrome: good surgical outcome after abrupt neurological decline. Br J Neurosurg 1995;9(5):659–66.

[104] George TM, Fagan LH. Adult tethered cord syndrome in patients with postrepair myelomeningocele: an evidence-based outcome study. J Neurosurg 2005;102(Suppl 2):150–6.

[105] Iskandar BJ, Fulmer BB, Hadley MN, et al. Congenital tethered spinal cord syndrome in adults. J Neurosurg 1998;88(6):958–61.

[106] Craig JJ, Gray WJ, McCann JP. The Chiari/hydrosyringomyelia complex presenting in adults with myelomeningocoele: an indication for early intervention. Spinal Cord 1999;37(4):275–8.

[107] McDonnell GV, McCann JP, Craig JJ, et al. Prevalence of the Chiari/hydrosyringomyelia complex in adults with spina bifida: preliminary results. Eur J Pediatr Surg 2000;10(Suppl 1):18–9.

[108] Berven S, Bradford DS. Neuromuscular scoliosis: causes of deformity and principles for evaluation and management. Semin Neurol 2002;22(2):167–78.

[109] Sawatzky BJ, Slobogean GP, Reilly CW, et al. Prevalence of shoulder pain in adult-versus childhood-onset wheelchair users: a pilot study. J Rehabil Res Dev 2005; 42(3 Suppl 1):1–8.

[110] Crandall RC, Birkebak RC, Winter RB. The role of hip location and dislocation in the functional status of the myelodysplastic patient. A review of 100 patients. Orthopedics 1989;12(5):675–84.

[111] Snela S, Parsch K. Follow-up study after treatment of knee flexion contractures in spina bifida patients. J Pediatr Orthop B 2000;9(3):154–60.

[112] Nagarkatti DG, Banta JV, Thomson JD. Charcot arthropathy in spina bifida. J Pediatr Orthop 2000;20(1):82–7.

[113] Valtonen KM, Goksor LA, Jonsson O, et al. Osteoporosis in adults with meningomyelocele: an unrecognized problem at rehabilitation clinics. Arch Phys Med Rehabil 2006;87(3): 376–82.
[114] Stepanczuk BC, Dicianno BE, Webb TS. Young adults with spina bifida may have higher occurrence of prehypertension and hypertension. Am J Phys Med Rehabil 2014;93(3): 200–6.
[115] Wilson R, Lewis SA, Dicianno BE. Targeted preventive care may be needed for adults with congenital spine anomalies. PM R 2011;3(8):730–8.
[116] Crytzer TM, Dicianno BE, Kapoor R. Physical activity, exercise, and health-related measures of fitness in adults with spina bifida: a review of the literature. PM R 2013;5(12): 1051–62.
[117] Cardenas DD, Topolski TD, White CJ, et al. Sexual functioning in adolescents and young adults with spina bifida. Arch Phys Med Rehabil 2008;89(1):31–5.
[118] Sawyer SM, Roberts KV. Sexual and reproductive health in young people with spina bifida. Dev Med Child Neurol 1999;41(10):671–5.

Advances in Pediatrics 61 (2014) 75–125

ADVANCES IN PEDIATRICS

ELSEVIER
MOSBY

Update in Pediatric Imaging

Brian Dunoski, MD[a,b], Thomas L. Slovis, MD[a,*]

[a]Children's Hospital of Michigan, 3901 Beaubien Drive, Detroit, MI 48301, USA; [b]Children's Mercy Hospital, 2401 Gillham Road, Kansas City, MO 64108, USA

Keywords
- Update • Pediatric imaging • Future trends

Key points
- The need for an ongoing partnership between the pediatric radiologist and pediatrician to insure the appropriate selection of examination is crucial.
- More emphasis should be placed on enhancing the pediatrician's skill in interpretation of the common examinations and knowing age-related variants.
- The benefit/risk ratio must be considered when ordering imaging procedures. This demands knowledge of the pathophysiology of disease.
- New techniques (eg, MR special sequences and MR musculoskeletal indications) and controversial aspects of diagnosis (eg, child abuse) are discussed.

INTRODUCTION
Recently, there has been a shift in emphasis in the ordering of pediatric imaging examinations. We have become more aware of the risks (radiation and sedation) and benefits whenever a study is suggested. We have appropriate criteria to help us select the best test to make the diagnosis least invasively [1–3]. A more complete knowledge of the natural history of disease allows us to reevaluate our imaging workup (eg, for urinary tract infection) [4]. In an era of cost containment, in which imaging accounts for 9% of medical care, we need to consider not only whether a test is necessary but also whether a cheaper test can be performed with the same outcome.

The emphasis on teaching imaging interpretation to the pediatrician has diminished, and few pediatric training programs have routine sessions on reading the image. It is perceived to be more important to order the correct test and then obtain a report on an electronic medical record (EMR) or a picture archiving communication system (PACS), sometimes without an image.

*Corresponding author. E-mail address: tslovis@med.wayne.edu

0065-3101/14/$ – see front matter
http://dx.doi.org/10.1016/j.yapd.2014.03.010
© 2014 Elsevier Inc. All rights reserved.

Although EMR and PACS have forever changed medical practice, it is less than optimal to accept results without reviewing the images and knowing how to interpret them within the framework of the patient's clinical condition. This observation is especially true when many examinations are read off site. In many instances, the reader knows little about the patient. If the radiologist reads few pediatric examinations, they know even less about pediatric diseases.

The rapid advances in technology, particularly magnetic resonance (MR) and computed tomography (CT), have made it difficult for all of us to keep up. Despite this gap, many pediatricians and pediatric subspecialists do not seek consultation with the pediatric imager. The pediatric health care provider and the pediatric imager with both the clinical information and the child's images and reports can decide together which test (or no test) would be best toward solving the child's problem.

This update discusses these issues and emphasizes examinations that are most frequently used by the practicing pediatrician. We also predict the most important advances in pediatric imaging over the next 5 years.

Appropriate examination plus risk-to-benefit consideration equals decreased imaging costs

Many tests are ordered without a full understanding of the pathophysiology of the disease. For example, skull radiographs are requested for head trauma in young infants when 50% of epidural/subdural hematomas occur in babies who do not have a skull fracture or abnormality visible on the skull examination. Ninety-five percent of pneumonia in infants and toddlers younger than 2 years is viral. The radiographic findings show peribronchial cuffing, subsegmental atelectasis, and sometimes, hyperexpansion: the same findings as in spasmodic airway disease (Fig. 1). Yet, we frequently obtain chest radiographs and treat the patients with antibiotics. We must understand that the radiologic resolution of pneumonia or empyema lags behind the clinical changes, so we must avoid unnecessary, nonproductive short-interval imaging. In the unusual case of pneumonia when it is necessary to reimage, the repeat examination should not occur until 21 days after diagnosis (assuming that the child responds appropriately). In empyema, complete resolution may take months, and interval radiographs are necessary only for clinical worsening (Fig. 2). Another blatant example of overuse of imaging is in the child who presents with abdominal pain and constipation. Constipation is a clinical symptom and does not need radiographic confirmation or quantification [5].

Ideally, the use of imaging should add value to clinical care and help determine the proper therapy or next step. For this reason, the American Academy of Pediatrics and American College of Radiology guidelines for imaging exist. Some of the most useful guidelines are on the workup of urinary tract infection, nonfebrile seizures, and chronic headaches (discussed later) [1,3,4,6]. There is a large, multi-institutional study regarding head trauma that suggests when imaging is helpful and can give a high sensitivity and negative predictive value so you know when not to image [7]. By using these guidelines, we can reduce

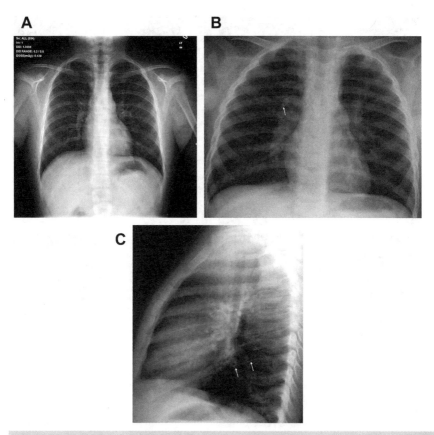

Fig. 1. Chest radiography. (A) Normal chest radiograph with the radiation metrics expressed in milliGrays in the right upper corner. To convert to millirads, move the decimal point 2 places to the right (0.129 mGy = 12.9 mrad). The dose varies by age, but for single-view chest examinations, it should be 3 to 15 mrad. Both Grays and rads are units of absorption, and in this instance, skin entrance dose. The heart and liver are transparent, so you can see the vessels through them. (B, C) Small airways disease. Frontal (B) and lateral (C) radiographs show peribronchial cuffing: doughnuts with a black center of air and thickened bronchial walls and secretions (*white cuff*), (*arrows*). The lungs are mildly hyperexpanded, and there are focal areas of atelectasis.

imaging by 25% in children with acute head trauma with a Glasgow coma score of 14 and 15 and achieve the same favorable outcomes.

There can be a considerable savings (eg, time, cost, unnecessary invasive tests) by not performing an imaging test. The best example is a young child with hip pain/gait disturbance. The disease that needs to be excluded immediately is septic arthritis, but the differential diagnosis is great. When we can trust our physical examination and laboratory tests, we find that the child with full range of motion, normal sedimentation rate, and white blood cell count does not have a septic hip and there is no need to perform an ultrasonography

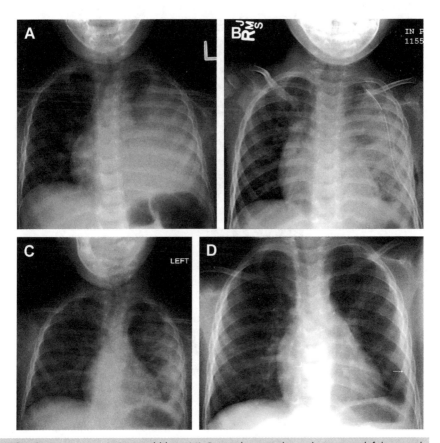

Fig. 2. Empyema in a 2-year-old boy. (A) Original image shows the opaque left lung, with slight mediastinal shift to the right. (B) Two days later, after chest tube drainage, there is improved aeration, but mediastinal shift remains. (C) Six days after the original image, the boy shows clinical improvement; he was put on intravenous antibiotics for 6 weeks (peripherally inserted central catheter). Note the normal position of the mediastinum. (D) The boy continued to be clinically well (but treated). Another image more than 1 month after diagnosis still shows pleural reaction (arrow). The examinations in images (C) and (D) did not contribute to the boy's care, and it takes months for the chest film to become normal.

test for the presence of fluid. Finding fluid might precipitate the need for joint aspiration; in the described child, aspiration is not necessary, because the child most likely has toxic synovitis, not septic arthritis (Fig. 3). We must learn to trust our physical examination. At our hospital, by working with the emergency department physicians and orthopedic subspecialists, we do not perform ultrasonography until consultation has occurred.

When it is decided that a test is appropriate, we must look at the risk/benefit ratio to choose the right test.

The major risks to the pediatric patient from imaging are those from radiation and sedation/anesthesia [8–10]. The radiation-producing tests and metrics

A   B

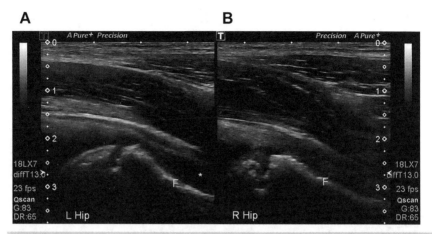

Fig. 3. Left hip pain and limping in a 6-year-old. (*A*) Ultrasonography of the left hip shows a large hip effusion (*asterisk*). (*B*) Ultrasonography of the right hip is normal. F, femur.

are listed in Box 1. These tests differ in radiation dose by a significant magnitude; for each appropriate test, we should use a dose as low as reasonably achievable to obtain diagnostic images: the ALARA principle.

We now use exclusively digital imaging (as opposed to analogue). With digital imaging, postprocessing of the image is possible, and almost any image can be made to look good. However, by viewing the final product (the image), we no longer know whether the appropriate radiation dose was used to obtain the picture (Fig. 4). Therefore, it is imperative that, whenever possible, a radiation

---

Box 1: Non–radiation-producing and radiation-producing tests

A. Non–radiation-producing imaging modalities

  1. MRI or MR

  2. Ultrasonography

B. Radiation-producing imaging modalities

  1. Radiographs

  2. Fluoroscopy

  3. CT

  4. Angiography

  5. Nuclear medicine

  6. Positron emission tomography

C. Interventional procedures such as insertion of vascular lines, drainage of abscesses, or biopsies. These can be performed either with radiation (fluoroscopy or CT) or without radiation (ultrasonography or MR). Sometimes, several kinds of imaging are used.

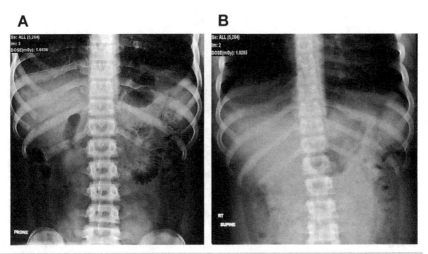

Fig. 4. Value of having a radiation metric on examination. (A, B) Prone (A) and supine (B) images of the abdomen in a 15-year-old with abdominal pain look good (images not shown in entirety), but the prone dose of 1.66 mGy (166 mrad) and supine dose of 1.92 mGy (192 mrad) are excessive (prone should be 35–55 mrad and the supine 35–70 mrad). This child received almost 3 times the maximum expected dose. Without the metrics and knowledge of the normal range, one would not be able to correct the technologist's error and prevent it from happening again.

metric be placed on the examination, so we know that the examination was tailored for the child (ie, <10 mrad for a young child's chest single view) (Table 1) [11].

Perhaps it is better at this point to explain why radiation burden is an issue. There are 2 types of radiation effects: deterministic and stochastic. The former includes effects solely related to dose (determined by the dose) (Box 2) [12,13]. The latter are effects that occur by chance (ie, randomly) and are not produced by dose. However, the more the radiation is absorbed, the greater the chance of a random effect.

There is agreement that doses of radiation that cause deterministic effects (>2 Gy) are harmful. There is also considerable evidence that doses of radiation lower than 10 mGy may cause cancer [9]. These are the doses (10 mGy–100 mGy) of higher-dose CT and cumulative dose of multiple CT examinations. We do know that the younger the age at radiation exposure, the greater the lifetime risk of excess cancers [14]. However, the question of whether a safe dose of radiation exists is probably not answerable [15]. It is obvious that we should take a conservative approach to the use of any radiation test.

The effect of radiation that we are most concerned with is that of cancer. Radiation causes cancer by altering the DNA of irradiated cells and their progeny (Fig. 5) [16]. Radiation-induced leukemia takes 10 years to manifest and solid tumors 20 to 30 years [9]. These solid tumors are the same tumors that occur in

Table 1
Radiation metrics and dose ranges

A. Radiation units (metrics)
  1. Absorbed dose (ie, absorbed by the patient)
    Units: the Gray (Gy) and the rad (rad)
      1 Gy = 100 rad
      1 cGy = 1 rad (cGy is a centiGray)
      10 mGy = 1 rad (mGy is a milliGray)
      1 mGy = 100 mrad
  2. Equivalent dose: a measured or calculated dose
    Units: the Sievert (Sv) and the rem (rem)
      1 Sv = 100 rem[a]
      10 mSv = 1 rem[a]
B. Background radiation
  1. The total background radiation is 300–350 mrad/y, about 1 mrad/d
  2. 50% is environmental, with radon accounting for 37% of that 50%
  3. 50% is man-made and almost all of it is medical. CT accounts for 24% of that 50%, even although it is <15% of all medical imaging. The CT dose index of a brain CT varies with age but is between 1500 and 3500 mrad in a child younger than 15 y. Compare this figure with the table below for abdomen and chests radiographs
C. Charts of the dose ranges for abdomen and chest radiographs at various ages accepted at the Children's Hospital of Michigan. These dose ranges are reviewed and altered as lower techniques are devised

Abdomen dose image chart			
Dose range (mrad)	Supine	Prone	Upright
Age 0–2 y	20–35	20–28	30–50
Age 3–5 y	30–50	30–45	45–70
Age 6–10 y	40–55	40–60	45–90
Patient weight exceeding 45 kg (100 lb) = use adult protocol			
Age 11–18+ y	35–70	30–55	40–85

Chest dose image chart		
Dose range (mrad)	Anteroposterior/Posteroanterior	Lateral
Age 0–2 y	5.0–8.0	6.0–10.0
Age 3–5 y	8.0–11.0	8.0–11.0
Age 6–10 y	8.0–13.0	10.0–22.0
Patient weight exceeding 45 kg (100 lb) = use adult protocol		
Age 11–18+ y	6.0–12.0	12.0–22.0

[a]For practical purposes, with γ rays (radiographs), a rem equals a rad.
 Data from T. Slovis, L. Baird, C. Suggs, personal communication, 2011.

the adult population, only in greater numbers. For these reasons, it is difficult to show a significant but small increase of cancer unless huge populations are studied for an extended period [9,17].

INTERPRETIVE SKILLS

The radiologist adds value by evaluating the entire radiograph or cross-sectional study. Most nonimagers look at the region in which they expect to

Box 2: Types of radiation effects

A. Deterministic effects

1. Determined by the dose (acute exposure >2 Gy and chronic exposure >5 Gy)

2. Examples of these effects:

   Erythema of the skin

   Epilation of the skin

   Cataracts

   Acute radiation toxicity

B. Stochastic effects

1. This is a random effect that can be caused by any dose. It is the effect we worry about with diagnostic radiation. It causes changes in DNA. The more the radiation, the more likely the random effect will occur.

2. The younger the child at exposure, the greater the risk.

3. There is a small individual risk of cancer but a greater public health issue, with more than 11 million CT examinations being performed on children in the United States (2011).

find disease (eg, in a wheezing child, look at the lungs and airway). However, there is more information on the radiograph. We use the catchphrase ABCs to alert the physician to look at the abdomen, bones, chest, and soft tissues on all examinations [18]. Look at the nonprimary anatomic regions first and the primary region last. When you look at the chest, be sure to do so in a specific manner: airway, mediastinum, and then, lungs. You must know the normal appearances (Fig. 6) and variations by age (Fig. 7). You must know which tests are nonspecific (Fig. 8) and which without a plausible history or abnormal laboratory work strongly suggest a specific diagnosis (Fig. 9).

The pediatrician must be conversant with the appropriate imaging examination for the most common clinical complaints (eg, ultrasonography for suspected intussusception, not plain radiographs) (Fig. 10). However, the next step in the imaging workup is more challenging. Each more advanced test may have several components. Ultrasonography may be ordered with color Doppler or with resistive indices (peak systolic velocity–end-diastolic velocity/peak systolic velocity), velocities, and wave forms. Most pediatric radiologists and nephrologists agree that resistive indices do not add value in the diagnosis of renal artery stenosis. The gold standard remains angiography.

CT may be ordered with or without contrast agent; performing both is double the radiation dose. Submillimeter contiguous CT slices (volumetric) can be performed, as we do in craniostenosis. MR is perhaps the most difficult to order, because there are so many different protocols, depending on what is considered the problem to be solved. Having MR spectroscopy (MRS) to help elucidate the biochemical evaluation of tumors or MR susceptibility

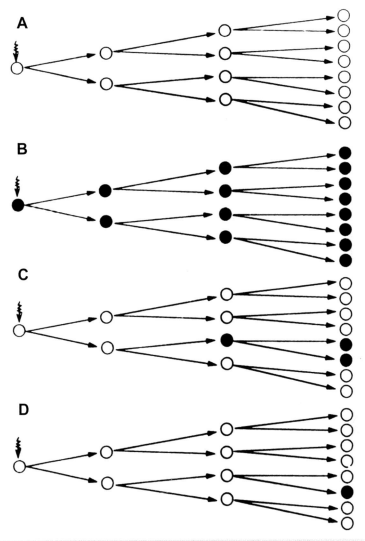

Fig. 5. Radiation-induced mutagenesis. Open circles represent normal wild-type cells, whereas closed circles represent mutated cells. (A) Most of the cells in an irradiated population retain the wild-type phenotype. (B) Example of a cell directly mutated by radiation exposure; the mutation is transmitted to all of its progeny. (C, D) Examples of mutations arising as a result of mutation-induced genomic instability. The irradiated cell and its immediate progeny are wild type, but the frequency with which mutations arise among the more distant descendants of the irradiated cell is increased. (*From* Little JB. Ionizing radiation. In: Kufe DW, Pollock RE, Weichselbaum RR, et al, editors. Holland—Frei cancer medicine. 6th edition. Ontario (Canada): BC Decker; 2003. p. 289–301.)

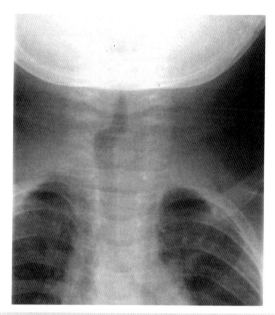

Fig. 6. Normal buckled airway of a 6-month-old in the expiratory phase of respiration. The airway is fixed at the larynx and the carina. Because on expiration the thoracic volume is too low for the entire airway to fit, it buckles away from the aortic arch and to the right, away from the normal left arch.

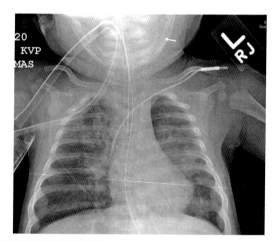

Fig. 7. Chest radiograph in an infant with fever and severe respiratory symptoms. The baby is intubated. Incidentally noted was the absence of tooth buds (*arrow*). All fetuses after 20 weeks' gestation should have tooth buds, and therefore, there is delayed bone age, suggesting the correct diagnosis of ectodermal dysplasia.

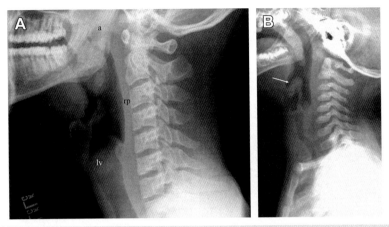

Fig. 8. Nonspecific radiographic findings. (A) Normal lateral neck examination shows the adenoids (a), retropharyngeal space (rp) and laryngeal ventricle (lv). The arrow is on the epiglottis, which is normal but difficult to see. (B) This 15-month-old has an enlarged, swollen epiglottis (arrow) but does not have epiglottitis. Rather, this is an abused child, who was made to drink scalding water. The epiglottis is burned and swollen. Most findings have a significant differential diagnosis.

sequences for finding hemosiderin or inversion recovery sequences for joint fluid and a gradient-echo image for cartilage are all important steps that must be considered.

Children with inflammatory bowel disease (IBD), or in whom you need to exclude IBD as a diagnosis, need small bowel evaluation. We used to perform the upper gastrointestinal small bowel examination, but this has radiation and is nonspecific. CT examination can be performed and is exquisite, but it too

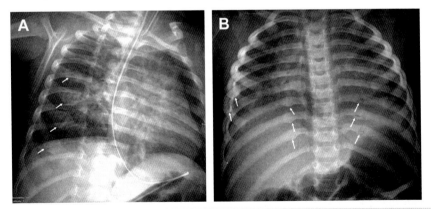

Fig. 9. Multiple fractures without an appropriate explanation: a more specific diagnosis. Coronal oblique view of the chest (A) and frontal chest (B) show multiple healing fractures (arrows) of different ages in a 1-year-old. There was no medical explanation for these injuries, and the medical causes of multiple fractures had been ruled out. This was an abused child.

A   B

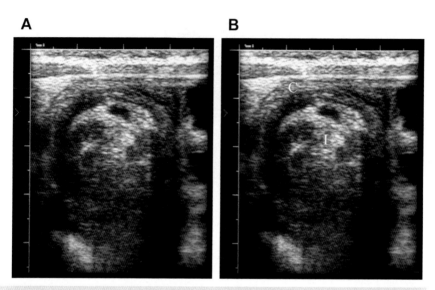

Fig. 10. Ultrasonographic study in a 1-year-old with crampy abdominal pain. (A, B) Unlabeled (A) and labeled (B) ultrasonographic images show the target sign of intussusception. The outer echogenic circle (C) is the colonic wall and the inner echogenic circle (I) in the intussuscipiens is the small bowel.

has radiation exposure. In children's hospitals, we now use MR enterography (MRE), which provides the most information without the dangers of radiation.

Without belaboring all the choices, in a complex problem, it is best to consult with the imager as to what is the right test performed the right way. Having to perform sedation twice for the wrong or incomplete examination is disconcerting for everyone.

The imager is continually pushed in specialized paths, and many adult population imagers are not as familiar with pediatric diseases as the pediatrician. A conversation allowing for both pediatrician and imager to know the correct history and differential diagnosis of the imaging findings provides for the most efficient optimal diagnosis and treatment of our patients.

Imaging choices in chest evaluation

Chest radiographs provide information not only of the lung parenchyma, airway, heart, and mediastinum but also the bones and upper abdomen. The usual radiation dose varies by patient age and size. Subjecting hospitalized children, including those in the intensive care unit, to daily radiographs and following a disease to radiographic resolution offer little benefit compared with the risks of radiation exposure [19]. To avoid unnecessary exposure to ionizing radiation, the use of radiographs should be limited to cases in which the results of the imaging study make the diagnosis or affect the treatment plan, cases in which the clinical presentation is confusing, or in children who are not responding to appropriate therapy.

Most children with a cough are not febrile or actively sick. In the child with chronic or persistent cough, a radiograph might be indicated, because this is a symptom of small airways disease. The first time a child wheezes, it may be appropriate to obtain a radiograph to rule out foreign body, vascular ring, and so forth. When a diagnosis of spasmodic airway disease is made, radiographs for wheezing children should be obtained only when the symptoms are unusual or severe or if the disease remains unresponsive to therapy. However, inflammation of the small peripheral airways results in lung opacities, which can make radiographic differentiation between asthma, bronchiolitis, viral pneumonia, and bacterial pneumonia challenging.

Cross-sectional imaging is useful when a child does not respond to appropriate therapy or when complications of a disease are suspected. Although the choice of imaging modality is often evident, discussion with the radiologist has become increasingly important to ensure the most effective choice, given the continual advancement of cross-sectional imaging techniques.

Ultrasonography is readily available and lacks ionizing radiation; its main limitations are dependency on the skill of the sonographer and attenuation of the ultrasound beam by structures superficial to the area of interest. Ultrasonography allows for easy evaluation of a pleural effusion (Fig. 11), masses close to the chest wall in the anterior or posterior mediastinum (Fig. 12), or congenital heart disease (echocardiography). Its portability means that the imaging study can come to the patient. Augmentation of grayscale still images with cine clips or color Doppler interrogation provides information on the motion of a structure (eg, the diaphragm when a child cannot be weaned from mechanical ventilation) or blood flow in vascular structures, respectively [20,21].

When ultrasonography is inadequate for directing clinical care of a sick child, MR imaging (MRI) or CT may be used to further define chest disease, including but not limited to infectious processes, chest masses (Fig. 13), and congenital heart and great vessel anomalies (Fig. 14). MRI has the advantage of producing high-quality images without ionizing radiation, but accessibility and the need for sedation or general anesthesia to limit patient motion remain limitations. Therefore, appropriate use of CT is a viable alternative, and it remains superior to MRI when evaluating the lungs (Fig. 15); correctly performed chest CT may have a dose less than 300 mrad.

Detailed images of the lung parenchyma in children with suspected interstitial lung disease can be obtained with high-resolution CT (HRCT); however, the imaging findings in diffuse lung disease are often nonspecific, and CT may add little practical information [22]. HRCT obtains thin-slice images through selected regions of the lung parenchyma as opposed to contiguous images of the chest obtained with a standard spiral or helical CT technique (which is better suited to all other applications of the modality).

One should take into consideration the necessity of immediate imaging versus delaying MRI or CT of the chest; this is especially true in infants with congenital pulmonary masses (bronchopulmonary foregut malformations). In infants who are clinically stable, cross-sectional imaging should be

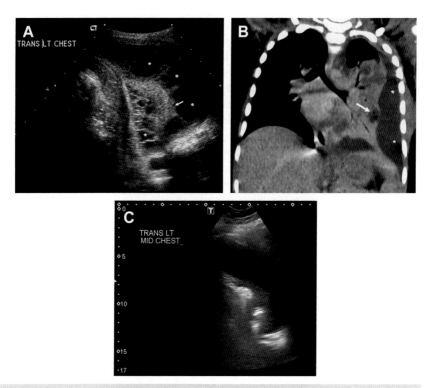

Fig. 11. Necrotizing pneumonia and empyema in a 2-year-old boy. (A) Ultrasonographic image shows normal lung (*arrow*) surrounded by a septated pleural effusion (*asterisk*), consistent with empyema. (B) Coronal contrast-enhanced CT image shows left lung pneumonia with a small abscess (*arrow*) in addition to the large parapneumonic effusion (*asterisk*). (C) For comparison with (A), this ultrasonographic image of a 9-year-old boy shows a simple pleural effusion.

reserved for preoperative planning closer to the time of surgical resection, because the image quality is generally better in larger children, and this practice avoids earlier exposure to radiation with CT or the risks of sedation with MRI (Fig. 16).

IMAGING DECISIONS IN GASTROINTESTINAL AND GENITOURINARY WORKUPS

Abdominal radiographs use bowel gas as an intrinsic contrast agent, which not only provides information about the gastrointestinal tract but also outlines solid structures. Despite the diagnostic usefulness of the distribution of bowel gas on a radiograph, its pattern is often nonspecific and may have poor correlation with clinical symptoms. Although radiographs are often the first-line imaging study in a child with symptoms referable to the abdomen, daily or progress studies are rarely indicated in children because of the cumulative radiation exposure and relative low diagnostic yield. The complex anatomy of the

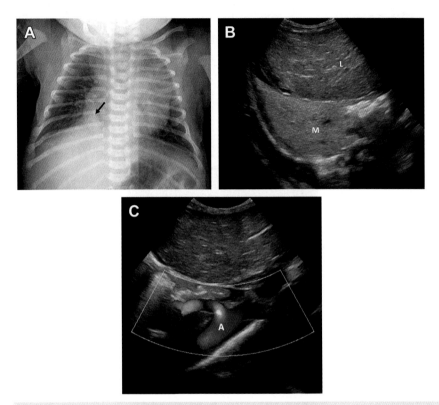

Fig. 12. Ultrasonography of a bronchopulmonary foregut malformation in a newborn. (*A*) Frontal chest radiograph shows opacity in the inferior medial right chest (*arrow*), correlating with the prenatal ultrasonographic findings of a pulmonary abnormality. (*B*) Grayscale ultrasonography of the right chest shows a posterior-inferior echogenic mass (M). L, liver. (*C*) Color Doppler interrogation of the same mass showed a systemic feeding artery arising from the aorta (A), suggesting pulmonary sequestration.

abdomen benefits from cross-sectional imaging, of which ultrasonography is most commonly used in children. The use of MRI has also steadily increased in the pediatric population; this is not only for its lack of ionizing radiation but also for its exquisite depiction of soft tissues and development of specific sequences, allowing for evaluation of the biliary tree, bowel wall, and urinary tract, described in greater detail later.

The diagnostic yield of imaging studies to explain vomiting is low, particularly in the young infant, and especially when gastroesophageal reflux is associated with overfeeding or when the infant has appropriately been gaining weight. However, the lack of an anatomic cause for vomiting has diagnostic usefulness, because it allows for medical treatment of the symptoms. Appropriate imaging study selection in the vomiting or refluxing infant is largely dependent on whether the emesis is bilious or nonbilious. When bilious, an upper gastrointestinal study is most appropriate and urgent to exclude

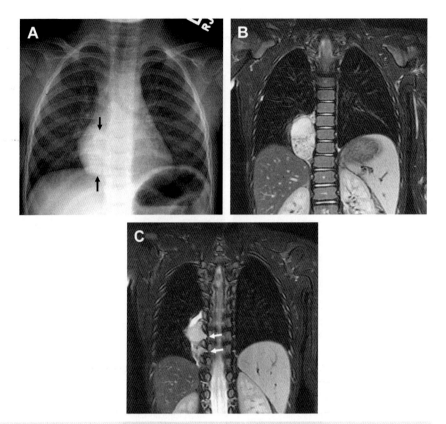

Fig. 13. Incidental discovery of a neuroblastoma in a 2-year-old girl presenting to the emergency department with fever. (A) Frontal chest radiograph shows a posterior mediastinal mass (*arrows*) with flecks of calcification. (B) Coronal MR images confirm a paraspinal soft tissue mass. The flecks of dark signal correlate with the calcification seen on radiography. (C) MRI is well suited to evaluating intraforaminal extension of tumor (*arrows*), as shown by this coronal MR image.

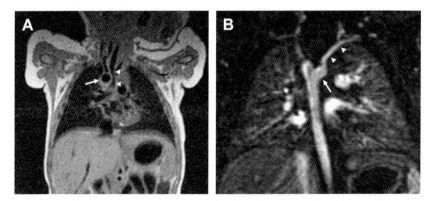

Fig. 14. Noisy breathing and multiple episodes of apnea in a 4-month-old girl discovered to have a vascular ring. (A) Coronal MR image of the chest shows a right-side aortic arch (*arrow*), exerting mass effect on the trachea (*arrowheads*). (B) Coronal MR angiography of the chest shows the left subclavian artery (*arrowheads*) arising from a large diverticulum of Kommerell (*arrow*).

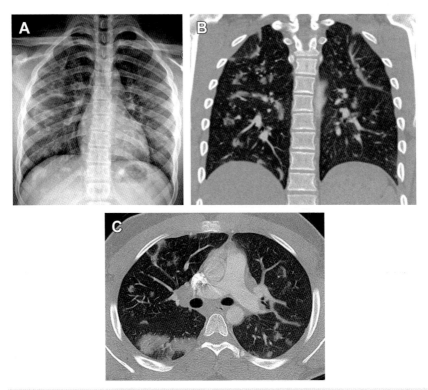

Fig. 15. Abnormal chest radiograph in a 15-year-old boy who presented for dyspnea. (A) Frontal chest radiograph show curvilinear opacities in both lungs. (B, C) Coronal (B) and axial (C) CT images of the chest show the same curvilinear opacities. The appearance is highly suggestive of cryptogenic organizing pneumonia, which was subsequently confirmed with lung biopsy.

malrotation (Fig. 17) and midgut volvulus. Infants with nonbilious emesis benefit most from targeted abdomen ultrasonography to answer specific questions (eg, does the child have pyloric stenosis or intussusception?) (Fig. 18) [23,24].

In children and adolescents, ultrasonography supplants radiographs and fluoroscopy as the best initial screening test for vomiting or abdomen pain. In addition to bowel-related causes of abdominal pain, cholecystitis, pancreatitis, and renal disease are readily shown by ultrasonography [25,26].

Classically, the upper gastrointestinal study with small bowel follow-through has been used to define the distribution and extent of IBD. MRE has emerged as an alternative to fluoroscopy; in many cases, MRE provides superior diagnostic information. Specific MR sequences sensitive to inflammation and the use of intravenous contrast agents allow for differentiation between acute and chronic changes of IBD (Fig. 19) [27,28].

MRI is also gaining traction in the evaluation of congenital and acquired biliary disorders formerly evaluated primarily with ultrasonography and nuclear

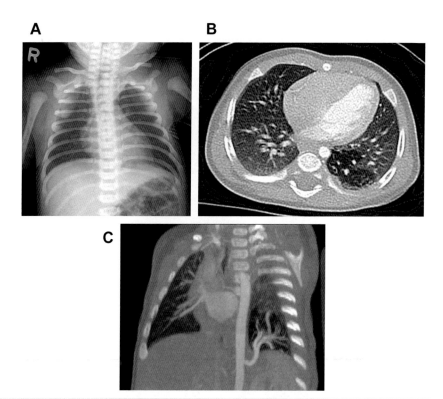

Fig. 16. Imaging in a full-term girl with prenatal ultrasonographic diagnosis of sequestration. (A) Frontal chest radiograph shows no visible abnormality. The child was clinically stable, so further cross-sectional imaging evaluation was planned for closer to the time of surgical resection. (B, C) Axial (B) and coronal (C) reformatted contrast-enhanced CT images obtained at 4 months of age show a lucent mass lesion in the posterior medial left lower lobe, with a systemic feeding artery arising from the aorta, consistent with sequestration.

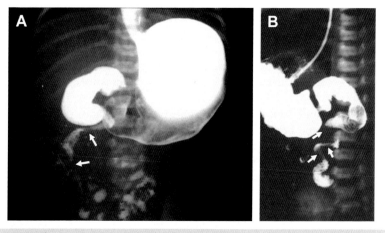

Fig. 17. Malrotation in an 8-month-old with bilious vomiting. (A) Frontal image from an upper gastrointestinal examination shows malpositioning of the duodenum with extrinsic compression from the Ladd bands (*arrows*). (B) Lateral image shows the corkscrew appearance of the duodenum.

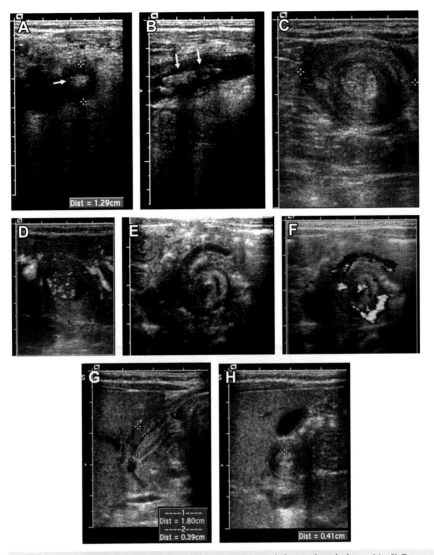

Fig. 18. The usefulness of ultrasonography in pediatric abdominal pathology. (*A, B*) Transverse (*A*) and longitudinal (*B*) ultrasonographic images in an 11-year-old boy with right lower quadrant abdominal pain show a thick-walled 1.3-cm-wide tubular structure in the right lower quadrant, containing an echogenic shadowing structure (*arrows*), confirmed at surgery to be an inflamed appendix, containing a calcified fecalith. The normal appendix has a diameter less than 0.6 cm. (*C, D*) Transverse grayscale (*C*) and power Doppler (*D*) ultrasonographic images in a 2-year-old boy with colicky abdominal pain show the target or bull's-eye appearance of an ileocolic intussusception. On color Doppler, there is vascular supply to the bowel, signifying viability. (*E, F*) Transverse grayscale (*E*) and color Doppler (*F*) ultrasonographic images in an infant with bilious vomiting. The whirlpool appearance of the swirling mesenteric vessels is concerning for midgut volvulus. The child was immediately taken to surgery, which confirmed malrotation with midgut volvulus. (*G, H*) Longitudinal (*G*) and transverse (*H*) grayscale images in a 1-month-old girl with projectile vomiting confirm hypertrophic pyloric stenosis as the cause. In (*G*), the channel length is 1.8 cm (18 mm) and wall thickness is 0.39 cm (3.9 mm). In (*H*), the wall thickness is 0.41 cm (4.1 mm). The normal pyloric muscle thickness should be less than 3 mm and channel length less than 15 mm.

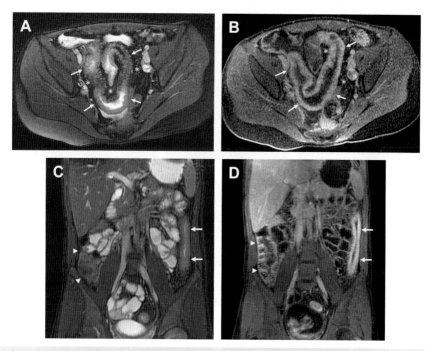

Fig. 19. MRE in 2 children with Crohn disease. (*A*, *B*) Axial fluid-sensitive (*A*) and contrast-enhanced (*B*) MR images in a 12-year-old girl show marked terminal ileal wall thickening and enhancement (*arrows*). Adjacent mesenteric fat hypertrophy and hyperemia (*asterisk*) are also present. (*C*, *D*) Coronal fluid-sensitive (*C*) and contrast-enhanced (*D*) MR images in a 17-year-old boy show left-side colonic wall thickening and hyperenhancement (*arrows*). Contrast this finding with the cecum, which is normal in appearance (*arrowheads*).

medicine hepatobiliary iminodiacetic acid scans. MR cholangiopancreatography (MRCP) acquires high-resolution images of the biliary system and pancreatic duct, which can easily be reconstructed in 3 dimensions (Fig. 20), avoiding the more invasive endoscopic retrograde cholangiopancreatography [29].

To better characterize a suspected abdominal mass (Fig. 21), ultrasonography remains the best first imaging study, because of its availability and lack of ionizing radiation or need for sedation. Identification of the origin of the mass and whether it is cystic or solid guides the need for further imaging evaluation, ideally with MRI. Unless there is a specific contraindication, intravenous contrast material should be administered, because it improves tumor detection and characterization as well as the relation of the tumor to adjacent blood vessels. The use of new liver-specific contrast agents (mangafodipir, gadobenate, gadoxetate) increases the diagnostic sensitivity and specificity for liver masses, although these agents are not yet approved for use in children in the United States [30]. In time, whole-body MRI may rival tomography (positron emission tomography [PET]/CT) for tumor surveillance, avoiding

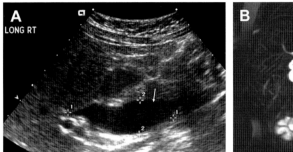
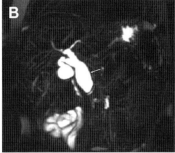

Fig. 20. Choledochal cyst in an 8-year-old girl with increased transaminase levels. (A) Grayscale ultrasonographic image of the abdomen right upper quadrant shows a fusiform cystic structure (arrow) in the expected position of the common bile duct. (B) Three-dimensional reformatted MRCP image confirms fusiform enlargement of the common bile duct (arrow), consistent with type 1 choledochal cyst.

the cumulative radiation exposure from repeat PET/CT studies required by oncology therapy protocols and clinical trials [31,32]. When MRI is not available or practical for further characterization of an abdominal mass, contrast-enhanced CT is a viable alternative and should be optimized to limit radiation exposure [33].

Appropriate imaging evaluation for a child experiencing their first urinary tract infection (UTI) has been a long-standing area of uncertainty, because vesicoureteral reflux does not cause infection and is frequently not associated with pyelonephritis or progressive renal scarring. Current imaging recommendations include ultrasonography of the kidneys and urinary bladder to screen for congenital or acquired genitourinary abnormalities, which may predispose a child to urinary stasis, pyelonephritis, progressive renal scarring, and end-stage renal disease. Voiding cystourethrography (VCUG) and renal

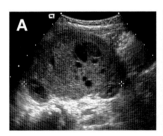
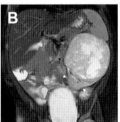
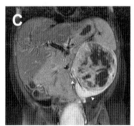

Fig. 21. Wilms tumor in a 5-month-old girl presenting with a palpable left flank mass. (A) Grayscale ultrasonographic image shows a large, heterogeneous solid-cystic mass arising from the left kidney. (B, C) Coronal fluid-sensitive (B) and contrast-enhanced (C) MR images of the abdomen show the complex solid-cystic mass arising from the left kidney, of which only a small portion of the inferior pole is recognizable (arrowheads). No tumor thrombus was seen by MRI (not shown).

scintigraphy should be reserved for children with abnormal ultrasonography findings or recurrent febrile UTIs [4]. MRI, especially MR urography (MRU), is increasingly being used, because of its superior visualization of the kidneys, ureters, and bladder and its ability to assess kidney function through quantification of renal parenchymal enhancement and contrast excretion (Fig. 22).

Complex congenital anomalies of the genital tract (eg, cloacal) often require multiple modalities to define anatomy. Initial evaluation with ultrasonography of the kidneys, bladder, and pelvis usually requires additional information from fluoroscopy (VCUG, pressure fistulogram), which may be augmented with MRI or MRU.

Advances in musculoskeletal imaging

Imaging evaluation of the pediatric musculoskeletal structures is challenging because of their constant evolution with growth. The bones, muscles, and ligaments change not only in imaging appearance but also in relative strength and composition. Although radiographs offer the best initial evaluation of the musculoskeletal system, certain structures are radiographically occult and may require other imaging modalities.

Most traumatic injuries in children can be completely evaluated with radiographs, because the relative strength of a younger child's tendons usually results in fractures of the weaker bone. Although CT is accompanied by a higher radiation dose than radiographs, it is better for defining complex fractures before surgical fixation. Children involved in sports or other high-level physical activity often require MRI to evaluate for subtle osseous and nonosseous injury (ie, injury to cartilage, tendons, and ligaments, internal derangement of joints, and bone contusions) (Fig. 23). Ultrasonography is useful when investigating soft tissue injuries (eg, hematoma, radiolucent foreign

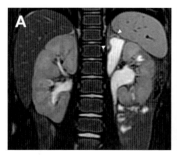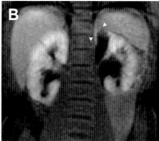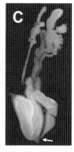

Fig. 22. Four-year-old girl with known left duplex kidney and upper pole obstruction who presented for MRU evaluation. (A) Coronal fluid-sensitive MR image shows marked atrophy of the left kidney upper pole parenchyma (*arrowheads*). (B) Postcontrast coronal MR image shows enhancement of the upper pole parenchyma, despite the atrophy (*arrowheads*). (C) Three-dimensional MRU reconstruction shows ectopic insertion of the left upper pole moiety to the bladder neck (*arrow*).

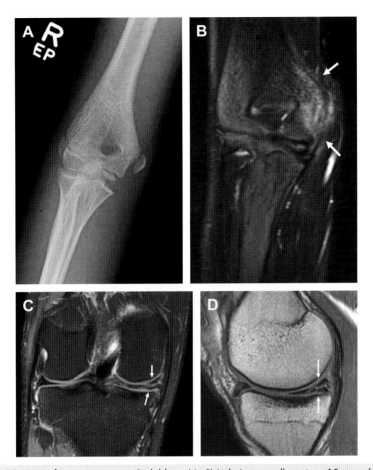

Fig. 23. MRI of sports injuries in 2 children. (*A, B*) Little League elbow in a 10-year-old boy with medial elbow pain. Frontal radiograph (*A*) of the right elbow shows no abnormality. Persistent pain prompted MRI (*B*), which shows edema (white or high signal) in the medial epicondyle and surrounding soft tissues (*arrows*). (*C, D*) Meniscus tear in a 17-year-old boy with severe knee pain after a basketball injury. The boy had negative radiographs (*not shown*). Coronal fluid-sensitive (*C*) and sagittal (*D*) MR images show a complex tear of the medial meniscus posterior horn. The arrows outline the meniscus, and the tear is in the middle of the meniscus.

body) and in experienced hands can be used to evaluate tendon and ligament injuries.

In children with inflammatory muscular and neuromuscular disorders, MRI has been increasingly used as a noninvasive diagnostic method. Imaging sequences sensitive to water content in the muscle allow for detection of myositis without need for biopsy. T2 mapping techniques allow for quantification of muscle edema, even before it is visibly apparent [34]. This technique can also be used to track the efficacy of therapy and in the future may allow for earlier initiation of therapy in subclinical disease, delaying the onset of symptoms [35].

Radiographs are generally adequate for evaluating congenital limb and skeletal anomalies. However, the use of MRI can be important to detect cartilaginous anomalies or when there is significant soft tissue involvement. In such cases, MRI is superior, because of its exquisite depiction of preossified cartilage and soft tissue structures (Fig. 24). Fetal MRI, which is already used to further characterize anomalies detected on prenatal ultrasonography, may become more useful in prenatal evaluation of skeletal dysplasias [36].

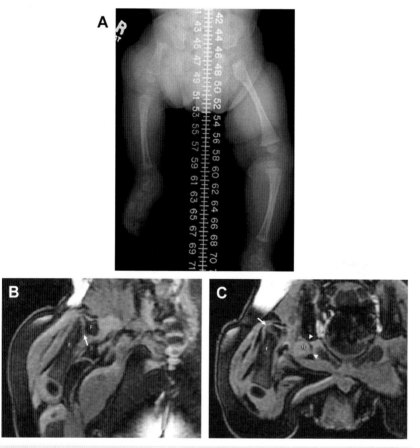

Fig. 24. Proximal femoral focal deficiency in a 5-month-old boy with leg-length asymmetry. (A) Radiographs show markedly short and dysmorphic proximal right femur (contrast to the normal left femur). (B, C) Cartilage-sensitive coronal oblique MR images of the femur (B) and the pelvis (C) show multiple anomalies, including pseudoarthrosis (*arrow*) of the ossified femur (F) and presence of a primarily cartilaginous femoral head (H) normally located in the right acetabulum (*arrowheads*).

MRI allows for earlier detection and characterization of acquired bone disease that is radiographically occult until late in the disease process. Osteomyelitis and osteonecrosis (Fig. 25) are 2 such entities, although differentiation between these processes can be difficult, even with contrast-enhanced MRI. Bone marrow changes in children with metabolic disorders, such as Gaucher disease, and these changes can be followed with MRI to assess the efficacy of treatment. The sensitivity of MRI for bone marrow and soft tissues has made it mandatory in the workup for malignant bone tumors, evaluating both the intramedullary and soft tissue extent (Fig. 26). Radiographs remain the most reliable imaging measure of the biological nature of a bone tumor (ie, aggressive vs nonaggressive) and thus are complementary to MRI.

Soft tissues tumors in children may be vascular malformations, most of which can be adequately imaged using ultrasonography (Fig. 27). MRI may be required when ultrasonography findings are inconclusive or when the mass has aggressive features. Advances in MR angiography (MRA) technique

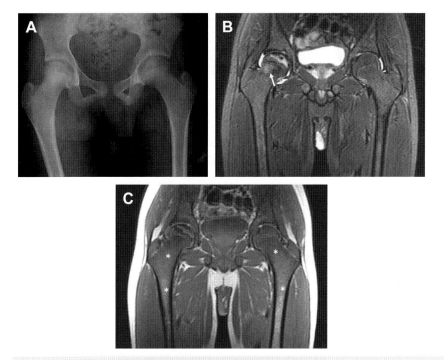

Fig. 25. Avascular necrosis of the hip in a 17-year-old boy with sickle cell disease and persistent right hip pain. (A) Frontal radiograph of the pelvis shows minimal increased sclerosis of the proximal right femur. (B, C) Coronal MR images of the pelvis show geographic signal abnormality in the right femoral head consistent with avascular necrosis with reactive edema (white) in the femoral neck (arrow). Note exuberant red marrow (asterisk) in the femoral necks and shafts as a consequence of this child's extramedullary hematopoeisis.

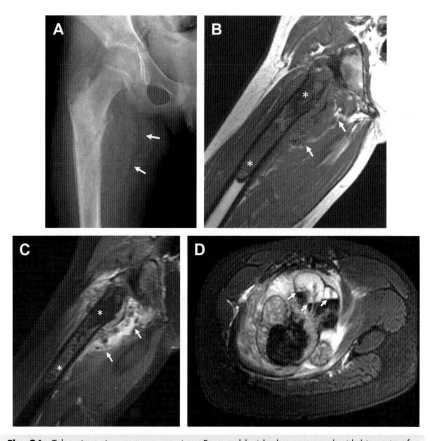

Fig. 26. Telangiectatic osteosarcoma in a 5-year-old girl who presented with hip pain after falling at the playground. Many children present with apparent accidents but have underlying congenital anomalies or tumors. (A) Radiograph of the right hip shows permeative destruction of the proximal right femur. Bowing of the fat planes in the medial thigh suggests an associated soft tissue mass (*arrows*). Radiographs offer the best chance at differential diagnosis of bone disease, because this modality is most accurate for showing biological behavior of the process. (B, C) Coronal non–fat-saturated (B) and fat-saturated (C) MR images show tumor replacement of the bone marrow (*asterisk*) and an associated juxtacortical soft tissue mass (*arrows*). Joint-to-joint imaging (not shown) did not show skip lesions. (D) Axial MR image shows fluid-fluid levels (*arrows*) within the soft tissue mass. Although fluid-fluid levels are more often seen in aneurysmal bone cysts, the destructive bone process shown on radiographs is consistent with telangiectatic osteosarcoma. This finding emphasizes the need for the radiograph.

allow for better definition of the vascular supply of a mass and may obviate formal angiography. Although radiography and CT are not first-line imaging studies for soft tissue masses, they may narrow the differential diagnosis when calcifications or destruction of adjacent bone are seen.

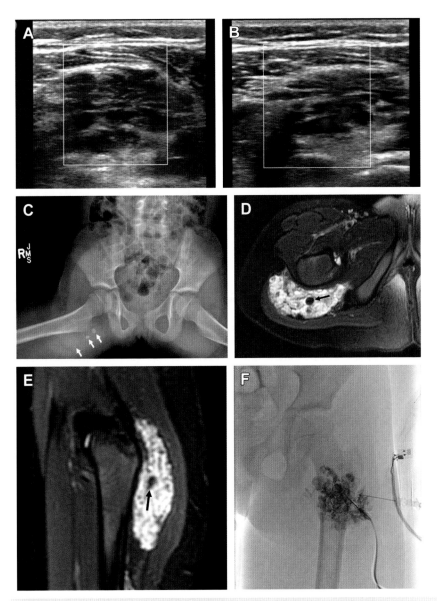

Fig. 27. A 6-year-old girl who had right buttock swelling after a gymnastics injury. She was discovered to have a venous malformation. (*A, B*) Grayscale (*A*) and color Doppler-enhanced (*B*) ultrasonographic images of the right buttocks show a lobulated, septated cystic mass with internal vascular flow, suggesting a venous malformation. (*C*) Frog-leg radiograph of the pelvis shows soft tissue asymmetry in the region of the mass, which contains round calcified phleboliths (*arrows*). (*D, E*) Axial (*D*) and sagittal (*E*) fluid-sensitive MR images show the cystic, septated mass containing phleboliths (*arrows*), consistent with a venous malformation. (*F*) Fluoroscopic spot image shows sclerotherapy injection of the venous malformation.

NEUROIMAGING

The most frequent indications for neuroimaging studies include patients with (1) seizures, (2) headaches, (3) neurologic developmental delays/congenital anomalies, and (4) trauma. Imaging of preterm infants or term babies with hypoxic/ischemic injury (HII) has also become important. In trauma and in instances of acute neurologic dysfunction without immediate availability of MR, CT is the premier imaging test. However, because of its great imaging detail and lack of radiation, MR is the most appropriate imaging modality in almost all other instances [37–40].

Seizures

There remains general agreement that children with febrile seizures need no routine imaging but rather an effective workup and treatment of the cause of the fever [6]. There is also agreement that most children with an afebrile unprovoked seizure and normal history and neurologic examination should have neuroimaging, although not as an urgency [41]. The reason for the MR is 2-fold: to detect the cause and to plan future treatment and, if necessary, follow-up imaging (Fig. 28) [42]. Most children, even infants younger than 24 months, with unprovoked seizure have a normal MR result, but 17% have findings influencing medical care (Fig. 29) [43]. The percentage of positivity varies with the age of presentation, the type of seizure, neurologic findings, and electroencephalography results.

Headaches

The need to image the child/adolescent with headaches is dependent on the history and the physical examination [44]. Although seizures or headaches frequently occur in patients with central nervous system (CNS) neoplasms, they are rarely the only sign or symptom [45]. In general, the child/adolescent with chronic recurring headaches and normal neurologic evaluation and no signs of intracranial pressure should not receive a CT scan [46]. However, imaging might be important and appropriate in the child/adolescent with persistent headaches greater than 6 months in duration and unresponsive to treatment [45]. When there are no neurologic findings but worrisome clinical data (eg, morning headaches, awakening from sleep, change in the character of the headaches, migraines without family history), MRI is indicated [47]. Of course, in cases of neurologic signs or symptoms or increase in symptoms of cranial pressure (vomiting and headaches), imaging becomes urgent. MR is clearly the modality of choice, because of its greater ability to define the brain parenchyma and find small lesions. The ability to note old bleeds and areas of restricted diffusion (vascular insufficiency or inflammation) is readily attainable. The use of MRA might be helpful in children with a positive family history of stroke or vascular abnormalities (Fig. 30).

In those rare instances of sudden severe headache (thunderclap), urgent neuroimaging should be performed, and the choices in this instance include immediate CT angiography or MR and MRA. The incidence of arteriovenous

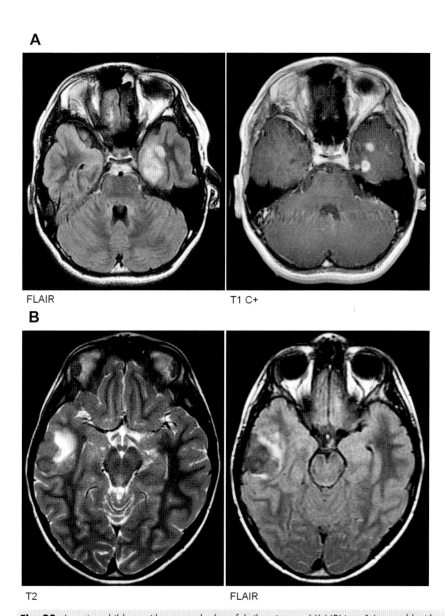

A

FLAIR   T1 C+

B

T2   FLAIR

Fig. 28. Imaging children with unprovoked nonfebrile seizures. (A) MRI in a 14-year-old with first seizure. Axial T2-weighted (T2W) fluid-attenuated inversion recovery (FLAIR) and T1-weighted contrast-enhanced MR images show a left temporal lobe partially enhancing lesion. The lesion was a cortical hamartoma. (B) MRI in a 10 year old with first seizure. Axial T2W and T2 FLAIR images show a large extra-axial lesion in the right middle cranial fossa. Enhanced coronal and axial images (C) show florid enhancement. The lesion, convex to the brain, was a meningioma. (D) Axial T2W FLAIR image in a 6-year-old shows a posterior fossa right cerebellar lesion proved to be an astrocytoma.

C

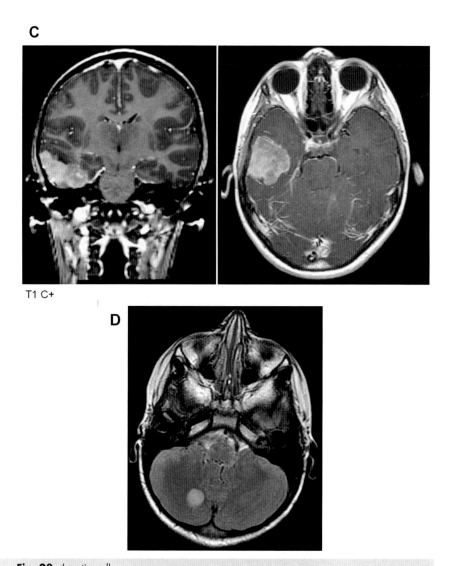

T1 C+

Fig. 28. (continued).

malformations is 4 times greater than aneurysms in children younger than 15 years [1].

Neurodevelopmental/Congenital anomalies

Most children with a neurodevelopmental/congenital anomaly (including macrocephaly) undergo MRI to help determine the cause of the problem [2,48–51]. The precise anatomic detail allows for the diagnosis of malformations of all types (Fig. 31). In some instances, the clinical presentation of the child suggests an inherited metabolic brain disorder or neurodegenerative disease. Clinical

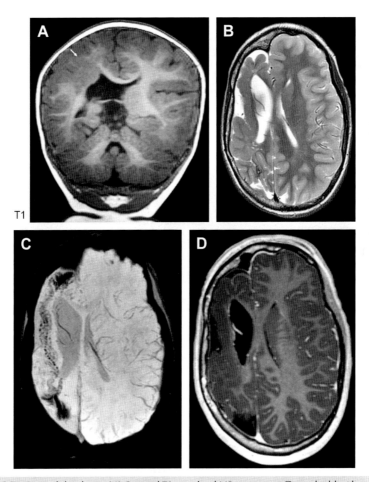

Fig. 29. Cortical dysplasia. (A) Coronal T1-weighted MR image in a 7-month-old with seizures shows asymmetry of the cortex, with thickened cortex (arrow) in the right parietal region and larger ventricle on this side (B–D) MRI in a 2-year-old with Sturge-Weber syndrome. Axial T2-weighted image (B) shows loss of volume in the right frontal parietal region with dysplastic cortex. The ventricle is larger ex vacuo. Susceptibility-weighted imaging sequence (C) shows excessive vessels (black) within the cortex. Enhanced axial T1-weighted image (D) shows excess enhancement in the right ventricular wall and on the surface of the cortex compared with the other side.

clues to these diagnoses include regression of development, basal ganglion signs, and progressive encephalopathy. In these instances, it might be advisable to perform both MRI and MRS. MRS is a biochemical evaluation of the brain (Fig. 32) [52]. Many metabolic and neurodegenerative disorders are associated with increased lactate or decreased N-acetylaspartate levels, or increased levels of other metabolites such as choline or myoinositol. The value of these findings suggests metabolic workup, which might not be otherwise considered (see Fig. 32).

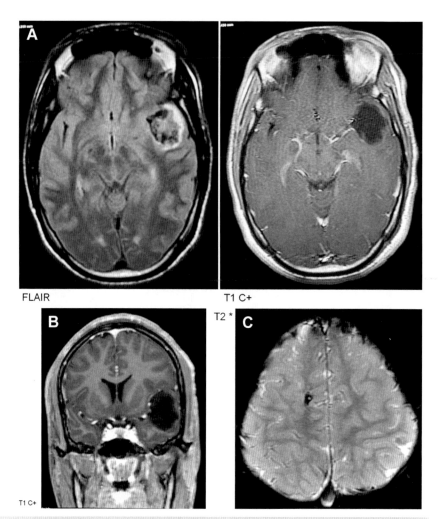

FLAIR   T1 C+

T2 *

Fig. 30. Imaging children with headaches. (A) MRI in a 17-year-old. Axial T2-weighted fluid-attenuated inversion recovery (FLAIR) and contrast-enhanced T1-weighted (T1W) images and coronal contrast-enhanced T1W image (B) show a left temporal lobe epidermoid. (C, D) Two patients who presented with headaches and had positive susceptibility-weighted imaging (SWI) sequences. Axial image (C) shows a cavernous angioma in the first patient. Axial SWI in the second patient (D) shows an arteriovenous malformation. (E–I) The value of MRA. The appearance of normal MRA (E) and MR venography (F). Compare that with MRA in a teenager with a migraine (G, I). The arteries are constricted on the left side (G), and the SWI sequence (H) shows venous engorgement. The patient returned to normal on follow-up examination (I).

    MRS is complex and normative peaks and ratios vary by the patient's age as well as the location in the brain. MRS has an important role in helping define focal CNS lesions (ie, tumors with increased choline levels) (Fig. 33). Relative increases of metabolites other than choline may give a hint to the histologic

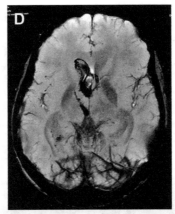

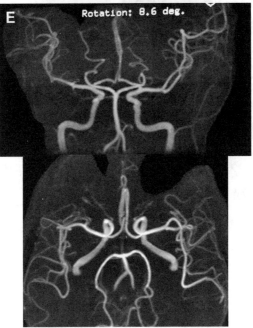

Fig. 30. (continued).

nature of the tumor (ie, taurine in medulloblastoma) [52]. MRS has been shown to be valuable in cases of cerebral abscess (see Fig. 33) [53].

It is appropriate to discuss diffusion tensor imaging (DTI) when imaging a child with a congenital brain malformation. This is a technique in which white matter microstructural integrity can be demonstrated, thus showing the white matter tracts. These color maps show the size and orientation of the white matter tracts in normal and abnormal states and help us understand the exact

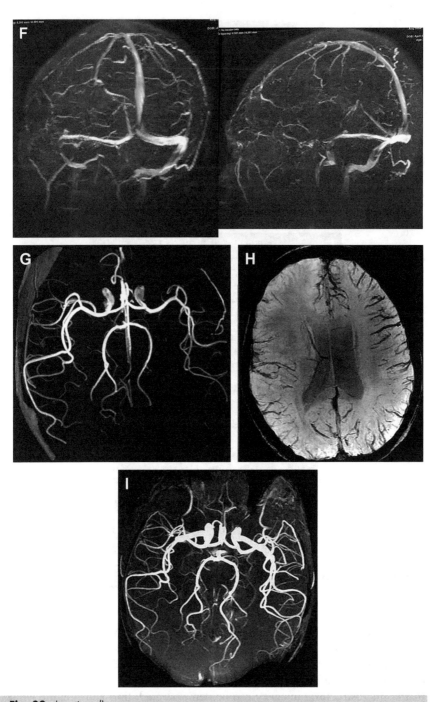

Fig. 30. (continued).

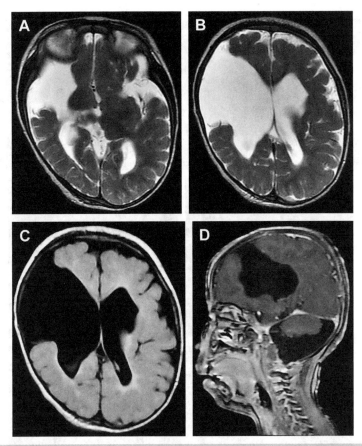

Fig. 31. Congenital anomalies. Open-lip schizencephaly and posterior fossa arachnoid cyst. (A, B) Axial T2-weighted (T2W) MR images at 2 different levels show the large fluid-filled defect lined with gray matter. The large defect communicates with the ventricle. (C) Similar findings are noted on this axial T2W FLAIR image. (D) Enhanced T1-weighted sagittal MR image shows both the schizencephaly and the posterior fossa arachnoid cyst.

defects in the congenital anomalies (Fig. 34). For example, in a rare disease called pontine tegmental cap dysplasia, DTI has shown the absence of superior and middle cerebellar peduncle decussation and an ectopic fiber tract causing the tegmental bulge [54].

When fiber tract maps are used in children with tumors, the neurosurgeon gains greater knowledge of which tracts are affected by the lesion (Fig. 35). The surgeon then can achieve more appropriate resection with less morbidity.

Trauma

The greatest overuse of CT imaging is in the child with minor trauma. Kuppermann and colleagues [7] have shown that in the proper clinical situation, we

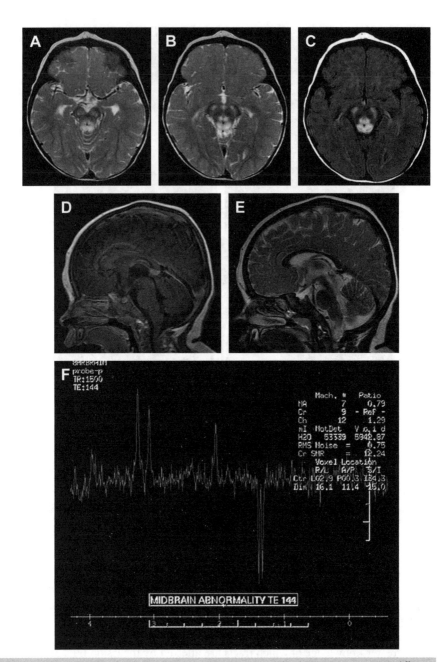

Fig. 32. (A–E) Multiple axial MR images (*top row*, T2-weighted [T2W] imaging at 2 different levels and T1-weighted [T1W] contrast-enhanced axial image; *bottom row*, 2 sagittal images, T1W contrast-enhanced and T2W). Abnormal high signal in the brainstem and periaqueductal enhancement. (F) MRS shows a huge lactate peak, doublet at 1.3 (the metric is the bottom line in parts/million).

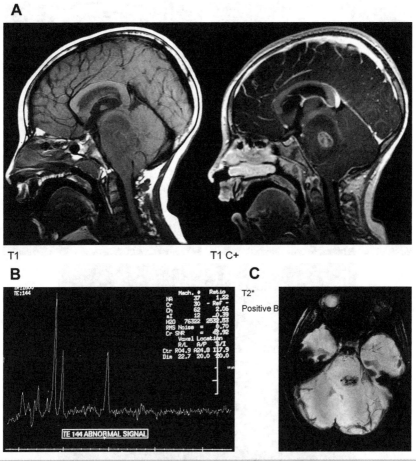

Fig. 33. Examples of where MRS is helpful: tumors and abscesses. (A–C) Six-month-old with vomiting and ataxia. Sagittal T1-weighted (T1W) images without and with contrast agent (A) show a large enhancing brainstem glioma. (B) MRS shows a large choline peak at 3.2. This finding is secondary to myelin breakdown and is characteristic of tumors and inflammation. (C) Axial MR susceptibility-weighted image shows bleeding (*black*) within the tumor. (D–F) A 4-month-old who presented with encephalopathy. Diffusion-weighted image shows restricted diffusion (*white*), with a large mass effect and shift of brain structures from left to right. (E) Axial T1W contrast-enhanced image shows rim enhancement consistent with necrotic tumor or abscess. (F) However, MRS shows multiple peaks between 0.9 and 1.3, representing amino acids and lactate, characteristic of brain abscess.

need not image but can still feel confident that we have not missed anything (Box 3). In their study of 42,412 children with a Glasgow coma scale of 14 to 15, of whom 14,969 received CT examinations, these investigators determined the need for CT. In children younger than 2 years, there was 100% negative predictive value and 100% sensitivity, and those older than 2 years

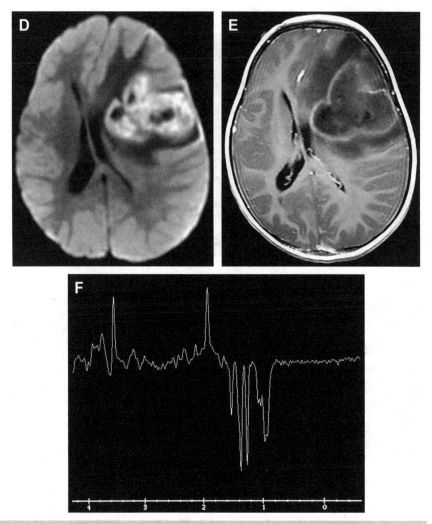

Fig. 33. (continued).

had a negative predictive value of 99.9% and a sensitivity of 96.8% [7]. Given that these data were from a large series, it seems that in minor trauma we can perform less imaging by about 25% without any risk of missing a lesion. Discussion of nonaccidental trauma is included in the section on child abuse.

Neonatal cerebral imaging

Imaging of the neonate has changed dramatically over the last 5 years. It is rare (only in acute birth trauma) to use CT. Ultrasonography remains the first test for most indications in the premature infant. However, the rapid technical advances (eg, diffusion, faster scans) have made MR the most important and best

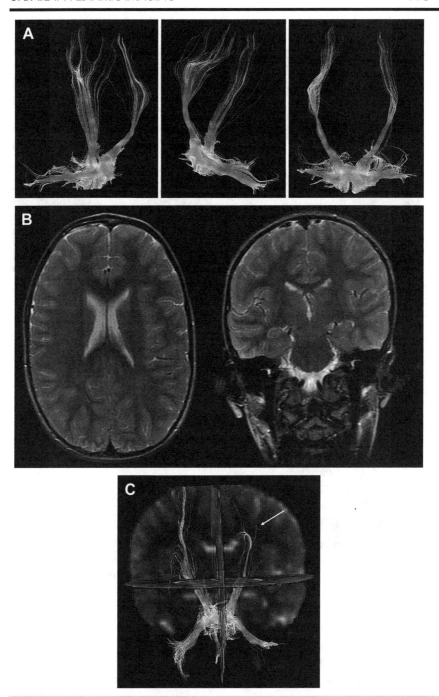

Fig. 34. DTI and fiber tractography. (A) Normal fiber tracts of the pyramidal pathways. (B) Child with congenital spastic diplegia. Axial and coronal MR views are normal. (C) However, tractography shows that the pyramidal tracts are grossly atrophic (arrow), left worse than right, compared with normal.

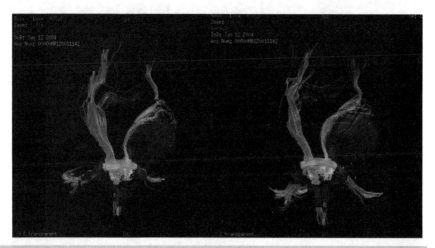

Fig. 35. Tractography in defining the effect of the tumor. Tractography in this child shows the left thalamic tumor deviating the left pyramidal tract.

Box 3: Evaluation of children with Glasgow coma scores of 14 to 15 after head trauma

A. Children younger than 2 years with the following clinical/historical evaluation had a negative predictive value of 100% and a sensitivity of 100% for clinically important brain injury.

1. Normal mental status

2. No scalp hematoma except for frontal

3. No loss of consciousness or loss of consciousness for less than 5 seconds

4. Nonsevere injury mechanism

5. No palpable fracture

6. Acting normally according to parents

B. Children 2 years and older with the following clinical/historical evaluation had a negative predictive value of 99.95% and a sensitivity of 96.8% for clinically important brain injury.

1. Normal mental status

2. No loss of consciousness

3. No vomiting

4. Nonsevere injury mechanism

5. No signs of basilar skull fracture

6. No severe headache

Data from Kuppermann J, Holmes JF, Dayan PS, et al. Identification of children at very low risk of clinically-important brain injuries after head trauma: a prospective cohort study. Lancet 2009;374:1160–70.

tool to evaluate neonates for the diagnosis and prognosis of such diseases as HII, for follow-up of intracranial hemorrhage, and for complete diagnosis of congenital anomalies (see earlier discussion).

Perinatal/prenatal stroke accounts for 25% of all pediatric strokes and has an incidence of 1 in 2300 to 5000 live births. The cause/risk factors include maternal thrombotic states, infections, and genetic factors, as well as fetal/neonatal genetic/thrombotic and congenital abnormalities and problems of delivery [55]. However, in most neonates, the cause is never found. The best MR sequence for diagnosing ischemia is diffusion-weighted imaging (DWI) (Fig. 36). It can be completed in 40 seconds or less, it shows ischemic lesions within the first hours, and it stays positive for up to 1 week (2–3 days in older children). The brain changes of ischemia restrict diffusion of water molecules; this then appears as high signal (white) on DWI and low signal (black) on apparent diffusion coefficient images. Another important sequence on MR is

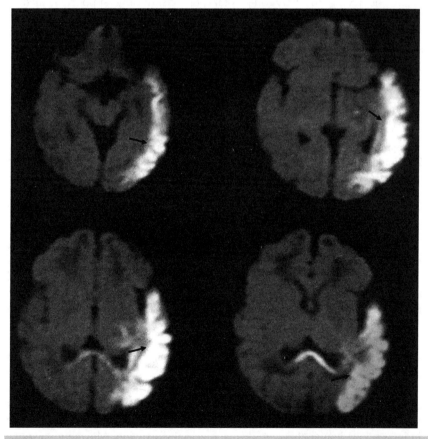

Fig. 36. Positive axial diffusion sequence in a neonate with ischemia. Edema prevents fluid diffusion and appears white on the images (*arrows*). The posterior corpus callosum is involved.

the susceptibility image to define hemosiderin. It can be either a T2* gradient-echo sequence or another susceptibility-weighted imaging (SWI) sequence (the gradient-echo proprietary sequence is called susceptibility-weighted angiography). It has been shown to be predictive of cerebral palsy [56].

Evaluation of the child suspected of having nonaccidental trauma

In the last several years, 2 topics have altered the imaging landscape of the diagnosis of nonaccidental trauma: (1) the role, if any, of vitamin D insufficiency/deficiency in the cause of skeletal fractures and (2) the role of cerebral sinovenous thrombosis and hypoxia in causing some of the imaging characteristics found in cerebral abusive head trauma [57].

The reason for the contrived discussion of both topics is to cast the diagnosis of child abuse in doubt. This is a legal ploy, because when there is no diagnosis of abusive head trauma, the defendant or already incarcerated individual did not commit a crime. The legal community, abetted by a few physicians, is trying to deny 50+ years of scientifically supported medical literature.

The relationship of vitamin D insufficiency/deficiency is best summarized in the following manner:

1. "There is no scientific evidence to connect vitamin D levels to fractures in the fetus or neonate. Calcium and phosphorus are transferred against a concentrations gradient from mother to fetus and placental parathyroid-related protein (PTHrP) up-regulates active placental calcium transfer" [58]. Intestinal absorption of calcium is passive in the neonate, not vitamin D dependent. Vitamin D becomes more important with maturity [58,59].
2. Congenital rickets (in infants younger than 6 months) is only found in infants whose mother has severe disease. These cases are mainly premature infants and show the radiographic findings of rickets [58,60].
3. Multiple articles describe infants with vitamin D insufficiency who do not have fractures or rickets [61].

The conclusions should be obvious: without biochemical evidence (altered calcium, phosphorus, and parathyroid hormone levels) or radiographic evidence of rickets, any fracture sustained by the baby is not caused by abnormalities of vitamin D. The National Institute of Medicine has reported that more than 20 ng/mL of 25-hydroxy vitamin D is adequate for bone health in 97.5% of the population [62].

The Appropriateness Criteria (last reviewed in 2012) of the American College of Radiology clearly present the approach to imaging a child with suspected abuse [3].

The second issue concerns the cause of subdural hematoma, retinal hemorrhages, and parenchymal findings in abusive head trauma. Because the highest mortality in nonaccidental injury occurs secondary to head trauma, particularly in infants and young children, this is a crucial discussion. Mortality varies between 10% and 50%, but even more discouraging is that more than 90% of survivors have significant disability [63].

The medical literature has documented that the unexplained findings of subdural hematoma and retinal hemorrhage strongly suggest child abuse [64–66]. However, for the same legal reasons as noted earlier, a hypothesis has evolved that cerebral sinovenous thrombosis or hypoxia-asphyxia can cause large subdural hematomas [67,68]. There is again no medical evidence to support either of these theories [69]. Concerning cerebral sinovenous thrombosis:

1. There are no cases in the literature in which cerebral sinovenous thrombosis caused subdural hematomas. This finding was shown again by McLean and colleagues [69] in 36 children.
2. Hedlund reported trauma as the major precipitating cause of cerebral sinovenous thrombosis and noted the absence of subdural hematomas [70].
3. It is the presence of ruptured cortical veins (showing trauma) that are thrombosed that is associated with subdural hematomas. These infants suffered abusive head trauma [71,72].

The second hypothesis without medical evidence is that HII causes macroscopic subdural hematomas such as those seen in abusive head trauma [68]:

1. It is now believed that both rupture of bridging veins as well as the rupture of the rich plexus of intradural vessels can play a role in the formation of subdural hematomas [73].
2. However, the subdural hematomas found post mortem in neonates with hypoxic-ischemic injury are small, only thin films, and not in any way similar to findings in abusive head injury.
3. This theory of the pathophysiology was retracted before the High Court of Justice in England and Wales in June, 2005 [74].

Several other concepts have evolved concerning imaging when evaluating a child suspected of sustaining abuse and abusive head trauma. We have learned

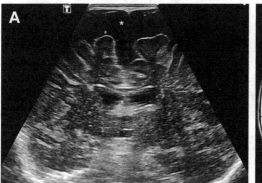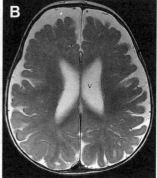

Fig. 37. An increase in extra-axial fluid or enlarged ventricles can rarely predispose children to subdural hematomas with minor trauma. (A) Ultrasonography of the brain in a 6-month-old with moderate extra-axial fluid (*asterisk*). He presented with macrocephaly. (B) MR of the same infant at 9 months shows even greater extra-axial fluid (*asterisk*) and now enlarged ventricles (V). Infants like this are at a small risk of serious injury from seemingly minor injury.

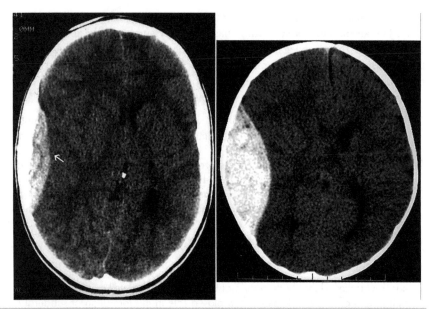

Fig. 38. Acute epidural hematoma on CT after an automobile accident. The lesion is hyperdense (acute) and convex to the brain (*arrow*). Epidural hematomas occur almost always after accidental trauma and are less common after child abuse.

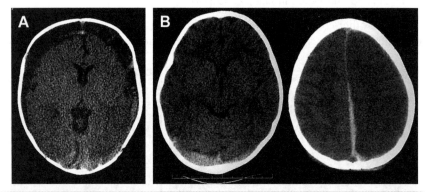

Fig. 39. Evaluation of subdural hematoma on CT. (*A*) Timing of mixed-attenuation subdural hematomas. The lesion is concave to the brain. It may be hyperdense (*white*), which means acute blood. It may be isodense (*gray-black*), which means subacute and occurring within 2 to 3 weeks, or it can be hypodense (*black*), which means most of the blood has been absorbed and is mostly cerebral spinal fluid (chronic). However, when it is mixed, as in this case, one cannot be sure. The isodense or hypodense component can occur in an acute injury when the arachnoid membrane is torn and cerebral spinal fluid dilutes the blood in the subdural space (hematohygroma). For these reasons, it is difficult to time bleeds on CT. (*B*) Bright subdural hematoma on axial CT. This is an acute injury with blood in the subdural space, in the left interhemispheric fissure and posteriorly on the tentorium.

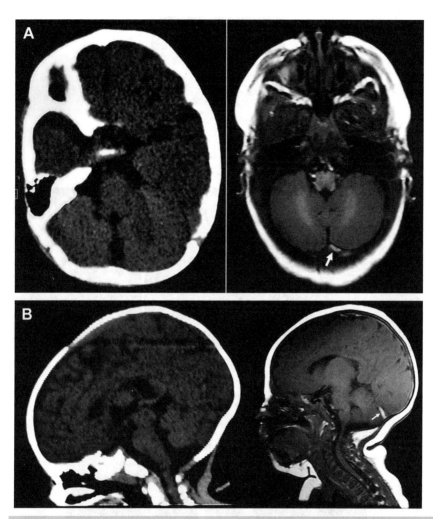

Fig. 40. The value of MR as opposed to CT in the evaluation of subdural hematomas. (A–C) CT in a 3-month-old who presented with an acute life-threatening experience (ALTE). (A) CT on the left does not show blood, but the MR shows some subdural blood (*arrow*). (B) Lateral comparisons again show blood only on the MR (*arrow*). (C) Susceptibility-weighted MR image shows blood (*black*) in the left subdural space. (D) Imaging in a different infant, who presented with sepsis and clotting disorder. These axial images show multiple areas of medullary vein thrombosis. This finding emphasizes the importance of MR and its multiple sequences in defining disease. (E–G) Imaging in these 3 infants shows how MR, except in acute conditions, gives the most information. Sagittal T1-weighted MR image (E) shows mixed subdural hematoma and clear subarachnoid space (*black*). Axial T2-weighted MR image (F) shows subdural membranes (*arrow*), showing the chronicity of the lesion. Axial diffusion-weighted image (G) shows restricted diffusion (*white*) secondary to abuse damage and ischemia.

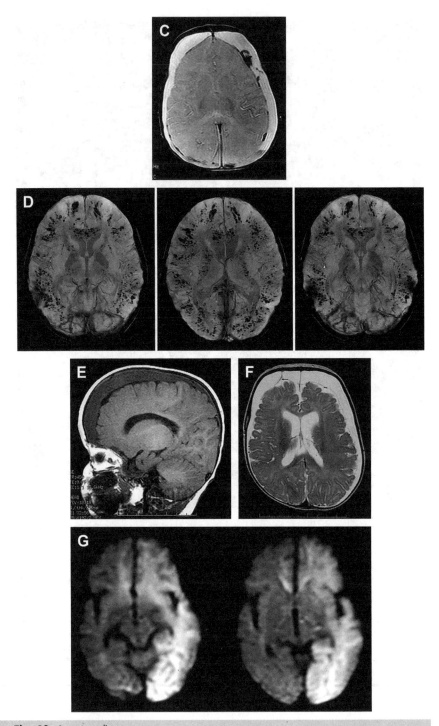

Fig. 40. (continued).

that infants with large extra-axial fluid collections (the benign subdural of infancy) have a small predilection for subdural hematomas with minor trauma (Fig. 37) [75,76]. In these infants, the social service investigation of the home situation becomes even more important.

We have learned that most acute epidural hematomas occur in accidental trauma (Fig. 38). We have also learned that the dating of subdural hematomas by CT is not accurate [77,78]. If there is only blood (white on the CT), we know that the trauma occurred within 7 to 10 days. However, any mixture of fluid and blood can be of various ages (the hematohygroma) (Fig. 39). Therefore, it is most important to understand that MR is more sensitive in detecting old blood and parenchymal injuries and in dating lesions (Fig. 40). Except in the clinically acutely ill state, MR would be the preferable imaging study. In general, MR is more sensitive for detecting parenchymal disease (Fig. 41).

We are learning that subdural blood can flow into the spinal subdural space. Studies have shown that 60% of children with abusive head trauma have spinal subdural hematomas from this cause [79]. Injury to the spine by nonaccidental trauma can also cause a primary spinal subdural hematoma as a separate injury.

FUTURE TRENDS

During the next 5 years, we might see the continuation of trends mentioned earlier and the following newer innovations:

1. Technical improvements will continue to significantly reduce CT doses and improve image quality. If this trend can produce doses approximate to those of a plain radiograph series (ie, the abdominal series), then CT might appropriately be used in cases in which radiographs would be the current first choice [80].
2. Radiation metrics will be required on each radiation-producing test.
3. MR will continue to be faster and more accessible. There will be a dramatic increase in technology to improve the patient's experience, such as reduced noise and scanning feet first to reduce claustrophobia.

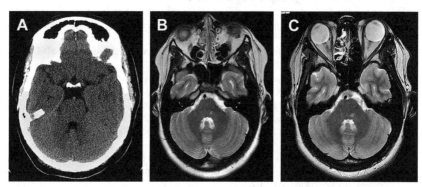

Fig. 41. The sensitivity of MR is greater than that of CT. (A) CT imaging is not usually performed in a teenager for developmental delay. It is clearly not the best test for this indication, and this CT was normal. (B, C) MR shows a left pontine high-signal lesion on T2-weighted axial images.

4. MR and CT vascular studies will improve and replace in many instances digital angiographic examinations.
5. Specific disease and site-specific treatment will progress, with improvement of molecular imaging. Molecular imaging is defined by Peter Brader as "combining the disciplines of molecular-cell biology, chemistry and multimodality optical radiotracer and MRI. Molecular imaging is the in vivo characterization and measurement of biological processes that occur at cellular and molecular levels at a macroscopic level of resolution" [81].
6. There will be a time when a child will be sent initially to the imaging department and entire batteries of tests tailored to their complaints will be rapidly performed, after consultation with the referring physician. The diagnosis will be made, and the child will be treated or admitted. The entire process will save a great deal of time and money and, most important, it will improve patient care through efficiency [82].

References

[1] American College of Radiology. ACR appropriateness criteria. Headache–child. Reston (VA): American College of Radiology; 1999. p. 1–8.

[2] Ashwal S, Russman BS, Blasco PA, et al. Practice parameter: diagnostic assessment of the child with cerebral palsy: report of the quality standards subcommittee of the American Academy of Neurology and the Practice Committee of the Child Neurology Society. Neurology 2004;62:851–63.

[3] Flaherty EG, Perez-Rossello JM, Levine MA, et al. Evaluating children with fractures for child physical abuse. Ped 2014;133:e477–89.

[4] Subcommittee on Urinary Tract Infection, Steering Committee on Quality Improvement and Management, Roberts KB. Urinary tract infection: clinical practice guideline for the diagnosis and management of the initial UTI in febrile infants and children 2 to 24 months. Pediatrics 2011;128:595–610.

[5] Berger MY, Tabbers MM, Kurver MJ, et al. Value of abdominal radiography, colonic transit time, and rectal ultrasound scanning in the diagnosis of idiopathic constipation in children: a systematic review. J Pediatr 2012;161:44–50.

[6] American College of Radiology. ACR appropriateness criteria. Seizures–child. Reston (VA): American College of Radiology; 1995. p. 1–8.

[7] Kuppermann J, Holmes JF, Dayan PS, et al. Identification of children at very low risk of clinically-important brain injuries after head trauma: a prospective cohort study. Lancet 2009;374:1160–70.

[8] Cauldwell C. Anesthesia risks associated with pediatric imaging. Pediatr Radiol 2011;41: 949–50.

[9] Slovis TL. Conference on the ALARA (as low as reasonably achievable) concept in pediatric CT intelligent dose reduction. Pediatr Radiol 2002;32:217–317.

[10] Linet MS, Slovis TL, Miller DL, et al. Cancer risks associated with external radiation from diagnostic imaging procedures. CA Cancer J Clin 2012;62:75–100.

[11] Slovis TL, Strauss KJ, Frush DP. How many strikes does it take till we are out? Pediatr Radiol 2011;41:547–8.

[12] Slovis TL, Frush DP, Berdon WE, et al. Biologic effects of diagnostic radiation on children. In: Slovis TL, editor. Caffey's pediatric diagnostic imaging. 11th edition. St Louis (MO): Mosby Elsevier; 2008. p. 3–13.

[13] Slovis TL. Biologic effects of radiation on children. In: Kliegman RM, Stanton BM, St Geme J, et al, editors. Nelson textbook of pediatrics. 19th edition. Philadelphia: Elsevier Saunders; 2011. p. 7557.

[14] Hall EJ. Lessons we have learned from our children: cancer risks from diagnostic radiology. Pediatr Radiol 2002;32:700–6.

[15] Upton AC. Report No. 136–evaluation of the linear-nonthreshold dose-response model for ionizing radiation. Bethesda (MD): NRCP Publications; 2001.

[16] Little JB. Ionizing radiation. In: Kufe DW, Pollock RE, Weichselbaum RR, et al, editors. Holland-Frei cancer medicine. 6th edition. Ontario (Canada): BC Decker; 2003. p. 289–301.

[17] Pearce MS, Salotti JA, Little MP, et al. Radiation exposure from CT scans in childhood and subsequent risk of leukaemia and brain tumours: a retrospective cohort study. Lancet 2012;380:499–505.

[18] Haller JO, Slovis TL, Joshi A, editors. Pediatric radiology. 3rd edition. Heidelberg (Germany), New York: Springer; 2005.

[19] Valk JW, Plotz FB, Scheurman FA, et al. The value of routine chest radiographs in a paediatric intensive care unit: a prospective study. Pediatr Radiol 2001;31:343–7.

[20] Mong A, Epelman M, Darge K. Ultrasound of the pediatric chest. Pediatr Radiol 2012;42: 1287–97.

[21] Newman B. Ultrasound body applications in children. Pediatr Radiol 2011;41:555–61.

[22] Schneebaum N, Blau H, Soferman R. Use and yield of chest computed tomography in the diagnostic evaluation of pediatric lung disease. Pediatrics 2009;124:472–9.

[23] Foley LC, Slovis TL, Campbell JB, et al. Evaluation of the vomiting infant. Am J Dis Child 1989;143:660–1.

[24] Blumer SL, Zucconi WB, Cohen HL, et al. The vomiting neonate: a review of the ACR appropriateness criteria and ultrasound's role in the workup of such patients. Ultrasound Q 2004;20:79–89.

[25] Hayes R. Abdominal pain: general imaging strategies. Eur Radiol 2004;14:123–37.

[26] Sivit CJ. Imaging the child with right lower quadrant pain and suspected appendicitis: current concepts. Pediatr Radiol 2004;34:447–53.

[27] Paolantonio P, Ferrari R, Vecchietti F, et al. Current status of MR imaging in the evaluation of IBD in a pediatric population of patients. Eur J Radiol 2009;69:418–24.

[28] Dillman JR, Ladino-Torres MF, Adler J, et al. Comparison of MR enterography and histopathology in the evaluation of pediatric Crohn disease. Pediatr Radiol 2011;41:1552–8.

[29] Fitoz S, Erden A, Boruban S. Magnetic resonance cholangiopancreatography of biliary system abnormalities in children. Clin Imaging 2007;31:93–101.

[30] Emery KH. Cross-sectional imaging of pediatric biliary disorders. Pediatr Radiol 2010;40: 438–41.

[31] Punwani S, Taylor SA, Bainbridge A. Pediatric and adolescent lymphoma: comparison of whole-body STIR half-Fourier RARE MR imaging with an enhanced PET/CT reference for initial staging. Radiology 2010;255:182–90.

[32] Schmidt GP, Reiser MF, Baur-Melnyk A. Whole-body MRI for the staging and follow-up of patients with metastasis. Eur J Radiol 2009;70:393–400.

[33] Strauss KJ, Goske MJ, Kaste SC, et al. Image gently: ten steps you can take to optimize image quality and lower CT dose for pediatric patients. AJR Am J Roentgenol 2010;194: 868–73.

[34] Kim HK, Laor T, Horn PS, et al. Mapping in Duchenne muscular dystrophy: distribution of disease activity and correlation with clinical assessments. Radiology 2010;255:899–908.

[35] Kim HK, Laor T, Horn PS, et al. Quantitative assessment of the T2 relaxation time of the gluteus muscles in children with Duchenne muscular dystrophy: a comparative study before and after steroid treatment. Korean J Radiol 2010;11:304–11.

[36] Krakow D, Lachman RS, Rimoin DL. Guidelines for the prenatal diagnosis of fetal skeletal dysplasias. Genet Med 2009;11:127–33.

[37] Gaillard WD, Chiron C, Cross JH, et al. Guidelines for imaging infants and children with recent-onset epilepsy. Epilepsia 2009;50:2147–53.

[38] McDonald BC, Hummer TA, Dunn DW. Functional MRI and structural MRI as tools for understanding comorbid conditions in children with epilepsy. Epilepsy Behav 2013;26(3): 295–302.

[39] Woodward LJ, Anderson PJ, Austin NC, et al. Neonatal MRI to predict neurodevelopmental outcomes in preterm infants. N Engl J Med 2006;355:685–94.

[40] Provenzale JM. Advances in pediatric neuroradiology: highlights of the recent medical literature. AJR Am J Roentgenol 2009;192:19–25.

[41] Mikati MA. Seizures in childhood. In: Kliegman RM, Stanton BM, St Geme J, et al, editors. Nelson textbook of pediatrics. 19th edition. Philadelphia: Elsevier Saunders; 2011. p. 2019–21.

[42] Hsieh DT, Chang T, Tsuchida TN, et al. New-onset afebrile seizures in infants: role of neuroimaging. Neurology 2010;74:150–6.

[43] Bernal B, Altman NR. Evidence-based medicine: neuroimaging of seizures. Neuroimaging Clin N Am 2003;13:211–24.

[44] Abend NS, Younkin D, Lewis DW. Secondary headaches in children and adolescents. Semin Pediatr Neurol 2010;17:123–33.

[45] Medina S, D'Souza B, Vasconcellos E. Adults and children with headache: evidence-based diagnostic evaluation. Neuroimaging Clin N Am 2003;13:225–35.

[46] Lateef TM, Grewal M, McClintock W, et al. Headache in young children in the emergency department: use of computed tomography. Pediatrics 2009;124:12–7.

[47] Lewis DW. New practice parameters: what does the evidence say? Curr Pain Headache Rep 2005;9:351–7.

[48] Himmelmann K, Uvebrant P. Function and neuroimaging in cerebral palsy: a population-based study. Dev Med Child Neurol 2011;53:516–21.

[49] Korzeniewski SJ, Birbeck G, DeLano MC, et al. A systematic review of neuroimaging for cerebral palsy. J Child Neurol 2008;23:216.

[50] Kulak W, Sobaniec W, Goscik M, et al. Clinical and neuroimaging profile of congenital brain malformations in children with spastic cerebral palsy. Adv Med Sci 2008;53: 42–8.

[51] Ashwal S, Michelson D, Plawner L, et al. Practice parameter: evaluation of the child with microcephaly (an evidence-based review). Report of the quality standards subcommittee of the American Academy of Neurology and the Practice Committee of the Child Neurology Society. Neurology 2009;73:887–97.

[52] Panigrahy A, Nelson MD Jr, Bluml S. Magnetic resonance spectroscopy in pediatric neuroradiology: clinical and research applications. Pediatr Radiol 2010;40:3–30.

[53] Pal D, Bhattacharyya A, Husain M, et al. In vivo proton MR spectroscopy evaluation of pyogenic brain abscesses: a report of 194 cases. AJNR Am J Neuroradiol 2010;31:360–6.

[54] Barkovich AJ, Raybaud C. Congenital malformations of brain and skull. In: Barkovich AJ, Raybaud C, editors. Pediatric neuroimaging. 5th edition. Philadelphia: Wolters Kluwer Lippincott Williams & Wilkins; 2012. p. 489.

[55] Schwartz ES, Barkovich AJ. Brain and spine lesions in infancy and childhood. In: Schwartz ES, Barkovich AJ, editors. Pediatric neuroimaging. 5th edition. Philadelphia: Wolters Kluwer Lippincott Williams & Wilkins; 2012. p. 243–61.

[56] De Vries LS, van Haastert IC, Benders MJ, et al. Myth: cerebral palsy cannot be predicted by neonatal brain imaging. Semin Fetal Neonatal Med 2011;16:279–87.

[57] Slovis TL, Strouse PJ, Coley BD, et al. The creation of non-disease: an assault on the diagnosis of child abuse. Pediatr Radiol 2012;42:903–5.

[58] Slovis TL, Chapman S. Vitamin D insufficiency/deficiency–a conundrum. Pediatr Radiol 2008;38:1153.

[59] Kovacs CS. Fetus, neonate and infant. In: Feldman D, Pike JW, Adams JS, editors. Vitamin D. 3rd edition. London: Elsevier Academic Press; 2011. p. 625–46.

[60] Kovacs CS. Bone development in the fetus and neonate: role of the calciotropic hormones. Curr Osteoporos Rep 2011;9:274–83.

[61] Perez-Rossello JM, Feldman HA, Kleinman PK, et al. Rachitic changes, demineralization, and fracture risk in healthy infants and toddlers with vitamin D deficiency. Radiology 2012;262:234–41.

[62] Ross AC, Manson JE, Abrams SA, et al. The 2011 report on dietary reference intakes for calcium and vitamin D from the Institute of Medicine: what clinicians need to know. J Clin Endocrinol Metab 2011;96:53–8.

[63] Palusci VJ. Introduction. In: Palusci VJ, Fischer H, editors. Child abuse and neglect. London: Manson; 2011. p. 1–10.

[64] Caffey J. Multiple fractures in the long bones of infants suffering from chronic subdural hematoma. AJR Am J Roentgenol 1946;56:163–73.

[65] Silverman FN. The roentgen manifestations of unrecognized skeletal trauma in infants. AJR Am J Roentgenol 1953;69:413–27.

[66] Kempe CH, Silverman FN, Steele BF, et al. The battered-child syndrome. JAMA 1962;181: 105–12.

[67] Barnes PD. Imaging of nonaccidental injury and the mimics: issues and controversies in the era of evidence-based medicine. Radiol Clin North Am 2011;49:205–9.

[68] Geddes JF, Tasker RC, Hackshaw AK. Dural haemorrhage in non-traumatic infant deaths: does it explain the bleeding in 'shaken baby syndrome'? Neuropathol Appl Neurobiol 2003;29:14–22.

[69] McLean LA, Frasier LD, Hedlund GL. Does intracranial venous thrombosis cause subdural hemorrhage in the pediatric population? AJNR Am J Neuroradiol 2012;33:1281–4.

[70] Hedlund GL. Cerebral sinovenous thrombosis in pediatric practice. Pediatr Radiol 2013;43(2):173–88.

[71] Adamsbaum C, Rambaud C. Abusive head trauma: don't overlook bridging vein thrombosis. Pediatr Radiol 2012;42:1298–300.

[72] Ehrlich E, Maxeiner H, Lange J. Postmortem radiological investigation of bridging vein ruptures. Leg Med (Tokyo) 2003;5:225–7.

[73] Mack J, Squier W, Eastman JT. Anatomy and development of the meninges: implications for subdural collections and CSF circulation. Pediatr Radiol 2009;39: 200–10.

[74] Jenny C. The intimidation of British pediatricians. Pediatrics 2007;119:797–9.

[75] Hellbusch LC. Benign extracerebral fluid collections in infancy: clinical presentation and long-term follow-up. J Neurosurg 2007;107:119–25.

[76] McNeely PD, Atkinson JD, Saigal G. Subdural hematomas in infants with benign enlargement of the subarachnoid spaces are not pathognomonic for child abuse. AJNR Am J Neuroradiol 2006;27:1725–8.

[77] Vezina G. Assessment of the nature and age of subdural collections in nonaccidental head injury with CT and MRI. Pediatr Radiol 2009;39:586–90.

[78] Zouros A, Bhargava R, Hoskinson M, et al. Further characterization of traumatic subdural collections of infancy. J Neurosurg 2004;100:512–8.

[79] Choudhary AK, Bradford RK, Dias MS, et al. Spinal subdural hemorrhage in abusive head trauma: a retrospective study. Radiology 2012;262:216–22.

[80] Singh S, Kalra MK, Shenoy-Bhangle AS. Radiation dose reduction with hybrid iterative reconstruction for pediatric CT. Radiology 2012;263:537–46.

[81] Brader P. Minisymposium: molecular imaging. Pediatr Radiol 2011;41:139–40.

[82] Thrall JH. What will radiology look like twenty-five years from now? J Thorac Imaging 2010;25:268–9.

Advances in Pediatrics 61 (2014) 127–148

ADVANCES IN PEDIATRICS

Conduction Defects/ Cardiomyopathies

Enid Gilbert-Barness, MBBS, MD, FRCPA, FRCPath

Laboratory Medicine, Pediatric, Obstetrics and Gynecology, Department of Pathology, College of Medicine, Tampa General Hospital, University of South Florida Morsani, 1 Tampa General Circle, Tampa, FL 33606, USA

Keywords
- Cardiomyopathies • Conduction disorders • Cardiac arrhythmias
- Inherited diseases • Sudden death

Key points
- Congenital heart block is frequently associated with maternal lupus.
- Carnitine arrhythmias may result in sudden death.
- Histiocytoid cardiomyopathy frequently results in death by the first 2 years of life.
- Barth syndrome is X-linked and is a mutation of Xq28-linked *G4.5 (TAZ)*.

INTRODUCTION

Conduction disorders result in cardiac arrhythmias that may be fatal and are inherited with arrhythmias and sudden death that are prominent features and include histiocytoid cardiomyopathy, arrhythmogenic right ventricular dysplasia, isolated noncompaction of the left ventricular myocardium, long QT syndrome, Brugada syndrome, congenital short QT syndrome, catecholaminergic polymorphic ventricular tachycardia, and carnitine deficiency. Although the histologic appearance of some of these disorders may be diagnostic, molecular analysis is necessary to clearly define the particular type of cardiomyopathy.

CONGENITAL HEART BLOCK

Congenital heart block (CHB) may be present in infants with both anatomically normal and malformed heart [1]. Most cases are sporadic; CHB occurs in 1 in 20,000 live births [2]. It may be a manifestation of neonatal lupus erythematosus (NLE).

The 2 most common neonatal manifestations of NLE are CHB and cutaneous lesions; approximately 50% of affected patients present with one or

E-mail address: egilbert@tgh.org

0065-3101/14/$ – see front matter
http://dx.doi.org/10.1016/j.yapd.2014.03.001 © 2014 Elsevier Inc. All rights reserved.

the other system involvement. The skin lesions most commonly appear on the infant's face, scalp, and upper trunk, resembling the lesions of discoid lupus erythematosus.

The manifestations of NLE result from the transplacental passage of maternal autoantibodies to the fetus. In more than 95% of the patients, the autoantibodies found in the mother and infant are anti-Ro, also known as Sjögren syndrome A antibodies (SSA) or anti-Ro/SSA, anti-La (SSB) antibodies, and antiribonucleoprotein (RNP) antibodies. Most mothers who have infants with this syndrome have no symptoms of collagen vascular disease; most infants of mothers with anti-Ro/SSA, anti-La, or anti-RNP antibodies do not develop NLE syndrome. The risk of a mother having a second child with NLE is about 25%.

CHB may be present in 50% of infants with neonatal systemic lupus erythematosus (SLE) [3]. Endocardial fibroelastosis (EFE) is commonly present; the Atrioventricular node is often absent or scarred, and the sino-atrial (SA) node and ventricular components may be calcified and fibrotic [4,5]. Complete heart block and other conduction defects with a high association with Ro antibodies implicate transplacental transfer of the antibody [6]. CHB develops in utero, usually during the second trimester. The heart block, unlike the other manifestations, is permanent. About one-quarter of infants with CHB have associated structural congenital cardiac anomalies, including atrial septal defect or ventricular septal defect, transposition of great arteries, and anomalous pulmonary venous drainage. Rarely, affected infants may have pericarditis, myocarditis, or a cardiomyopathy.

Because of the strong association of CHB with maternal lupus, every infant with CHB should undergo laboratory studies for anti-Ro/SSA, anti-SSB, and anti-RNP antibodies. Mothers of infants with CHB may have a detectable soluble tissue RNP antigen, anti-Ro/SSA, in their serum [7]. Immunoglobulins (Ig) IgG and IgA may be detected in the SA node, epicardium, and nerves [8].

Most infants with neonatal SLE have characteristic skin lesions and cardiac problems [9]. The characteristic annular erythematous macules, papules, or plaques of neonatal SLE may be present at birth, but they usually appear on the scalp and elsewhere by 2 months of age and disappear by 6 months of age.

LONG QT SYNDROME
Several genes that have been identified (Table 1) encode for cardiac ion channels for potassium ion channels or sodium ion channels. Mutations in these genes cause disturbed function of these channels which are called *channelopathies*. In each case, the altered ion channel function produces prolongation of the action potential and propensity to *torsade de pointes* ventricular tachycardia. Characteristic findings are prolongation of the QT interval and T-wave abnormalities on the electrocardiogram (EKG). However, the QT interval at presentation is normal about 10% of the time and just borderline prolonged another 30%, so diagnosis may be difficult. The symptoms are syncope and sudden death, typically occurring during exercise or emotional upset. The

manifestations vary, depending on the genotype present. The phenotype also probably varies, depending on the specific mutation involved. Phenotype heterogeneity is also caused by variable penetrance and expressivity. The Lange-Nielsen form is caused by novel mutations in the KVLQT1 gene [10]. The cardiac ion channel dysfunction and QT prolongation are inherited as an autosomal-dominant disease, like the Romano-Ward variant. The hearing deficit is inherited as an autosomal recessive trait. The Jervell, Lange-Nielsen phenotype occurs when both parents have the mutant KVLQT1 gene and an offspring inherits the abnormal gene from both parents. The child is, therefore, homozygous for the mutant gene and manifests severe long QT syndrome. The KVLQT1 gene also encodes for elements of the hearing mechanism, and deafness occurs when patients are homozygous but not heterozygous (ie, the parents are not deaf) for the mutant KVLQT1 gene. The Jervell, Lange-Nielsen syndrome, therefore, requires unusual circumstances; thus, it is rare.

The relative frequency of these genotypes is not known. At present, it seems that the potassium-channel genotypes cause 90% to 95% of genotype cases, with KVLQT1 and KLVQT2 (HERG) approximately equally represented. The SCN5A genotype accounts for about 5% to 10% of the cases. Potassium loading [11] and flecainide [12] may be of therapeutic benefit in the CQT2 (HERG) genotype, and potassium channel-opener drugs [13–15] and verapamil [16] may assist all K+ genotype patients. In the SCN5A genotype, experimental [17] and clinical studies [18] suggest that the sodium channel-blocker drug mexiletine may prevent the repetitive opening of the channel. Currently, it is not known whether these new therapies will be as effective as or more effective than beta-blockers.

BARTH SYNDROME

In 1981 and 1983, Barth and colleagues [19,20] described a large pedigree showing X-linked inheritance of a disorder characterized by dilated cardiomyopathy, neutropenia, skeletal myopathy, abnormal mitochondria, cristae, and occasional inclusion bodies. In 1987, Hodgson and colleagues [21] reported the same disorder in another kindred. Many boys in at least 3 generations and 7 sibships connected through women died of sepsis caused by agranulocytes or of cardiac failure between 3 days and 31 months of age. Endocardial fibrosis was documented in 2 cases. Granulocytopenia was found early in cord blood samples; differentiation in the bone marrow was arrested at the myelocyte stage, and mitochondrial abnormalities were demonstrated in granulocyte precursors. Neustein and colleagues [22] had earlier reported on an infant with cardiomyopathy and chronic congestive heart failure who may have had the same disorder with abnormal mitochondria on electron microscopy from an endomyocardial biopsy. Kelly and colleagues [23] reported similar cases with increased levels of urinary 3-methylglutaconic acid (3MGC) and 2-ethylhydracrylic acid and called the disorder Barth syndrome.

Table 1
Inherited LQTS

Locus name	Chromosomal locus	Gene symbol	Protein (symbol)	Current	In vitro characterization	Gene-specific therapy[a]
LQT1	11P15.5	KCNQ1	I_{Ks} Potassium channel α-subunit (KvLQT1)	↓ IKs	Dominant negative suppression, trafficking defect, abnormal response to β-AR signal	β-blockers,[b] potassium channel openers[b]
LQT2	7q35-q36	KCNH2	I_{Kr} Potassium channel α-subunit (HERG)	↓ IKr	Dominant negative suppression, trafficking defect, abnormal gating	β-blockers,[b] potassium supplement,[b] potassium channel openers, fexofenadine, and thapsigargin
LQT3	3p21	SCN5A	Cardiac sodium channel α-subunit (Nav 1.5)	↑ INa	Abnormal gating: sustained current, slower inactivation, faster recovery, increased window current	Sodium channel blockers (mexiletine)[b]
LQT4	4q25-q27	ANK2	Ankyrin B, (ANKB)	↓ Ncx1, Na/K ATPase, InsP3	Loss of expression and mislocalization	None proposed
LQT5	21q22.1-q22.2	KCNE1	I_{Ks} Potassium channel β-subunit (MinK)	↓ IKs	Dominant negative suppression, abnormal gating, reduced response to β-AR signal	β-blockers, potassium supplement, potassium channel openers

LQT6	21q22.1-q22.2	KCNE2	I_k Potassium channel β-subunit (MiRP)	↓ IKr	Reduced current density and abnormal channel gating	β-blockers, potassium supplement, potassium channel openers, fexofenadine, and thapsigargin
LQT7/Andersen	17q23.1-q24.2	KCN12	I_{K1} Potassium channel (Kir2.1)	↓ IK1	Dominant negative suppression, nonfunctional channels, trafficking defect, abnormal gating	None proposed
LQT8/Timothy	12p13.3	CACNA1c	Voltage-gated calcium channel (CaV1.2)	↑ ICa	Loss of inactivation	Calcium channel blockers[b]
LQT9	3p25	CAV3	Caveolin-3	↑ INa	Increased late INa	Sodium channel blockers (mexiletine)
LQT10	11q23	SCN4B	Cardiac sodium channel β-4 subunit	↑ INa	Increased late INa	Sodium channel blockers (mexiletine)
LQT11	7q21-22	mAKAP	A-kinase anchoring proteins	↓ IKs	Reduced phosphorylation of the IKs channel	β-blockers
LQT12	20q11.2	SNTA1	Syntrophin	↑ INa	Increased late INa	Sodium channel blockers (mexiletine)

Abbreviations: InsP3, inositol 3-phosphate receptor; Na/K ATPase, sodium potassium ATP pump; NCx, sodium calcium exchanger; β-AR, β-adrenergic receptor; IKr, current through cardiac rapid delayed rectifier; IKs, current through cardiac slow delayed rectifier; INa, current through sodium channel; ICa, current through calcium channel.

[a]Possible gene/mechanism-specific therapies are reported based on known pathophysiology.

[b]Experimentally or clinically tested therapies.

From Ruan Y, Liu N, Napolitano C, et al. Therapeutic strategies for long-QT syndrome: does the molecular substrate matter? Circ Arrhythm Electrophysiol 2008;1:290.

Later Kelley and colleagues [24] more clearly described this disorder in 7 affected boys with dilated cardiomyopathy, growth retardation, neutropenia, and persistently elevated urinary levels of 3-methyglutaconate, 3-methylglutarate, and 2-ethylhydracrylate. The clinical course of the disorder was characterized by severe cardiac disease and recurrent infections during infancy and early childhood but relative improvement in later childhood. The initial presentation of the syndrome varied from congenital dilated cardiomyopathy and congestive heart failure to isolated neutropenia without clinical evidence of heart disease. EFE with neonatal death has also been reported [25].

By means of linkage studies in the family reported by Barth and colleagues [26], Bolhuis and colleagues [27] demonstrated the BTHS locus on Xq28.

In patients with Barth syndrome, Bione and colleagues [28] identified mutations in the *G4.5 (TAZ)* gene, which introduced stop codons in the open reading frame, aborting translation of most of the putative proteins.

Barth and colleagues [29] updated information on Barth syndrome following the prediction that the *G4.5 (TAZ)* gene encodes one or more acyltransferases [30]. Lipid studies in patients with Barth syndrome have been shown to have deficiency of cardiolipin, especially the tetralinoleoyl form (L4-CL) [31]. Deficiency of L4-CL was subsequently demonstrated in a variety of tissues from patients with Barth syndrome [32], but determination in platelets or cultured skin fibroblasts was the most specific biochemical test. Barth syndrome was the first identified inborn error of metabolism that directly affects cardiolipin, a component of inner mitochondrial membrane necessary for proper functioning of the electron transport chain. Barth and colleagues [33] also found that some patients with Barth syndrome have deficient docosahexaenoic acid and arachidonic acid.

Pantothenic acid, a precursor of coenzyme A, produced a dramatic and sustained improvement in myocardial function and in growth, neutrophil cell count, hypocholesterolemia, and hyperuricemia. Digoxin may result in dramatic improvement.

Diagnostic criteria for Barth syndrome
There are 4 principal diagnostic criteria for Barth syndrome:

Dilated cardiomyopathy
Growth retardation
Neutropenia, chronic or cyclic
3-Methylglutaconic aciduria

Additional cardinal characteristics (Box 1) include skeletal muscle weakness and hypotonia, underdevelopment of skeletal muscle, cardiac left ventricular noncompaction with deep trabeculation, multiple septal defects, EFE and delayed motor development in early childhood.

Diagnostically important laboratory findings (Box 2) include 3-methylglutaconic aciduria and acidemia, increased urinary excretion of citric acid cycle intermediates and 2-ethylhydracrylic acid, hypocholesterolemia, low level of

---

Box 1: Additional criteria for Barth syndrome

In addition to the cardinal characteristics of Barth syndrome, other important findings include

Skeletal weakness and hypotonia

Underdevelopment of skeletal muscle

Cardiac left ventricular noncompaction, deep trabeculation, multiple septal defects

Endocardial fibroelastosis

Delayed motor development in early childhood

Exercise intolerance unrelated to cardiac disease; rapid fatigue

Recurrent focal or systemic bacterial infections

Recurrent severe aphthous ulcers

Cognitive disabilities, especially in math and tasks requiring visual-spatial skills

Increased frequency of isolated congenital malformations

Hypoglycemia during the perinatal period or early infancy

Family history of similarly affected boys

From Gilbert-Barness E, Barness LA. Research review: pathogenesis of cardiac conduction disorders in children genetic and histopathologic aspects, festschrift for Dr John M. Opitz. Am J Med Genet A 2006;140A:1993–2006; with permission.

---

tetralinoleoyl cardiolipin in muscle, platelets or cultured fibroblasts, and mutation of Xq28-linked *G4.5 (TAZ)* gene.

Barth syndrome varies in different families and in the same family; 80% have all 4 principal criteria or all 4 may be absent in a male with the mutation. Some patients may rarely have another mitochondrial genetic disorder. There have been no proven affected females but the carrier has skewed X-inactivation (ie, preferential expression of the normal 4.5 gene), which has been found in all of the women with Barth mutations who have been studied.

Box 2: Diagnostically important laboratory findings in Barth syndrome

3-Methylglutaconic aciduria and academia

Increased urinary excretion of citric acid cycle intermediates and 2-ethylhydracrylic acid

Hypocholesterolemia

Low level of tetralinoleoyl cardiolipin in muscle, platelets, or cultured cells

Mutation of Xq28-linked *G4.5 (TAZ)* gene

From Gilbert-Barness E, Barness LA. Research review: pathogenesis of cardiac conduction disorders in children genetic and histopathologic aspects, festschrift for Dr John M. Opitz. Am J Med Genet A 2006;140A:1993–2006; with permission.

Diagnosis of Barth syndrome should be based on the cardinal clinical features and evaluation of the following:

1. Quantitative urine organic acid analysis should be obtained including 3MGC quantitation. (This can be increased in other mitochondrial disorders, but in Barth syndrome it is usually 5 to 20 higher.)
2. If 3MGC is increased in patients with cardiomyopathy, the diagnosis of Barth syndrome should be considered.

Specific laboratory testing for Barth syndrome

1. 3-Methylglutaconic aciduria and acidemia should be documented. Blood 3MGC testing is more meaningful than urinary analysis, but must be done by isotope dilution gas chromatography-mass spectrometry.
2. The Barth G4.5 (TAZ) gene mutation that clearly disables protein synthesis or function is the most definitive test for X-q28-linked Barth syndrome. In addition, the finding of a severely depressed level of tetralinoleoyl cardiolipin in platelets, cultured cells, or muscle tissue seems to be specific for Barth syndrome caused by mutations in the G4.5 (TAZ) gene. Genetic testing for Barth syndrome involves several steps: (1) DNA preparation, (2) amplification of the G4.5 (TAZ) gene by polymerase chain reaction (PCR), (3) DNA sequencing of the PCR products, (4) comparison of patients' G4.5 (TAZ) sequence to the normal reference sequence, and (5) check of sequence differences in the coding segments against the mRNA sequence and its translation product (protein sequence) to determine possible effects of the mutation on the function of the G4.5 (TAZ) protein.
   DNA can be obtained from blood cells, buccal swabs, tissue culture cells, pathology tissue samples, or blood spots (eg, from newborn metabolic screening). For blood, a sample of at least 3 mL is needed to provide adequate DNA for testing. For infants who often have a higher white blood cell count, 1 to 3 mL may be sufficient. For prenatal testing, DNA from cultured amniocytes obtained from amniocentesis or from a chorionic villus biopsy can be used.
   Adult female family members can be tested for carrier status. Such carrier testing is faster because one only needs to test for the specific mutation.
3. Complete blood count: Neutropenia is one of the more variable features of Barth syndrome and can be chronic, cyclic, or absent. When cyclic, the duration of the cycle for most patients falls between 21 and 28 days. Peak absolute neutrophil counts (ANC) are often normal (>2000), and the lows are often zero. Thus, serial blood counts may be necessary to determine if a patient suspected to have Barth has neutropenia. For diagnostic purposes, the ANC should not be determined when a patient is acutely ill because the ANC is typically normal or increased during a bacterial infection after the first or second day. In addition to neutropenia, patients with Barth often have relatively or even absolutely increased monocyte counts, without apparent cyclic changes.
4. Echocardiogram: In a few monitored Barth pregnancies, dilated cardiomyopathy has developed in utero during the last trimester, but often it is not clinically manifest until sometime in the first 6 months. In a few patients, the heart function may be normal throughout childhood or may become abnormal for the first time at any age during childhood. The echocardiogram typically shows mild ventricular hypertrophy and more left ventricular dilatation with abnormally low

shortening and ejection fractions. In addition, occasionally trabeculation is severe enough to warrant the diagnosis of left ventricular noncompaction. Arrhythmias and ventricular tachycardia are frequent.

5. Analysis of growth parameters: The mean length of infants with Barth syndrome at birth is normal, but weight for length (height) is often mildly decreased, most likely because of muscle hypoplasia. Typically, the growth velocity of children with Barth in the first 2 years gradually decreases. Thereafter, growth velocity is normal, and the length or height remains parallel but less than the third centile until puberty. At puberty, a prolonged growth spurt begins, often lasting until late teenage years until normal final adult height is attained.

Pathology of Barth syndrome

Skeletal muscle biopsy shows lipid accumulation in type I fibers and degenerative changes (Fig. 1), and electron microscopy of skeletal muscle shows abnormal bizarre mitochondria (Fig. 2) and frequently mitochondrial inclusions (Fig. 3).

ISOLATED NONCOMPACTION OF LEFT VENTRICLE

Isolated noncompaction of the left ventricular myocardium (persistence of spongy myocardium) (Fig. 4) is a rare form of congenital cardiomyopathy in which the left ventricular wall fails to become flattened and smother than it normally would during the first 2 months of embryonic development. It can be diagnosed prenatally by ultrasound (Fig. 5). This developmental arrest results in decreased cardiac output with subsequent left ventricular hypertrophy. According to the extent of the damage, patients may be asymptomatic or may exhibit symptoms of heart failure, systemic emboli, or various forms of arrhythmia. The EKG is usually abnormal in both children and adults with noncompacted myocardium and may show a right or left axis deviation, left or right bundle branch block, or even nonspecific ST segment changes. Various types of arrhythmia have been described in these patients, such as atrial fibrillation, paroxysmal supraventricular tachycardia in the context of

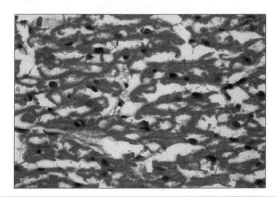

Fig. 1. Vacuolization of the myocardial fibers in Barth syndrome (HE stain, original magnification 400x).

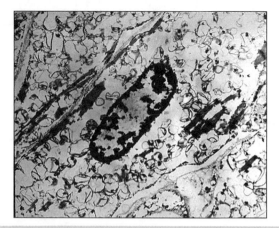

Fig. 2. Bizarre and fragmented mitochondria.

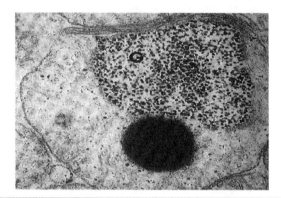

Fig. 3. EM showing granular deposits of glycogen in the cytoplasm in Barth syndrome.

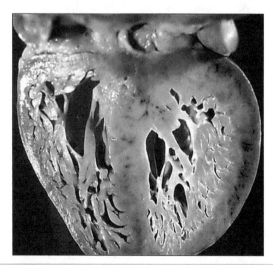

Fig. 4. The gross appearance of the right and left ventricles. The left ventricle is coarsely trabeculated resembling the right ventricle. The invaginations of the noncompaction predisposed to thrombi and arrhythmia.

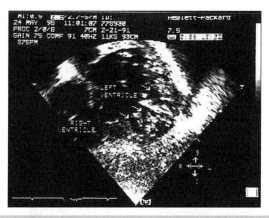

Fig. 5. Noncompaction by ultrasound showing the trabeculation of the left ventricle (*arrows*).

Wolff-Parkinson-White syndrome, ventricular arrhythmias, and sudden cardiac death [33–36].

Some cases are isolated, although familial distribution of the disease has been described. Inheritance may be either dominant or recessive. A severe, sex-linked form of noncompacted myocardium has also been described, caused by the mutation of the G4.5 gene in the q28 region of the X chromosome, allelic with the gene responsible for Barth syndrome. Some patients have a characteristically dysmorphic appearance, with a projecting forehead, low-set ears, high-arched palate, and micrognathia. Noncompacted myocardium has been described in infants with severe obstructive diseases of the left and right ventricles, in cases of anomalous origin of the coronary arteries from the pulmonary artery, or even in combination with more complex congenital heart disease. The aberrant left ventricular trabeculae predispose to cardiac conduction abnormalities and potentially fatal cardiac arrhythmias. The interstices within the trabeculated left ventricle predispose to thrombus formation with secondary systemic embolic events. Fibroelastosis of the adjacent ventricular endothelium is a secondary phenomenon, resulting from an abnormal blood flow pattern in the left ventricular chamber [33,37].

ARRHYTHMOGENIC RIGHT VENTRICULAR DYSPLASIA

Arrhythmogenic right ventricular dysplasia I (ARVD) is occasionally present in infants. Ventricular tachycardia, left bundle branch block, and right ventricular dilatation characterize the clinical features. A recent infection frequently precedes the onset of symptoms [38]. The principal histologic findings in a biopsy of the right ventricle of an affected patient are fatty infiltration (Fig. 6) with or without interstitial fibrosis of the myocardium. Cardiac enlargement is mostly localized to the right ventricle, although similar abnormalities may be present on the left side of the heart [39]. There are more than 200 reported cases, with a mean presentation of 30 years and a 2:1 to 3:1 male preponderance. At least 30% of cases

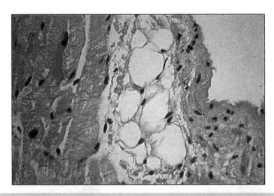

Fig. 6. Arrhythmogenic right ventricular dysplasia (HE stain, original magnification 100x). Microscopic section showing lipid deposits in the myocardium. (*From* Gilbert-Barness E, editor. Potter's pathology of the fetus, infant and child. 2nd edition. Elsevier; 2007.)

are familial [40,41]. Two patterns of inheritance have been described in ARVD: an autosomal dominant form, which is most common, and an autosomal recessive form called *Naxos disease*, in which ARVD is part of a cardiocutaneous syndrome including hyperkeratosis of the palms and soles and woolly hair [42]. Disease loci for the autosomal dominant form have been mapped to chromosomes 14q23-q24 (ARVD1) [43], 1q24-q43 (ARVC2) [44], 14q12-q22 (ARVD3) [45], 2q32 (ARVD4) [46], 3p25 (ARVD5) [47,48] 10p12-p14 (ARVD6) [49]), 10q22, 6p24 (ARVD8) [41,50] and 12p11 (ARVD9) [51]. Desmoplakin was the first disease-causing gene identified in autosomal dominant ARVD; the affected family had a missense mutation linked to 6p24 (ARVD8) [41]. Desmoplakin is a key component of desmosomes and adherens junctions that is important for maintaining the right adhesion of many cell types, including those in the heart and skin. When these junctions are disrupted, cell death and fibrofatty replacement occur. Five established disease-causing genes in ARVC encoding desmosomal proteins, plakoglobin, desmoplakin, plakophilin-2, desmoglein, and desmocollin in autosomal dominant disease and plakoglobin and desmoplakin in Naxos disease, support a new model for the pathogenesis of ARVD [52]. Impaired desmosome function when subjected to mechanical stress causes myocyte detachment and cell death. The myocardial injury may be accompanied by inflammation as the initial phase of the repair process, which ultimately results in fibrofatty replacement of damaged myocytes.

In a study of 60 patients with sudden death in young northern Italians, at least 20% had histologic evidence of right ventricular dysplasia at autopsy. Although 10% of such patients are asymptomatic [53], they may present with palpitations, syncope, congestive heart failure, or even sudden death; these episodes are commonly precipitated by exertion. The classic electrocardiographic finding is ventricular tachycardia, often with left bundle branch block. The optimal strategies for preventing sudden cardiac death and the indications for implantable cardioverter-defibrillator therapy in patients with ARVC are not well defined [54].

BRUGADA

Brugada syndrome is an autosomal dominant characterized by right bundle branch block and ST segment elevation in leads V1 to V3. It may result in sudden death. The EKG is fast, with polymorphic ventricular tachycardia. The average age of onset of symptoms is 40 years, but it may occur in very young children. In some gene mutations and in cardiac sodium (Na) channels SCN5a (allelic with LQT3), the fast inactivation of the Na channel leaves the K transient outward current unopposed in phase 1 of the action potential resulting in reentrant arrhythmias. Pharmacologic therapy has been ineffective; implantable defibrillators have had some success.

HISTIOCYTOID CARDIOMYOPATHY

Histiocytoid (oncocytic) cardiomyopathy is characterized by cardiomegaly; incessant ventricular tachycardia; and, frequently, sudden death in the first 2 years of life [55–58]. Some reports have included children up to 4 years of age [59,60]. Female preponderance is approximately 4:1 [61]. Most cases (90%) occur in female children less than 2 years of age, leading to intractable ventricular fibrillation or cardiac arrest. The lesion resembles a hamartoma with histiocytoid or granular cell features [58]. It has clearly been defined as a mitochondrial disorder of complex III (reduced coenzyme Q-cytochrome c reductase) of the respiratory chain of cardiac mitochondria [58]. It has been associated with congenital cardiac defects [58,59,61]. The etiology favors either an autosomal recessive gene or an X-linked condition [62,63]. Female predominance may be explained by gonadal mosaicism for an X-linked mutation. An X-linked condition seems likely because of the reported association with another rare X-linked condition, microphthalmia with linear skin defects that is monosomic for Xp22 [62]. An X-linked dominant mutation has been associated with lethality in males. One sporadic case of A8344G and mtDNA mutation, best known for the myoclonic epilepsy, myopathy, and ragged red fibers (MERRF) phenotype, in an infant with histiocyoid cardiomyopathy and sudden death at 11 months of age has been reported [64].

Histopathologic findings in patients with histiocytoid cardiomyopathy include multiple flat to round, smooth, yellow nodules located beneath the endocardial surface of the left ventricle, the atria, and the 4 cardiac valves. The nodules are composed of demarcated, large, foamy, granular cells (Fig. 7). Glycogen, lipid, and pigment may be seen in these cells as well as a lymphocytic infiltrate. Immunostaining shows perimembranous immunoreactivity for muscle-specific actin but not for the histiocytic markers, S100 protein and CD69 (KP) [65–69]. These cells may be abnormal Purkinje cells, but a primitive myocardial precursor cannot be excluded. Radiofrequency ablation of a conduction defect may be an effective treatment of dysrhythmias [70]. Surgical intervention with prolonged survival has been reported [71].

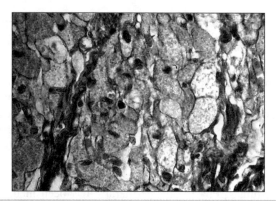

Fig. 7. Histiocytoid cardiomyopathy with large cells containing granular cytoplasm (HE stain, original magnification 400x).

CONGENITAL SHORT QT SYNDROME

Congenital short QT syndrome is a new familial primary electrical disease of the heart, which is characterized by abnormally short QT interval and paroxysmal atrial and ventricular tachyarrhythmias, including sudden cardiac death [72]. To date, only a few families have been identified [73,74]. Genetic mutations in KCNH2 in familial forms [75] and KCNQ1 in sporadic cases [76] have been identified. A missense mutation (C to G substitution at nucleotide 1764), which resulted in the amino acid change (N588K) in KCNH2, has been identified by Hong and colleagues [77] in 3 families with the disease; they concluded that codon 588 is a hot spot for this familial form of short QT syndrome. Biophysical analysis indicated that the mutation was creating a gain of function in the IKr current, causing a shortening of the action potential. This current is largely responsible for repolarization and thus the QT interval duration [78]. The mutation increases IKr, leading to a shortening of action potential duration and arrhythmias [75,77]. The gene map locus is 7q35-q36. In the reported families with short QT syndrome, the median age at diagnosis was 30 years [73]. Sudden death in the generations, in both male and female patients, suggests an autosomal dominant mode of inheritance [79]. Cardiac arrest may be the first clinical presentation and has been reported in patients from 3 months to 62 years of age [73,79]. From the clinical point of view, this syndrome has a broad clinical phenotype and a wide range of symptoms, even in families with the same mutation [77]. The optimal therapy for short QT syndrome has not been established [74].

CATECHOLAMINERGIC POLYMORPHIC VENTRICULAR TACHYCARDIA

Catecholaminergic polymorphic ventricular tachycardia (CPVT), also known as familial CPVT, occurs in the absence of structural heart disease or known associated syndromes [80–88]. It is an autosomal dominant, inherited disease with a relatively early onset and a mortality rate of approximately 30% by the age of 30 years [86]. It is characterized by episodes of syncope, seizures, or sudden death in response to physiologic or emotional stress [87]. The disorder typically presents in childhood or adolescence [80,81,83]. Mutations in the cardiac ryanodine receptor gene (RyR2), which encodes a cardiac sarcoplasmic reticulum (SR) Ca(2+) release channel [83,85,86,89] mapped to chromosome 1q42-q43 [84], have been identified in some families with the disease [83–86]. A second genetic form with autosomal recessive inheritance involves the calsequestrin 2 gene (CASQ2), mapped to chromosome 1p13-21 [87,90,91]. Polymorphic ventricular tachycardia may also present in patients with no significant structural heart disease and no family history [92]. Some, but not all, of these patients have de novo mutations similar to mutations observed in patients with familial disease [83,93,94]. Beta-blockers are the cornerstone of therapy, but some patients do not have a complete response to this therapy and receive an implantable cardioverter-defibrillator [93].

CARNITINE DEFICIENCY

Carnitine is metabolized through lysine and butyrobetaine that is hydroxylated in the liver (Fig. 8). Carnitine is an essential cofactor in the transfer of long-chain fatty acids across the inner mitochondrial membrane and carnitine deficiencies result in defective metabolism of long-chain fatty acids. Mutations in proteins that participate in carnitine transport and metabolism are heritable causes of dilated cardiomyopathy that are transmitted as recessive traits. Dilated cardiomyopathy is also a feature of mutations in the organic cation

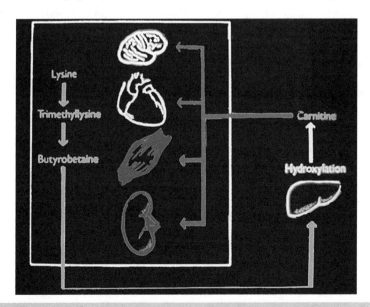

Fig. 8. Metabolism of carnitine.

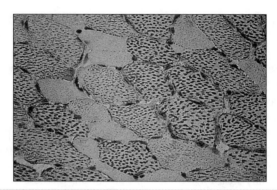

Fig. 9. Microscopic section of the skeletal muscle in carnitine deficiency showing accumulation of lipid vacuoles in type I fibers (Oil-red-O stain, original magnification 400x).

transporter protein, which transports carnitine into cells; it also occurs in translocase deficiency, which transports carnitine into cells and shuttles carnitine and acylcarnitine into the mitochondria. It also occurs in carnitine palmitoyltransferase II, which catalyzes carnitine derivatives into acyl coenzyme A. Cardiomyopathy can be the presenting manifestation of these carnitine-deficiency states. Cardiac function is normal in heterozygous carnitine deficiency. Carnitine deficiency results in the accumulation of neutral lipid within type I skeletal muscle fibers, (Fig. 9) the myocardium, and the liver. Skeletal muscle weakness, episodic weakness, episodic hypoglycemia, encephalopathy, dilated cardiomyopathy, and brady-dysrhythmic cardiac arrests are common [95,96]. The disease is diagnosed by muscle biopsy or by measurement of plasma carnitine concentrations.

Myopathic carnitine deficiency is a rare condition caused by either a defect of a muscle-specific carnitine transporter or to excessive leakage of carnitine from skeletal muscle. Carnitine palmityl transferase II deficiency is characterized by recurrent episodes of exercise-induced myoglobinuria.

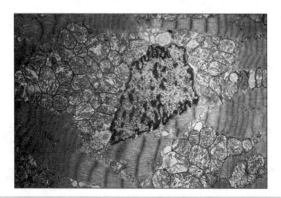

Fig. 10. Accumulation of large mitochondria.

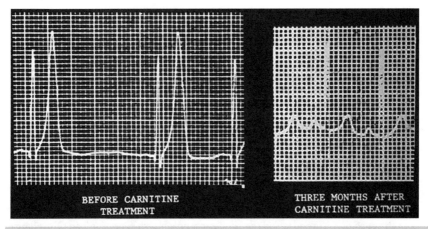

BEFORE CARNITINE
TREATMENT

THREE MONTHS AFTER
CARNITINE TREATMENT

Fig. 11. EKG in carnitine deficiency showing high-peaked T waves before carnitine treatment reverting to normal after carnitine treatment.

Systemic carnitine deficiency results in the accumulation of neutral lipid within type I skeletal muscle fibers (see Fig. 1), the myocardium, and the liver. Congestive and hypertrophic cardiomyopathy results, and brady-dysrhythmic cardiac arrests are common [95,96].

Two clinical subtypes are recognized: that associated with multiple episodes of acute encephalopathy, which resemble Reye syndrome [97–99], and that associated with cardiomyopathy characterized by cardiomegaly and congestive failure at an early age [95], with striking T-wave changes in the EKG. The heart is large and globular. The endocardium may show mild endocardial fibrosis. Ultrastructurally, myofibrils are disrupted, and there is an accumulation of large aggregates of mitochondria (Fig. 10). After treatment with L-carnitine, pathologic changes are resolved and the EKG reverts to normal (Fig. 11).

Acknowledgments

The editors greatly appreciate the generous assistance of Thora Steffensen, MD, for her expert editing of this document.

References

[1] Michaelsson M, Engle M. Congenital complete heart block: an international study of the natural history. Cardiovasc Clin 1972;4:85–101.

[2] Gruntheroth WG, Motolsky AG. Inherited disorders of cardiac rhythm and conduction. Prog Med Genet 1983;5:581.

[3] McCue CM, Mantakas ME, Tingelstad JB, et al. Congenital heart block in newborns of mothers with connective tissue disease. Circulation 1977;56(1):82–90.

[4] Lev M. Pathogenesis of congenital atrioventricular block. Prog Cardiovasc Dis 1972;15(2):145–57.

[5] Shenker L. Fetal cardiac arrhythmias. Obstet Gynecol Surv 1979;34(8):561–72.

[6] Bulkley BH, Roberts WC. The heart in systemic lupus erythematosus and the changes induced in it by corticosteroid therapy. A study of 36 necropsy patients. Am J Med 1975;58(2):243–64.

[7] Scott JS, Maddison PJ, Taylor PV, et al. Connective-tissue disease, antibodies to ribonucleo-protein, and congenital heart block. N Engl J Med 1983;309(4):209–12.

[8] Litsey SE, Noonan JA, O'Connor WN, et al. Maternal connective tissue disease and congenital heart block. Demonstration of immunoglobulin in cardiac tissue. N Engl J Med 1985;312(2):98–100.

[9] Petri M, Watson R, Hochberg MC. Anti-Ro antibodies and neonatal lupus. Rheum Dis Clin North Am 1989;15(2):335–60.

[10] Neyroud N, Tesson F, Denjoy I, et al. A novel mutation in the potassium channel gene KVLQT1 causes the Jervell and Lange-Nielsen cardioauditory syndrome. Nat Genet 1997;15(2):186–9.

[11] Compton SJ, Lux RL, Ramsey MR, et al. Genetically defined therapy of inherited long-QT syndrome. Correction of abnormal repolarization by potassium. Circulation 1996;94(5):1018–22.

[12] Hallman K, Carlsson L. Prevention of class III-induced proarrhythmias by flecainide in an animal model of the acquired long QT syndrome. Pharmacol Toxicol 1995;77(4):250–4.

[13] Chinushi M, Aizawa Y, Furushima H, et al. Nicorandil suppresses a hump on the monopha-sic action potential and torsade de pointes in a patient with idiopathic long QT syndrome. Jpn Heart J 1995;36(4):477–81.

[14] Vincent G, Fox J, Zhang L. Effects of potassium channel opener in KVLQT1 long QT gene carriers. J Am Coll Cardiol 1997;29:183A.

[15] Sato T, Hata Y, Yamamoto M, et al. Early afterdepolarization abolished by potassium chan-nel opener in a patient with idiopathic long QT syndrome. J Cardiovasc Electrophysiol 1995;6(4):279–82.

[16] Shimizu W, Ohe T, Kurita T, et al. Effects of verapamil and propranolol on early afterdepo-larizations and ventricular arrhythmias induced by epinephrine in congenital long QT syn-drome. J Am Coll Cardiol 1995;26(5):1299–309.

[17] Priori SG, Napolitano C, Cantu F, et al. Differential response to Na+ channel blockade, beta-adrenergic stimulation, and rapid pacing in a cellular model mimicking the SCN5A and HERG defects present in the long-QT syndrome. Circ Res 1996;78(6):1009–15.

[18] Schwartz PJ, Priori SG, Locati EH, et al. Long QT syndrome patients with mutations of the SCN5A and HERG genes have differential responses to Na+ channel blockade and to in-creases in heart rate. Implications for gene-specific therapy. Circulation 1995;92(12):3381–6.

[19] Barth PG, Vant Veer-korthof ET, Van Delden L, et al. An X-linked mitochondrial disease affecting cardiac muscle, skeletal muscle and neutrophil leukocytes. In: Busch HFM, Jennekens FGI, Schotte HR, editors. Beetsterzwaag (The Netherlands): Mefar; 1981. p. 161–4.

[20] Barth PG, Scholte JA, Berden JA, et al. An X-linked mitochondrial disease affecting cardiac muscle, skeletal muscle and neutrophil leukocytes. J Neurol Sci 1983;62:327–55.

[21] Hodgson S, Child A, Dyson M. Endocardial fibroelastosis: possible X linked inheritance. J Med Genet 1987;24(4):210–4.

[22] Neustein HB, Lurie PR, Dahms B, et al. An X-linked recessive cardiomyopathy with abnormal mitochondria. Pediatrics 1979;64(1):24–9.

[23] Kelly R, Clark B, Morton D, et al. X-linked cardiomyopathy, neutropenia and increased uri-nary levels of 3-methylglutaconic and 2-ethylhydracrylic acids. Am J Hum Genet 1989;45(Suppl).

[24] Kelley RI, Cheatham JP, Clark BJ, et al. X-linked dilated cardiomyopathy with neutropenia, growth retardation, and 3-methylglutaconic aciduria. J Pediatr 1991;119(5):738–47.

[25] Orstavik KH, Skjorten F, Hellebostad M, et al. Possible X linked congenital mitochondrial cardiomyopathy in three families. J Med Genet 1993;30(4):269–72.

[26] Barth PG, Scholte HR, Berden JA, et al. An X-linked mitochondrial disease affecting cardiac muscle, skeletal muscle and neutrophil leucocytes. J Neurol Sci 1983;62(1–3):327–55.

[27] Bolhuis PA, Hensels GW, Hulsebos TJ, et al. Mapping of the locus for X-linked cardioskeletal myopathy with neutropenia and abnormal mitochondria (Barth syndrome) to Xq28. Am J Hum Genet 1991;48(3):481–5.

[28] Bione S, D'Adamo P, Maestrini E, et al. A novel X-linked gene, G4.5. is responsible for Barth syndrome. Nat Genet 1996;12(4):385–9.

[29] Barth PG, Valianpour F, Bowen VM, et al. X-linked cardioskeletal myopathy and neutropenia (Barth syndrome): an update. Am J Med Genet A 2004;126A(4):349–54.

[30] Neuwald AF. Barth syndrome may be due to an acyltransferase deficiency. Curr Biol 1997;7(8):R465–6.

[31] Vreken P, Valianpour F, Nijtmans LG, et al. Defective remodeling of cardiolipin and phosphatidylglycerol in Barth syndrome. Biochem Biophys Res Commun 2000;279(2): 378–82.

[32] Schhlame M, Towbin J, Jehle R, et al. Deficiency of tetralinoleoyl-cardiolipin in Barth syndrome. Ann Neurol 2002;51:634–7.

[33] Chin TK, Perloff JK, Williams RG, et al. Isolated noncompaction of left ventricular myocardium. A study of eight cases. Circulation 1990;82(2):507–13.

[34] Ritter M, Oechslin E, Sutsch G, et al. Isolated noncompaction of the myocardium in adults. Mayo Clin Proc 1997;72(1):26–31.

[35] Jenni R, Oechslin E, Schneider J, et al. Echocardiographic and pathoanatomical characteristics of isolated left ventricular non-compaction: a step towards classification as a distinct cardiomyopathy. Heart 2001;86(6):666–71.

[36] Pignatelli RH, McMahon CJ, Dreyer WJ, et al. Clinical characterization of left ventricular noncompaction in children: a relatively common form of cardiomyopathy. Circulation 2003;108(21):2672–8.

[37] Michel RS, Carpenter MA, Lovell MA. Pathological case of the month. Noncompaction of the left ventricular myocardium. Arch Pediatr Adolesc Med 1998;152(7): 709–10.

[38] Gilbert-Barness E. Review: metabolic cardiomyopathy and conduction system defects in children. Ann Clin Lab Sci 2004;34(1):15–34.

[39] Manyari DE, Klein GJ, Gulamhusein S, et al. Arrhythmogenic right ventricular dysplasia: a generalized cardiomyopathy? Circulation 1983;68(2):251–7.

[40] Hermida JS, Minassian A, Jarry G, et al. Familial incidence of late ventricular potentials and electrocardiographic abnormalities in arrhythmogenic right ventricular dysplasia. Am J Cardiol 1997;79(10):1375–80.

[41] Rampazzo A, Nava A, Malacrida S, et al. Mutation in human desmoplakin domain binding to plakoglobin causes a dominant form of arrhythmogenic right ventricular cardiomyopathy. Am J Hum Genet 2002;71(5):1200–6.

[42] Protonotarios N, Tsatsopoulou A, Patsourakos P, et al. Cardiac abnormalities in familial palmoplantar keratosis. Br Heart J 1986;56(4):321–6.

[43] Rampazzo A, Nava A, Danieli P, et al. The gene for arrhythmogenic right ventricular cardiomyopathy maps to chromosome 14q23-q24. Hum Molec Genet 1994;3: 959–62.

[44] Rampazzo A, Nava A, Erne P, et al. A new locus for arrhythmogenic right ventricular cardiomyopathy (ARVD2) maps to chromosome 1q42-q43. Hum Mol Genet 1995;4(11): 2151–4.

[45] Severini GM, Krajinovic M, Pinamonti B, et al. A new locus for arrhythmogenic right ventricular dysplasia on the long arm of chromosome 14. Genomics 1996;31(2): 193–200.

[46] Rampazzo A, Nava A, Miorin M, et al. ARVD4, a new focus for arrhythmogenic right ventricular cardiomyopathy, maps to chromosome 2 long arm. Genomics 1997;45(2): 259–63.

[47] Ahmad F, Li D, Karibe A, et al. Localization of a gene responsible for arrhythmogenic right ventricular dysplasia to chromosome 3p23. Circulation 1998;98(25):2791–5.

[48] Hodgkinson KA, Parfrey PS, Bassett AS, et al. The impact of implantable cardioverter-defibrillator therapy on survival in autosomal-dominant arrhythmogenic right ventricular cardiomyopathy (ARVD5). J Am Coll Cardiol 2005;45(3):400–8.

[49] Li D, Ahmad F, Gardner MJ, et al. The locus of a novel gene responsible for arrhythmogenic right-ventricular dysplasia characterized by early onset and high penetrance maps to chromosome 10p12-p14. Am J Hum Genet 2000;66(1):148–56.

[50] Melberg A, Oldfors A, Blomstrom-Lundqvist C, et al. Autosomal dominant myofibrillar myopathy with arrhythmogenic right ventricular cardiomyopathy linked to chromosome 10q. Ann Neurol 1999;46(5):684–92.

[51] Gerull B, Heuser A, Wichter T, et al. Mutations in the desmosomal protein plakophilin-2 are common in arrhythmogenic right ventricular cardiomyopathy. Nat Genet 2004;36(11): 1162–4.

[52] Sen-Chowdhry S, Syrris P, McKenna WJ. Genetics of right ventricular cardiomyopathy. J Cardiovasc Electrophysiol 2005;16(8):927–35.

[53] Kullo L, Edwards W, Seward J. Right ventricular dysplasia: the Mayo Clinic experience. Mayo Clin Proc 1995;70:541–8.

[54] Wichter T, Breithardt G. Implantable cardioverter-defibrillator therapy in arrhythmogenic right ventricular cardiomyopathy. A role for genotyping in decision-making? J Am Coll Cardiol 2005;45:409.

[55] Prahlow JA, Teot LA. Histiocytoid cardiomyopathy: case report and literature review. J Forensic Sci 1993;38(6):1427–35.

[56] Witzleben CL, Pinto M. Foamy myocardial transformation of infancy: 'lipid' or 'histiocytoid' myocardiopathy. Arch Pathol Lab Med 1978;102(6):306–11.

[57] Suarez V, Fuggle WJ, Cameron AH, et al. Foamy myocardial transformation of infancy: an inherited disease. J Clin Pathol 1987;40(3):329–34.

[58] Franciosi RA, Singh A. Oncocytic cardiomyopathy syndrome. Hum Pathol 1988;19(11): 1361–2.

[59] Malhotra V, Ferrans VJ, Virmani R. Infantile histiocytoid cardiomyopathy: three cases and literature review. Am Heart J 1994;128(5):1009–21.

[60] Zangwill SD, Trost BA, Zlotocha J, et al. Orthotopic heart transplantation in a child with histiocytoid cardiomyopathy. J Heart Lung Transplant 2004;23(7):902–4.

[61] Shehata BM, Patterson K, Thomas JE, et al. Histiocytoid cardiomyopathy: three new cases and a review of the literature. Pediatr Dev Pathol 1998;1(1):56–69.

[62] Bird LM, Krous HF, Eichenfield LF, et al. Female infant with oncocytic cardiomyopathy and microphthalmia with linear skin defects (MLS): a clue to the pathogenesis of oncocytic cardiomyopathy? Am J Med Genet 1994;53(2):141–8.

[63] Baillie T, Chan YF, Koelmeyer TD, et al. Test and teach. Ill-defined subendocardial nodules in an infant. Histiocytoid cardiomyopathy. Pathology 2001;33(2):230–4.

[64] Vallance HD, Jeven G, Wallace DC, et al. A case of sporadic infantile histiocytoid cardiomyopathy caused by the A8344G (MERRF) mitochondrial DNA mutation. Pediatr Cardiol 2004;25(5):538–40.

[65] Heifetz SA, Faught PR, Bauman M. Pathological case of the month. Histiocytoid (oncocytic) cardiomyopathy. Arch Pediatr Adolesc Med 1995;149(4):464–5.

[66] Ferrans VJ, McAllister HA Jr, Haese WH. Infantile cardiomyopathy with histiocytoid change in cardiac muscle cells. Report of six patients. Circulation 1976;53(4): 708–19.

[67] Saffitz JE, Ferrans VJ, Rodriguez ER, et al. Histiocytoid cardiomyopathy: a cause of sudden death in apparently healthy infants. Am J Cardiol 1983;52(1):215–7.

[68] Zimmerman A, Diem P, Cottier H. Congenital "histiocytoid" cardiomyopathy: evidence suggesting a developmental disorder of the Purkinje cell system of the heart. Virchows Arch A Pathol Anat Histol 1982;396:187–95.

[69] Ferrans VJ. Pathologic anatomy of the dilated cardiomyopathies. Am J Cardiol 1989;64(6):9C–11C.

[70] Kauffman SL, Chandra N, Peress NS, et al. Idiopathic infantile cardiomyopathy with involvement of the conduction system. Am J Cardiol 1972;30(6):648–52.

[71] Van Hare GF. Radiofrequency catheter ablation of cardiac arrhythmias in pediatric patients. Adv Pediatr 1994;41:83–109.

[72] Gussak I, Brugada P, Brugada J, et al. Idiopathic short QT interval: a new clinical syndrome? Cardiology 2000;94(2):99–102.

[73] Giustetto C, Di Monte F, Wolpert C, et al. Short QT syndrome: clinical findings and diagnostic-therapeutic implications. Eur Heart J 2006;27(20):2440–7.

[74] Bjerregaard P, Gussak I. Short QT syndrome: mechanisms, diagnosis and treatment. Nat Clin Pract Cardiovasc Med 2005;2(2):84–7.

[75] Brugada R, Hong K, Dumaine R, et al. Sudden death associated with short-QT syndrome linked to mutations in HERG. Circulation 2004;109(1):30–5.

[76] Bellocq C, van Ginneken AC, Bezzina CR, et al. Mutation in the KCNQ1 gene leading to the short QT-interval syndrome. Circulation 2004;109(20):2394–7.

[77] Hong K, Bjerregaard P, Gussak I, et al. Short QT syndrome and atrial fibrillation caused by mutation in KCNH2. J Cardiovasc Electrophysiol 2005;16(4):394–6.

[78] Tseng GN. I(Kr): the hERG channel. J Mol Cell Cardiol 2001;33(5):835–49.

[79] Gaita F, Giustetto C, Bianchi F, et al. Short QT syndrome: a familial cause of sudden death. Circulation 2003;108(8):965–70.

[80] Wren C, Rowland E, Burn J, et al. Familial ventricular tachycardia: a report of four families. Br Heart J 1990;63(3):169–74.

[81] Leenhardt A, Lucet V, Denjoy I, et al. Catecholaminergic polymorphic ventricular tachycardia in children. A 7-year follow-up of 21 patients. Circulation 1995;91(5):1512–9.

[82] Fisher JD, Krikler D, Hallidie-Smith KA. Familial polymorphic ventricular arrhythmias: a quarter century of successful medical treatment based on serial exercise-pharmacologic testing. J Am Coll Cardiol 1993;94:2015–22.

[83] Priori SG, Napolitano C, Memmi M, et al. Clinical and molecular characterization of patients with catecholaminergic polymorphic ventricular tachycardia. Circulation 2002;106(1):69–74.

[84] Swan H, Piippo K, Viitasalo M, et al. Arrhythmic disorder mapped to chromosome 1q42-q43 causes malignant polymorphic ventricular tachycardia in structurally normal hearts. J Am Coll Cardiol 1999;34(7):2035–42.

[85] Priori SG, Napolitano C, Tiso N, et al. Mutations in the cardiac ryanodine receptor gene (hRyR2) underlie catecholaminergic polymorphic ventricular tachycardia. Circulation 2001;103(2):196–200.

[86] Laitinen PJ, Brown KM, Piippo K, et al. Mutations of the cardiac ryanodine receptor (RyR2) gene in familial polymorphic ventricular tachycardia. Circulation 2001;103(4):485–90.

[87] Lahat H, Pras E, Olender T, et al. A missense mutation in a highly conserved region of CASQ2 is associated with autosomal recessive catecholamine-induced polymorphic ventricular tachycardia in Bedouin families from Israel. Am J Hum Genet 2001;69(6):1378–84.

[88] Nof E, Lahat H, Constantini N, et al. A novel form of familial bidirectional ventricular tachycardia. Am J Cardiol 2004;93(2):231–4.

[89] Wehrens XH, Lehnart SE, Huang F, et al. FKBP12.6 deficiency and defective calcium release channel (ryanodine receptor) function linked to exercise-induced sudden cardiac death. Cell 2003;113(7):829–40.

[90] Lahat H, Eldar M, Levy-Nissenbaum E, et al. Autosomal recessive catecholamine- or exercise-induced polymorphic ventricular tachycardia: clinical features and assignment of the disease gene to chromosome 1p13-21. Circulation 2001;103(23):2822–7.

[91] di Barletta MR, Viatchenko-Karpinski S, Nori A, et al. Clinical phenotype and functional characterization of CASQ2 mutations associated with catecholaminergic polymorphic ventricular tachycardia. Circulation 2006;114(10):1012–9.

[92] Eisenberg SJ, Scheinman MM, Dullet NK, et al. Sudden cardiac death and polymorphous ventricular tachycardia in patients with normal QT intervals and normal systolic cardiac function. Am J Cardiol 1995;75(10):687–92.

[93] Wilde AA, Bhuiyan ZA, Crotti L, et al. Left cardiac sympathetic denervation for catecholaminergic polymorphic ventricular tachycardia. N Engl J Med 2008;358(19):2024–9.

[94] Tan JH, Scheinman MM. Exercise-induced polymorphic ventricular tachycardia in adults without structural heart disease. Am J Cardiol 2008;101(8):1142–6.

[95] Tripp ME, Katcher ML, Peters HA, et al. Systemic carnitine deficiency presenting as familial endocardial fibroelastosis: a treatable cardiomyopathy. N Engl J Med 1981;305(7): 385–90.

[96] Waber LJ, Valle D, Neill C, et al. Carnitine deficiency presenting as familial cardiomyopathy: a treatable defect in carnitine transport. J Pediatr 1982;101(5):700–5.

[97] Bremer J. Carnitine–metabolism and functions. Physiol Rev 1983;63(4):1420–80.

[98] Karpati G, Carpenter S, Engel AG, et al. The syndrome of systemic carnitine deficiency. Clinical, morphologic, biochemical, and pathophysiologic features. Neurology 1975;25(1): 16–24.

[99] Engel A, Rebouche C, editors. Pathogenetic mechanisms in human carnitine deficiency syndromes. New York: John-Wiley; 1982.

Advances in Pediatrics 61 (2014) 149–195

ADVANCES IN PEDIATRICS

Advances in Minimally Invasive Surgery in Pediatric Patients

Hope T. Jackson, MD[a], Timothy D. Kane, MD[a,b],*

[a]Department of Surgery, The George Washington University School of Medicine & Health Sciences, Washington, DC, USA; [b]Surgical Residency Training Program, Division of Pediatric Surgery, Department of Surgery, Sheikh Zayed Institute for Pediatric Surgical Innovation, Children's National Medical Center, 111 Michigan Avenue, Northwest, Washington, DC 20010-2970, USA

Keywords
• Minimally invasive surgery • Pediatrics • Technology

Key points

- The use of minimally invasive techniques for surgical conditions in pediatric patients has increased dramatically over the last several years.
- The emergence of minimally invasive surgery has allowed pediatric surgeons to manage critically ill neonates, children, and adolescents with improved outcomes in pain, postoperative course, cosmesis, and return to normal activity.
- New and emerging techniques, such as single-incision laparoscopy, endoscopy-assisted surgery, and robotic surgery, all reveal the potential for even further advancement in the management of pediatric patients.

INTRODUCTION

The first laparoscopic cholecystectomies were performed in 1985 and 1987 [1,2]. With the success of this procedure, minimally invasive general surgery emerged as arguably one of the most important advancements in the surgical field this century. Within 6 years of the first laparoscopic cholecystectomy, the procedure became the standard of care for the treatment of cholelithiasis and cholecystitis in the United States and industrialized countries. Over the past 30 years, the use of laparoscopy and minimally invasive techniques for surgical procedures that were previously treated with large open incisions has dramatically increased and continues to develop presently with even newer

Disclosures: None.

*Corresponding author. E-mail address: tkane@cnmc.org

0065-3101/14/$ – see front matter
http://dx.doi.org/10.1016/j.yapd.2014.03.011
© 2014 Elsevier Inc. All rights reserved.

techniques and approaches. Advantages of these techniques are thought to be the development of less adhesions and scar tissue, less postoperative pain, less disruption of anatomy and function, and better cosmesis [3]. Surgery for pediatric patients has also seen a sharp increase in the number of procedures being performed via a minimally invasive approach; this approach is now the standard of care for many surgical conditions affecting infants, children, and adolescents. This article provides an overview of the advances in minimally invasive surgery (MIS) in common surgical conditions of the thorax and abdomen in the pediatric patient and discusses the newest minimally invasive techniques that are emerging in the care of these patients.

ADOPTION OF MIS IN PEDIATRIC SURGERY

Although laparoscopic cholecystectomy revolutionized the practice of adult general surgery, initially this advancement had little impact on the practice of pediatric surgery. Uncertainty about additional costs, longer operative time, the use of instruments primarily designed for adults in children, and skepticism about applying the often-quoted benefits of smaller scars and shorter hospital stays to children are some of the main reasons pediatric surgeons were initially hesitant to accept laparoscopy as a more suitable alternative to traditional open surgery [4]. Several developments helped to change the way MIS techniques were viewed by pediatric surgeons. The development of smaller instruments (2- and 3-mm instruments vs the 5- to 10-mm instruments used in adult surgery); neonatal insufflators that deliver carbon dioxide in a manner that limits overinsufflation that could result in pulmonary complications in already fragile neonates; and, finally, published evidence that supported the notion that laparoscopy was a feasible alternative have all contributed to the dramatic shift in pediatric surgery over the last 15 years [3,5,6].

Before these developments, laparoscopic appendectomy and cholecystectomy remained the primary procedures performed in children because of the similarity of these procedures and technique to those performed in adults. However, the technological advances in instruments allowed pediatric surgeons to feel more comfortable attempting procedures that are specific to the pediatric population. Currently, complicated neonatal and pediatric surgical conditions can now be treated with MIS techniques. See Table 1 for a list of the most common procedures that are now being performed via minimally invasive techniques.

ADVANCES IN THORACIC PROCEDURES

Conventional thoracotomy has historically been performed by the posterolateral approach and now more recently with a muscle-sparing technique. Notable complications after thoracotomy include musculoskeletal deformities, scoliosis, winged scapula, and shoulder dysfunction [7]. Others complications include poor cosmesis as well as breast and chest wall deformities, particularly in children [8,9].

Rodgers and Talbert [10] first introduced thoracoscopy in children in 1976 when they described 9 children undergoing thoracoscopy for diagnostic purposes. The rapid progression and evolution of MIS in the 1990s complemented

Table 1
List of procedures that can now be performed via minimally invasive approaches (thoracoscopic/laparoscopic)

Nissen fundoplication	Appendectomy
Ladd procedure	Tracheoesophageal fistula repair
Cholecystectomy	Thymectomy
Splenectomy	Gastrostomy
Pyloromyotomy	Reduction of intussusception
Endorectal pull-through for imperforate anus and Hirschsprung disease	Resection of choledochal cyst
Congenital diaphragmatic hernia repair	Distal pancreatectomy
Duplication cyst resection	Inguinal/ventral hernia repair
Mediastinal teratoma resection	Pulmonary Lobectomy
Meckel diverticulectomy	Adrenalectomy
Pancreatic tumor resection	Colectomy
Heller myotomy	Oophorectomy
Bronchogenic cyst resection	Ambiguous genitalia evaluation
Aortopexy	Congenital cystic adenomatoid malformation resection

by the refinements in instrumentation and skill led to a dramatic increase in the use of thoracoscopy for multiple indications in neonates and children. Video-assisted thoracoscopic surgery (VATS) has become a major approach for thoracic surgical procedures performed by pediatric surgeons [11,12]. The safety and efficacy has been demonstrated by numerous studies, and the thoracoscopic approach to the pediatric thoracic cavity has been shown to be associated with a significantly better cosmetic outcome and less musculoskeletal sequelae than conventional thoracotomy [13–16].

Tracheoesophageal fistula repair

Tracheoesophageal fistula (TEF) is a common congenital anomaly that results in an abnormal connection between the trachea and esophagus that often results in pulmonary complications in neonates and children. It has an incidence of 1 in 3000 to 4500 live births. Esophageal atresia (EA) is a congenital anomaly that is commonly associated with TEF. EA, with or without TEF, is present in about 1 in 3000 live births. Repair of TEF depends on the location of the TEF and, if EA is present, also depends on the length of the esophagus. The traditional approach to TEF repair requires a large posterolateral right thoracotomy incision. See Box 1 for a review of the essential steps of procedure. The first thoracoscopic repair of an EA was performed in 1999 at the International Pediatric Endosurgery Group meeting [17]. Following this accomplishment, several small series of TEF repair with and without EA were reported [18–21]. In 2005, Holcomb and colleagues [11] performed a large multi-institutional review of outcomes for 104 newborns treated for EA/TEF thoracoscopically. Thoracoscopic outcomes were compared with historic controls (thoracotomies performed 20 years prior). They concluded that the minimally invasive approach was comparable with the standard open repair and

---

Box 1: Essential steps to TEF-EA repair

Transection of azygos vein[a] to appreciate proximal/distal esophagus and fistula

Division of the fistula and repair of tracheal defect

Mobilization of proximal and distal esophagus

Primary esophagoesophagostomy with transanastomotic nasogastric tube in place

These steps apply for both open and thoracoscopic repair.

[a] Some advocate leaving the azygos vein intact citing improvement in the vascularity of the area, which can decrease the leak rate. This point is still controversial.

---

suggested that the minimally invasive approach may have fewer musculoskeletal sequelae. In response to the major criticism that this study looked at historical controls, Burford and colleagues [22] conducted a review of 73 patients undergoing thoracotomy for EA/TEF repair from 1993 to 2008. These data were compared with Holcomb and colleague's thoracoscopic data to provide a more contemporary comparison between the two approaches. In their series, thoracoscopic repair yielded complication rates similar to the contemporary thoracotomy cases. There were no significant differences noted in terms of anastomotic leaks, stricture, recurrence, or need for fundoplication; however, trends toward an increase in anastomotic leak and need for fundoplication were noted in the thoracoscopic group. This review also questioned whether musculoskeletal sequelae were still prevalent as no patient developed musculoskeletal sequelae as a direct consequence of thoracotomy. Although no randomized prospective study has been conducted, subsequent studies still suggest that avoiding a posterolateral thoracotomy in a neonate should still be a priority to minimize the development of scoliosis and shoulder girdle weakness [23]. Although studies have advocated muscle sparing and/or lateral thoracotomies, with various skin incisions to improve on these problems [8], these incisions can be difficult to develop, still require spreading of the rib interspace, and offer more limited access and visualization but still may not eliminate the risk of scoliosis.

The most touted benefit of the thoracoscopic approach is the improved visualization of the anatomy and fistula secondary to the optical magnification (Fig. 1) [23,24]. This improvement allows for more precise identification of the fistula; easy mobilization of the esophagus; and minimal manipulation of the trachea, which may help diminish the occurrence of tracheomalacia [23]. Challenges associated with thoracoscopic TEF repair include single lung ventilation in neonates with poor lung compliance, suturing in the neonatal thorax (mainly the esophageal anastomosis), and technically managing long gap defects (>1.5 cm). The transpleural approach has been cited as the disadvantage of using the thoracoscopic approach as it may predispose to mediastinitis; however, several nonrandomized series have been published citing no difference in mortality and morbidity between the transpleural and retropleural approach

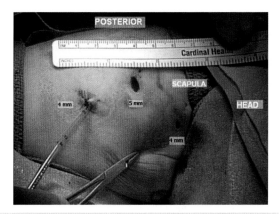

Fig. 1. Thoracoscopic port placement for TEF repair.

[25,26]. In terms of special considerations for the thoracoscopic approach, some researchers suggest a low threshold for conversion to an open procedure in patients with long gap defects as the risks of increased operative time may outweigh the benefits of the minimally invasive repair [24]. Outcomes from several series can be found in Table 2.

Thoracoscopic repair is feasible and safe in the neonates with TEF with and without esophageal atresia. Although more advances are necessary to address the challenges that exist with this approach, performance of this complex repair thoracoscopically is a positive contribution toward the pediatric surgeon's ultimate goal of surgical correction of disease processes with limited associated morbidity.

Table 2
Outcomes in thoracoscopic TEF-EA repair

Series	N	Operative time (min)	Leaks (%)	Strictures (%)	Recurrence (%)	Need for fundoplication (%)
Lovvorn [223], 2001	9/10	55–120	22.0	33.0	11.0	—
Martinez-Ferro [224], 2002	9	70–189 (105)	22.0	33.0	0	—
Bax et al [20], 2002	8	138–250 (198)	12.5	50.0	0	—
Holcomb et al [11], 2005	98/104	129.9	7.7	3.8	1.9	24.0
Nguyen et al [24], 2006	5/6	75–215 (152)	0	20.0	0	—
Rothenberg [23], 2013	51/52	50–120 (85)	1.9	19.6	0	29.9

Outcomes in several of the first series looking at thoracoscopic TEF repair. The dash (—) represents an area that was not specifically reported in the corresponding series.

Congenital diaphragmatic hernia repair

Congenital diaphragmatic hernia (CDH) is a condition in which a defect in the diaphragm allows abdominal organs to exist in the thoracic cavity. The abdominal organs compress the developing lungs that leads to pulmonary hypoplasia on the ipsilateral side. This defect occurs in about one in every 2500 to 3500 live births [27,28]. Much of the acute mortality associated with neonatal CDH is a consequence of pulmonary hypoplasia and persistent pulmonary hypertension [29,30]. Prenatal attempts to ameliorate pulmonary hypoplasia, including in utero repair of the defect and fetoscopic endoluminal tracheal occlusion, have been met with limited success [31–34]. Despite the advances in neonatal care that have improved survival rates, surgical management of neonatal CDH still remains controversial and has advanced more slowly. Classically, CDH repair was performed via transverse subcostal laparotomy or thoracotomy in pediatric patients and via thoracotomy in adults. Small videoscopic instrumentation has allowed pediatric surgeons to perform a minimally invasive approach to CDH repair that has been touted to lead to less morbidity, faster recovery, improved cosmesis and shorter hospitalization but concerns that this approach may precipitate complications such as pulmonary acidosis, hypoxemia and pulmonary hypertension has led to a more cautious adoption of this approach [35,36].

The first minimally invasive CDH repair was performed laparoscopically in a 6-month-old infant and reported in 1995 by van der Zee and Bax [37]. In 1998, Rothenberg and colleagues [38] reported 2 laparoscopic repairs of Bochdalek-type CDH in their article describing their experience with MIS in infants. In 2001, Becmeur and colleagues [39] published a report detailing the successful thoracoscopic repair in 3 cases of late-presenting CDH in infants. Following this report, many of the reports of minimally invasive CDH repair have been dominated by the thoracoscopic rather than laparoscopic approaches [40–44]. Gourlay and colleagues [44] published the first report to demonstrate improved outcomes for neonatal thoracoscopic repair when compared with the traditional open repair. This review was a retrospective review that compared the outcomes of patients who underwent thoracoscopic repair with a physiologically matched historical control group who underwent an open repair. From 2004 to 2007, 20 of 33 patients (61%) underwent successful thoracoscopic repair; from 1999 to 2003, 40 patients underwent open repair. The thoracoscopic group had a statistically and clinically significant faster return to full enteral feeds, shorter duration on the ventilator, decreased sedation requirement postoperatively, and developed less severe complications. They reported that the criteria associated with a successful thoracoscopic repair were (1) absence of significant congenital cardiac anomaly, (2) absence for the need for preoperative extracorporeal membrane oxygenation (3) peak inspiratory pressure less than or equal to 26 on the day of surgery, and (4) an oxygenation index less than or equal to 5 on the day of surgery.

Lansdale and colleagues [31] performed a meta-analysis of other studies that compared open and endosurgical CDH repairs and reported that neonatal thoracoscopic CDH repair has an increased recurrence risk (almost 3-fold) and operative time compared with open repair, though survival and prosthetic patch usage are comparable. The higher recurrence risk was explained as a potential expected consequence of the learning curve and technical difficulties of this procedure. These difficulties included intracorporeal suturing in the limited workspace of the neonatal thorax and the potential that the thoracoscopic approach may not allow for complete mobilization of the diaphragmatic tissue that is often more easily achieved via subcostal laparotomy. Inadequate mobilization may lead to thoracoscopically placed sutures and patches that are secured to less substantial tissue, increasing the risk for recurrence [31]. Although not reported, increased recurrence rates may be related to poor patient selection for this approach by surgeons with inexperience in advanced neonatal MIS. It is likely that this excess recurrence risk will reduce as surgeons progress along the learning curve and become more familiar with the technical steps involved. The increased operative time (>50 minutes) seen in the thoracoscopic group was consistent with other comparisons of pediatric minimally invasive procedures and open surgery [45,46]; however, this could discourage surgeons from choosing this approach as increased operative time is likely undesirable in physiologically labile newborns with CDH. What is encouraging from this is that if previous experience with MIS is indicative, operative times are likely to decrease as surgeons' expertise with endosurgical CDH repair improves [31,47]. When comparing the thoracoscopic and laparoscopic approaches, both are feasible [48]; but many researchers (the authors included) think the thoracoscopic approach offers more advantages in terms of ease of technique, physiologic consequences of carbon dioxide insufflation, and acceptable recurrence rates (Figs. 2–4, Table 3) [35,40,41,49].

Surgical management of CDH remains a challenge, particularly in the critically ill neonate. In neonates who have been optimized in terms of their pulmonary physiology, MIS techniques, particularly the thoracoscopic technique, have been shown to be a safe and feasible approach that both reduces the physiologic stresses of surgery and effectively closes the diaphragmatic defect. As surgeons continue to improve with this technique, the number of vulnerable newborns born with this condition who have successful outcomes following repair should continue to increase.

Pulmonary resection

As discussed at the beginning of this section, the evolution of MIS in the 1990s led to a dramatic increase in the use of thoracoscopy for multiple purposes in neonates and children. By the mid 1990s, thoracoscopy had become an accepted technique in the treatment of empyema; mediastinal masses; bleb resection; and, in many cases, the preferred technique for lung biopsies to obtain tissue in cases of interstitial lung disease or malignancy [50–52]. In comparison with transbronchial biopsies or the standard or mini-thoracotomy approach, with thoracoscopic biopsy, the entire surface of the lung and pleura can be evaluated through limited access ports, and biopsies from multiple areas

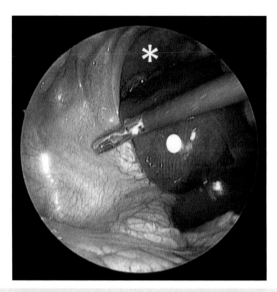

Fig. 2. Right-sided CDH with visible defect (*star*) and herniated abdominal contents-liver within the right chest (*circle*).

can easily be obtained. In addition, the postoperative pain and recovery associated with a thoracoscopic biopsy allows for some of these biopsies to be performed on an outpatient basis [53,54].

In 2003, Rothenberg [55] and Albanese and colleagues [56], respectively, described their experiences with thoracoscopic lobectomy in infants and

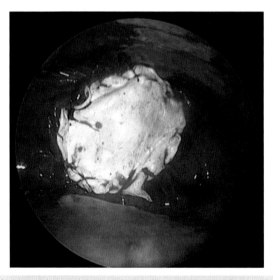

Fig. 3. Right-sided CDH repaired thoracoscopically with the use of a prosthetic patch.

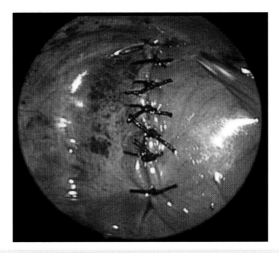

Fig. 4. Left-sided CDH repaired thoracoscopically with interrupted sutures.

children for congenital and acquired lung lesions. Rothenberg [55] reported on 45 patients who underwent a video-assisted thoracoscopic lobe resection from 1995 to 2002. Forty-three of the 45 patients underwent successful lobectomy via the thoracoscopic technique. They concluded that thoracoscopic lung resection is a safe and efficacious technique that is associated with the same decrease in postoperative pain, recovery, and hospital stay as seen in other commonly performed minimally invasive procedures. These conclusions remained with similar results when they reported a 10-year review of their experience with this procedure (97 thoracoscopic lobectomies) in 2007 [16]. The preoperative diagnoses of the patients treated included pulmonary sequestration/congenital

Table 3
Commonly cited advantages and disadvantages of the thoracoscopic and laparoscopic approaches for CDH repair

	Advantages	Disadvantages
Thoracoscopic	• Improved visualization with large working space • Only intermittent carbon dioxide insufflation needed • Easier reduction of intestine and repair of defect • Extended thoracic examination	• Inability to examine the intra-abdominal viscera to rule out malrotation and other abdominal anomalies • Increased risk of abdominal viscera puncture
Laparoscopic	• Abdominal viscera examination • Secure suturing without risk of visceral injury	• Limited workspace and visibility following reduction of hernia contents • Requires sustained carbon dioxide insufflation

pulmonary adenomatoid malformation, severe bronchiectasis, congenital lobar emphysema, and malignancy. Albanese and colleagues [56] reported on 14 consecutive patients with similar diagnoses from 1999 to 2002 who had a pulmonary lobectomy via the MIS technique shortly after Rothenberg. Using single lung ventilation and a controlled pneumothorax with low pressure to facilitate visualization, all lobectomies were completed successfully using 3 ports and the Ligasure (Ligasure Covidien, Mansfield, MA, USA) thermal energy device for vessel division and fissure completion when necessary. There were no intraoperative or postoperative complications in patients who were followed up to 35 months postoperatively.

Albanese and Rothenberg [57] subsequently combined their experiences to report the largest series with the longest period of follow-up (1–10 years) in pediatric patients receiving thoracoscopic lobectomies. All but 3 of the 144 procedures were performed thoracoscopically, with one intraoperative complication (compromise of a left upper lobe bronchus) and 4 postoperative complications: pneumonia, pneumothorax, empyema, and prolonged chest tube drainage. Long-term follow-up revealed no cases of musculoskeletal deformity or weakness.

In terms of comparing the thoracoscopic approach with open resection (Fig. 5), in 2008, Vu and colleagues [58] performed a retrospective chart review of consecutive congenital cystic adenomatoid malformations (CCAM) resections. Twelve patients had thoracoscopic resections and 24 had open resections. Their analysis found that although minimally invasive resection of CCAM resulted in a longer operative time, these patients had a significantly

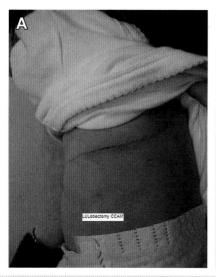 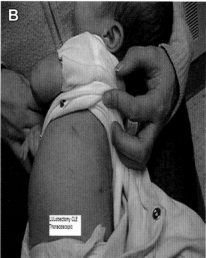

Fig. 5. Thoracotomy versus thoracoscopic incisions. (A) Thoracotomy incision following left upper lobectomy for congenital cystic adenomatoid malformations (CCAM). (B) Thoracoscopic incisions following left upper lobectomy for congenital lobar emphysema (CLE).

shorter hospital stay and reduction in complications. The researchers did mention that resection in patients with a history of pneumonia is challenging and should be considered a risk factor for conversion to thoracotomy.

These studies highlight that minimally invasive techniques can be applied to lung resections and are safe and feasible in the pediatric population.

Esophagectomy

Esophageal stricture following lye ingestion is a common indication for esophagectomy in children. Primary management consists of dilation of the stricture, but patients with strictures that persist despite dilatation (often secondary to severe lumen narrowing and stricture length) may require esophageal replacement. Esophageal replacement with reinstitution of oral feeding has been shown to be advantageous in children [59]. Minimally invasive esophagectomy and gastric pull-up techniques for esophageal cancer and benign esophageal disorders refractory to nonoperative management have been achieved for adults with improved postoperative quality-of-life scores, comparable morbidity, and equal or lower mortality rates when compared with standard open techniques [60,61]. Attempting these minimally invasive approaches in pediatric patients for the management of stricture secondary to caustic injury is limited and has been met with some concern as the mediastinum can be significantly scarred in these cases.

In 2001, Cury and colleagues [62] described 2 children who underwent thoracoscopic esophagectomy for benign esophageal strictures. Although the procedures were without complication, laparotomy was used to achieve the gastric conduit creation in both cases. In 2004, Nwomeh and colleagues [63] reported on the first completely minimally invasive esophagectomy through a combined thoracoscopic and laparoscopic approach in a 17-year-old patient with an intractable caustic esophageal stricture. Postoperatively, the patient tolerated a regular diet for 4 years until she developed a gastric ulcer that resulted in a gastrobronchial fistula that required thoracotomy for repair. In 2007, they reported on a second case performed via the combined thoracoscopic/laparoscopic approach in a 13-month-old child who had ingested lye and developed strictures that failed to respond to serial dilations [64]. Esophageal mobilization was performed thoracoscopically; the gastric conduit, pyloroplasty, and esophagogastric anastomosis were performed laparoscopically (Fig. 6). Because of the small thoracic inlet in this patient, a right minithoracotomy was performed to negotiate the gastric conduit safely into the chest and limit injury. At the last follow-up of 3 years, the patient has been doing well and had not developed any strictures or required dilations. The researchers reported that although creation of the gastric conduit laparoscopically was relatively straightforward, the most challenging aspects of this case proved to be esophageal mobilization and conduit negotiation in the thorax as this area is frequently scarred with fibrosis.

In 2007, Shalaby and colleagues [65] reported their experience performing 27 laparoscopic-assisted transhiatal esophagectomies over a 3-year period. The

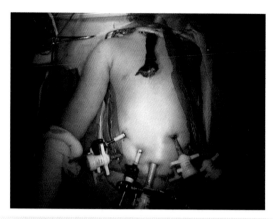

Fig. 6. Laparoscopic port placement for gastric pull-up for stricture following lye ingestion. The esophagus and attached proximal stomach are resected thoracoscopically and removed through a cervical incision.

transhiatal technique involves only laparoscopic access, and the esophageal mobilization is achieved via blunt dissection with the laparoscopic instruments. Their patients were followed from a range of 6 months to 3 years. Complications included anastomotic leak (3 patients [11.1%]) and stricture formation (4 patients [14.8%]). The authors have had similar results with minimally invasive esophagectomy with gastric pull-up in 5 additional patients (2 caustic strictures, 3 esophageal atresia; Kane TD, personal communication, 2013) (Fig. 7).

Although longer outcome data and additional comparative studies are needed, all of these studies support the notion that although technically challenging, minimally invasive esophagectomy can be performed, via multiple approaches, safely, effectively, and in the hands of surgeons with experience in both open esophageal surgery and advanced thoracoscopic and laparoscopic techniques.

Aortopexy

Tracheomalacia is generalized weakness and/or floppiness of the tracheal wall and may cause luminal obstruction, particularly at times of increased intrathoracic pressure, such as expiration, crying, or coughing. Although it usually presents at birth, it may develop later in life. Infants with concomitant EA and TEF have a high incidence (up to 40%) of feeding difficulties and respiratory infections and often require hospitalization during the first few years of life. Although most cases resolve over time with growth and development of the child, those patients with severe symptoms require surgical treatment. Aortopexy is the most commonly used surgical method for the treatment of severe tracheomalacia. The procedure takes advantage of the close anatomic relationship between the aortic arch and the trachea. The aortic arch lies immediately anterior to the trachea and posterior to the sternum. Elevation of the aorta against the posterior surface of the sternum lifts the anterior wall of the trachea

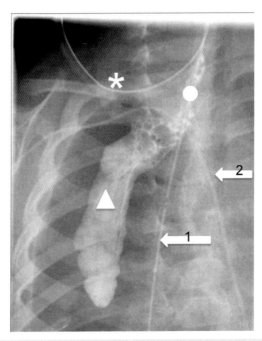

Fig. 7. Postoperative upper gastrointestinal series following gastric pull-up. Penrose drain extending from the cervical incision (*star*) with a radiopaque marker at the site of the esophagogastric cervical anastomosis (*circle*). Contrast enters the gastric pouch (*triangle*) without extravasation and settles and seems to taper abruptly. This patient did not undergo a pyloroplasty, so this is secondary to the patient experiencing pylorospasm at the time of the study. Midline chest tube (*arrow 1*) and PICC line (*arrow 2*) are shown in the midline and patient's left, respectively. PICC, peripherally inserted central catheter.

and relieves luminal narrowing with success rates in upwards of 90% [66–68]. Aortopexy previously has been performed by thoracotomy, median sternotomy, or the cervical approach; however, in 2000 and 2002, DeCou and Schaarschmidt [69,70] reported the first cases of thoracoscopic aortopexy, respectively. Perger and colleagues [71] also performed 5 of these cases and achieved resolution of symptoms in all patients. They proposed that the thoracoscopic approach offered improved exposure of the surgical field, was cosmetically more pleasing to patients and their families, and could result in less pulmonary complications and less narcotic requirement compared with open thoracotomy. Similarly, van der Zee and Bax [66] reported the largest thoracoscopic series to date of 6 patients. All procedures were performed thoracoscopically; after a follow-up period of 27 months, 2 patients had recurrences that were treated thoracoscopically without incident, whereas the others have had uncomplicated postoperative courses. All of these procedures were initially performed via a left-sided approach. In 2008, Kane and colleagues [72] showed that the procedure could be performed initially via either the left or right approach, and their 2 patients had no recurrences for 2 and 3 years, respectively. Although many of these reports are limited by sample size, tracheomalacia requiring operative intervention by aortopexy is an uncommon condition. These studies and several smaller studies support the notion that thoracoscopic aortopexy is feasible and safe in infants and children and may be of particular value in patients who have recurred after open repair (Figs. 8 and 9).

Pectus excavatum repair

Pectus excavatum (PE) is the most common congenital chest wall abnormality that results from posterior depression of the sternum and the inferior costal cartilages. It occurs in approximately 8 per 1000 live births [73]. Although the condition itself is rarely, if ever, life threatening, the most important aspect of the pathophysiology of PE is that the extent of sternal depression determines the degree of cardiac and pulmonary compression, which directly relates to the degree of incapacitation secondary to impaired cardiopulmonary function at high levels of cardiac output [74,75].

Indications for repair of PE include impaired cardiopulmonary function, pain, improved cosmesis, and recurrence after failed repair. Surgical repair of PE was first achieved in the early 1900s. In 1949, Ravitch [76] described a new technique that involved excision of all the deformed costal cartilages including the perichondrium, xiphoid excision, and sternal osteotomy with anterior fixation of the sternum. With minor modifications, this remained

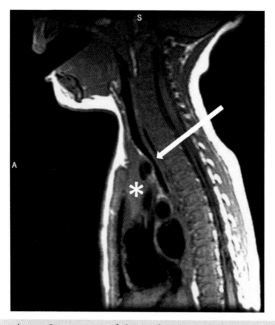

Fig. 8. Tracheomalacia. Compression of the trachea (*arrow*) posterior to the aortic arch (*star*).

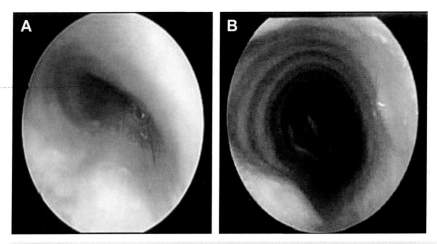

Fig. 9. Tracheomalacia. Bronchoscopy demonstrating tracheal compression preoperatively (A) and (B) postoperatively following minimally invasive aortopexy.

the procedure of choice for nearly 50 years. In 1997, Dr Donald Nuss introduced a minimally invasive approach to surgical repair that he had been performing since 1987. The following year, Nuss and colleagues [77] published their 10-year experience with this procedure in 42 patients younger than 15 years. The procedure differed from the Ravitch procedure in that it necessitated minimal dissection and required neither incision into nor resection of the costal cartilages. In brief, a convex steel bar is inserted under the sternum through small bilateral thoracic incisions. The steel bar is inserted with the convexity facing posteriorly; when it is in position, the bar is turned over, thereby correcting the deformity. Once permanent remolding has occurred, the bar is removed in an outpatient procedure approximately 2 to 3 years later. Following this publication, Nuss [78] reported on new modifications to the procedure that included the routine use of thoracoscopy, which allowed for direct visualization of the mediastinal structures, new instruments for tunneling and bar rotation, development of bar stabilizers, and placement of pericostal sutures around the bar to prevent bar displacement.

In 2008, Nuss [78] published a 20-year update on the outcomes of this procedure. Early and late complications (Table 4) have been markedly reduced by meticulous attention to preoperative clearance, bar stabilization, evacuation of the pneumothorax, incentive spirometry, and prophylactic antibiotics. In addition to Dr Nuss' results, many centers have also reported marked improvement in their complication rate after the early learning experience [79–83]. Of note, the rate of bar displacement decreased dramatically (~ 15% to less 1%) with the introduction of stabilizers and the use of pericostal sutures around the bar.

When comparing the Nuss with the Ravitch procedures, one recent meta-analysis by Nasr and colleagues [84] found that both procedures have similar rates of overall complications, length of stay, and time to ambulation. The

Table 4
Early and late postoperative complications of patients receiving Nuss procedure

Early	Pneumothorax with spontaneous resolution	60.4% (n = 613)
	Pneumothorax with chest tube	3.6% (n = 36)
	Horner syndrome (temporary)	17.7% (n = 179)
	Drug reaction	3.6% (n = 36)
	Pneumonia	0.6% (n = 6)
	Hemothorax	0.6% (n = 6)
	Pericarditis	0.5% (n = 5)
	Pleural effusion that required drainage	0.3% (n = 3)
	Cardiac perforation	0%
	Death	0%
Late	Bar displacement	5.8% (n = 58)
	Requiring revision	50% (28/58)
	Overcorrection	3.2% (n = 32)
	Bar allergy	2.9% (n = 29)
	Recurrence	0.8% (n = 8)
	Skin erosion	0.1% (n = 1)

Early postoperative complications encountered in 1015 primary operations performed between 1987 and 2008.

Ravitch procedure had a significantly longer time of operation; when looking at specific complications, the Nuss procedure had a higher rate of pneumothorax, hemothorax, and reoperation secondary to bar migration or persistent deformity. In terms of cardiopulmonary function, one recent study does suggest that there is greater improvement in pulmonary function following the Nuss procedure [85]. In addition, there is a suggestion that the Nuss procedure might provide better visualization in cases of recurrence (both Nuss and Ravitch), as these patients also require lysis of adhesions before bar placement [76,84].

Overall, what is clear from the literature is that the minimally invasive repair of PE is a feasible and safe alternative to the open Ravitch repair. This approach and other minimally invasive approaches will likely continue to evolve and develop as technology continues to advance.

ADVANCES IN ABDOMINAL PROCEDURES

Stephen Gans and Berci [86] reported the first case of laparoscopy in pediatric surgery in 1971. At the time of this publication, access into the peritoneal cavity was termed *peritoneoscopy*, which was soon replaced with *laparoscopy*. Gans and Berci's first case was successful confirmation of an inguinal hernia by placing the endoscope through the known contralateral hernia sac. Initially, the application of laparoscopy in children was for diagnostic purposes; however, much like thoracoscopy, the evolution of MIS in the 1990s led to a dramatic increase in the use of laparoscopy for multiple purposes in neonates and children. The incidence of complications in pediatric laparoscopy is reported to be around 4% to 5%; in most cases, the complications can be managed laparoscopically [87–89]. Complications may be related to the minimally invasive approach (access, equipment, insufflation) or specific to the actual procedure. Complications that are procedure specific may occur with an open technique as well as with a minimally invasive approach [87–91]. As with children who presented with thoracic surgical conditions, there was similar hesitation to apply minimally invasive techniques in children based only on the success in adult patients. However, after several studies showed laparoscopy to be feasible and safe, many pediatric surgeons have adopted this approach; it is now the standard of care for many pediatric surgical conditions [6,92–94].

Antireflux procedures

Gastroesophageal reflux (GER) is a common and often benign occurrence in the pediatric population that refers to the regurgitation of gastric contents into the esophagus. Most of these patients (>65%) will experience spontaneous resolution of their symptoms by 2 years of age [95–97]. Those who continue to have symptoms and develop complications, such as failure to thrive, secondary respiratory disease, laryngospasm, esophagitis, and esophageal strictures, are classified as having GER disease (GERD). Treatment options include dietary or behavioral modifications, pharmacologic intervention, and surgical therapy. Surgical management of GERD typically becomes necessary in the presence of GER complications and/or failed medical therapy. Over the years, laparoscopic antireflux procedures (first reported in children in 1992) have been shown to have comparable outcomes and lower complication rates compared with the open approach and have replaced the open approach as the primary surgical approach for the treatment of GERD (see Box 2 for the essential steps of the procedure and Figs. 10–12) [98–100].

Fundoplication provides definitive treatment of GERD and is highly effective in most circumstances. The fundus of the stomach can be wrapped around the distal esophagus either 360° (ie, Nissen fundoplication) or to lesser degrees (ie, Thal or Toupet fundoplication). Initially described in 1954 by Rudolph Nissen, the Nissen fundoplication has evolved to become the standard operation for the surgical treatment of GERD in children and adults [101]. Partial fundoplication procedures involve wrapping the distal esophagus to a lesser degree than required in the Nissen procedure (eg, 270°). Partial wraps are commonly performed in those patients with esophageal motility disorders to prevent dysphagia that may result from a complete fundoplication. Several studies comparing Nissen and partial fundoplications have overall reported similar results in outcomes in neurologically normal children [102–106],

---

Box 2: Essential steps to the laparoscopic Nissen procedure

Gastroesophageal junction mobilization with identification of main vagi trunks

Hiatal dissection and creation of retroesophageal window

Division of short gastric vessels/gastrosplenic ligament

Crural approximation

Creation of a 360° wrap with a bougie in place

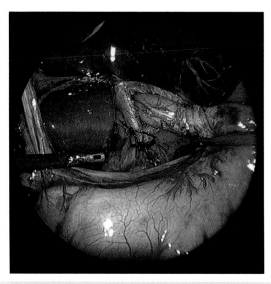

Fig. 10. Laparoscopic Nissen fundoplication technique. Esophageal mobilization with creation of a retroesophageal window and crural approximation (sutures).

though the Thal procedure has been shown to yield higher recurrence rates in children with neurologic impairments (Table 5) [107].

The laparoscopic approach for both complete and partial fundoplication requires intracorporeal suturing and specific dissection and mobilization techniques that can be challenging to even the most experienced surgeon. Several studies have examined the learning curve associated with performing these antireflux procedures in children. In children, Meehan and Georgeson [108] looked

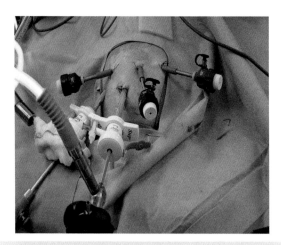

Fig. 11. Port placement for laparoscopic Nissen fundoplication.

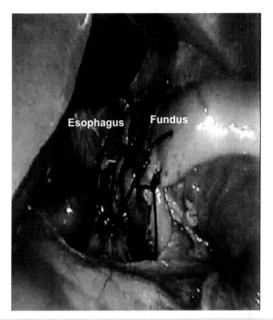

Fig. 12. Laparoscopic Nissen fundoplication technique. Completed 360° fundoplication.

at the learning curve in their first 160 cases of laparoscopic fundoplications and suggested a learning curve in terms of conversion to open and operative times between 20 and 25 cases. In his series of 220 procedures, Rothenberg [47] also reported an estimated learning curve for laparoscopic Nissen fundoplication to be between 20 and 50 cases. As this learning period is to be expected, the presence/consultation of a senior surgeon during this period may mitigate longer operative times and increased risk of surgical complications.

Achalasia

Achalasia is a primary motility disorder of the esophagus that results in poor relaxation of the lower esophageal sphincter (LES) and eventual loss of

Table 5
Outcomes in antireflux surgery

	Dysphagia (%)	Postoperative complications (%)	Recurrence rates (%)	Repeat surgical intervention (%)
Nissen	4–24	4–22	3–46	2–14
Toupet	2	3–8	1–25	~2–11
Thal	2–22	3	6–20	10–14

Ranges based on retrospective reviews by Esposito and colleagues [102,103], Chung and colleagues [104], Steyaert and colleagues [105], and Subramaniam and Dickson [106] and randomized prospective study by Kubiak and colleagues [107]. Those categories with only 1% value represent the only study that individually looked at a particular outcome category for Nissen, Toupet, or Thal.

esophageal peristalsis. Although this condition more commonly affects adults, children represent about 5% of all cases of achalasia, with an estimated incidence of 0.11 cases per 100,000 children [109–111]. The treatment of achalasia involves several therapies that include medical treatment to attempt to relax the LES, pneumatic dilation to stretch the LES, botulinum toxin injections to paralyze the LES, and surgical myotomy to disrupt the muscle fibers of the LES [112]. Although underlying disease cannot be eradicated, these interventions have improved the symptoms associated with achalasia in many children [112]. Performed in 1913 by Ernest Heller, cardiomyotomy originally involved anterior and posterior incisions in the outer longitudinal and inner circular muscle layers. The procedure was modified to just performing an anterior myotomy and is now the current procedure performed when referring to a Heller myotomy or cardiomyotomy. Since the development of minimally invasive approaches, there has been a significant shift in the treatment of achalasia; laparoscopic Heller myotomy has become the treatment of choice for achalasia in adults and now an accepted approach in children.

There have been reports of both laparoscopic and thoracoscopic repair in children [113,114]. Rothenberg and colleagues [115] reported their experience with 9 children who had Heller myotomies. Four children had a thoracoscopic Heller (TH), whereas the remaining 5 had a laparoscopic approach. They found that both procedures were safe in children but that TH yielded longer operating times and hospital stays. They also suggested that without the addition of a partial fundoplication, TH might result in silent GER, as 2 of these patients had postoperative pH studies consistent with mild reflux. Other researchers have preferred the laparoscopic technique citing that, although the thoracoscopic approach provided relief of dysphagia (>80%), the fundoplication was more technically difficult and greater than 50% of these patients had GER postoperatively [116,117].

Although it is clear that the minimally invasive Heller is an effective and safe procedure in children, debate still exists regarding the utility of a concomitant antireflux procedure and, if chosen, which antireflux procedure to select. Those who oppose the use of an antireflux procedure claim that avoiding excessive posterior dissection and any closure of the crura will help prevent reflux symptoms [118]. However, the adult and pediatric literature in general support the use of an antireflux procedure with a Heller myotomy, as the risk of developing GER has been reported to be as high as 48% in long-term follow-up [119,120]. Dor fundoplication has been combined with Heller myotomy in several series in the pediatric population with adequate results [117,121,122]. Patti and colleagues [117] reported no residual dysphagia and normal pH studies at 19 months of follow-up in 13 children with achalasia. Mattioli and colleagues [121] reported a 15% incidence in dysphagia (3 out of 20 children) and normal pH studies at a mean 45-month follow-up period (range 6–102 months). In the authors' own experience in 24 pediatric patients, they prefer laparoscopic Heller myotomy with Dor fundoplication and have had an 8% incidence of dysphagia (3 of 24), 2 requiring only single dilatation and one a laparoscopic

redo myotomy 2014 [123]. Posterior fundoplication (Toupet) has been successful in children, though recurrence rates greater than 25% have been reported
after the procedure (range of follow-up 1–66 months). Posterior partial fundoplication has been more effective in controlling postoperative dysphagia in the
adult literature than in children [112,120]. No prospective studies have been
performed that compares the various partial fundoplication procedures in patients receiving a Heller myotomy. Moving forward, there has been a report
of a single-incision laparoscopic Heller myotomy with Dor fundoplication
[124]. Although the procedure has been successful, more studies, including
long-term follow-up, is necessary before conclusions can be reached.

Pancreatic tumors

Pancreatic tumors are very rare in children and adolescents. In fact, reports
from large referral centers spanning 20 years of experience consist of less
than 10 patients each and the largest series from Memorial Sloan-Kettering
over 35 years consists of only 17 patients. Reported incidences in the United
States range from 1 case per 18,000 to 0.018 cases per 100,000 [125,126];
abroad, these tumors account for less than 0.2% of deaths from cancer in children [127]. Because of the small incidence of these tumors in children, most of
the available literature on the topic is represented in case reports and limited
literature reviews. Although most pancreatic cancers in adults are ductal adenocarcinoma, these tumors are extremely rare in children [128]. Pancreatoblasto-
mas, solid pseudopapillary carcinoma, acinar cell carcinoma, exocrine and
endocrine epithelial tumors, nonepithelial tumors, and sarcomas have all
been reported in children [129].

Surgical resection has been and continues to be the mainstay of treatment of
these tumors. However, the retroperitoneal location of the pancreas has delayed the application of minimally invasive techniques to pancreatic surgery.
Laparoscopic procedures for adult pancreatic tumors were first performed in
the late 1990s [130,131]. Since then, laparoscopic distal pancreatectomies
were reported in children with successful outcomes, including shorter hospital
stays and better cosmetic results [132–134]. Despite the greater magnification
and improved visualization the laparoscopic approach provides, pediatric surgeons have taken a more conservative approach to laparoscopic pancreatic procedures. Many surgeons favored an open approach to pancreatic tumor
resection to maximize splenic preservation because overwhelming postsplenec-
tomy infection is prevalent in the pediatric population [135]. As laparoscopic
techniques have advanced, however, various methods of vessel preservation
have become available; laparoscopic spleen-sparing pancreatic tumor resections
have been successfully performed in children [136–139].

The success of laparoscopic pancreatectomy in children can be best exemplified by the experience in children with solid pseudopapillary tumors (SPT).
Thirteen laparoscopic pancreatectomy procedures have been reported in pediatric patients with SPT. Ten of the tumors were located in the pancreatic tail, 2
were in the uncinate process, and one was in the central portion or body of the

pancreas [133,135,140–144]. Of the tumors resected with a laparoscopic distal pancreatectomy, only 2 included splenectomy, because the splenic vessels could not be separated from the neoplasm and pancreas [135]. Cavallini and colleagues [145] performed a retrospective review in 2011 of 10 patients (3 patients were children aged 11, 13, and 17 years) who received a laparoscopic pancreatectomy for SPT. They reported no tumor recurrence in all 10 patients with a median follow-up time of 47 months. They concluded that the laparoscopic approach is a safe approach but that application in pediatric patients is still under development. In terms of the authors' own center experience, they recently reported on their experience with 3 patients (2 patients aged 13 years and one 14 year old) who were found to have SPT and were managed with laparoscopic pancreatectomy. Two of the 3 patients required splenectomy because of the inability to separate the tumor from the spleen without risking spillage of tumor. However, the patient with the largest tumor was able to undergo laparoscopic distal pancreatectomy with splenic preservation because the tumor was located more proximally in the pancreas indicating that tumor size does not preclude splenic salvage (Fig. 13).

Several authors have raised concern about an increased risk of recurrence of SPT with the laparoscopic technique [132,140]. Fais and colleagues [140] described 3 children and one child, respectively, who developed recurrences; they were subsequently managed with open surgery. It is important to point out that each of these patients underwent initial laparoscopic biopsy either before or at the time of resection. The authors agree with Cavallini and colleagues [145] that even when one considers an open resection for these types of pancreatic masses in children, biopsy is not recommended preoperatively

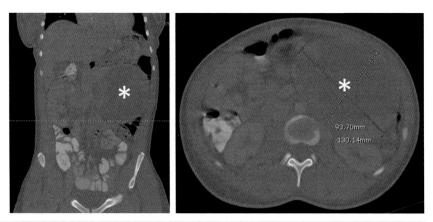

Fig. 13. Solid pseudopapillary pancreatic tumor. Computed tomography scan of a 13-year-old patient found to have a 13.0 × 11.0 × 9.4-cm solid pseudopapillary mass originating in the body with extension into the tail of the pancreas (*star*). The patient underwent laparoscopic distal pancreatectomy with splenic preservation and resection margin negative for tumor. Her postoperative course was uneventful and follow-up at 24 months showed no recurrent disease.

or perioperatively as this may have a direct impact on tumor recurrence and peritoneal dissemination.

Overall, laparoscopic resection of pancreatic tumors is an acceptable approach when applied in the appropriate clinical setting with frequent follow-up to monitor for recurrence. Splenic conservation may be possible depending on tumor proximity to the spleen and splenic vessel involvement with the tumor. As more pediatric surgeons report their experience with laparoscopic pancreatic tumor resection for all tumor types, the laparoscopic approach could become the preferred method of treatment of pediatric patients found to have pancreatic tumors.

Traumatic injuries

Intra-abdominal injury affects approximately 10% to 15% of pediatric patients [146,147]. Of this percentage, most of these injuries can be managed nonoperatively, though care must be taken as missed injury or delayed diagnosis can have devastating consequences [147–149]. Although the focused assessment with sonography for trauma ultrasound and computed tomography (CT) scans have improved decision making in the trauma bay, equivocal ultrasound results and concern for radiation exposure in the pediatric population still leave room for challenges when considering operative intervention in this group of patients.

In 1977, Carnevale and colleagues [150] first described MIS in pediatric trauma specifically as a diagnostic tool in abdominal trauma. In this report, 20 patients presenting with abdominal trauma (5 children aged 4–17 years) underwent diagnostic laparoscopy. All 5 children showed evidence of nonactive injury (eg, nonbleeding liver laceration) and were spared an open laparotomy. For unclear reasons, interest was not sustained after this report; but as minimally invasive techniques have increased in use and in some cases become the standard of care for certain pediatric surgical conditions, there has been increasing interest in the application of these techniques in the management of injured children [147]. Both laparoscopic and thoracoscopic techniques have become important diagnostic and therapeutic tools in the evaluation of blunt and penetrating abdominal and thoracic injuries.

The main proposed benefit of minimally invasive techniques is the avoidance of negative thoracotomies and laparotomies, which, in trauma patients, usually constitute generous incisions to allow for comprehensive exploration. As discussed throughout this article, these incisions can be associated with significant morbidity [149]. In 2006, Feliz and colleagues [148] conducted a retrospective review of a pediatric level 1 trauma center database. Of their 7127 trauma admissions, 113 had abdominal explorations for blunt and penetrating trauma. Thirty-two patients (28%) had laparoscopy performed, and the results were positive for injury in 23 patients (72%) and negative for injury in 9 (28%). In looking at the 23 patients found to have injuries, laparoscopy was diagnostic and nontherapeutic in 3 (10%) patients with nonexpanding hematomas. Laparoscopy was both diagnostic and therapeutic in 6 patients (19%). Finally, laparoscopy assisted in the diagnosis and subsequent open repair in 14 patients (44%). Laparotomy was avoided in 18 patients (56%). They reported no missed injuries or complications and concluded that laparoscopy reduces the morbidity of a negative laparotomy and is a safe method for the evaluation and treatment of traumatic injuries in hemodynamically stable pediatric patients. In 2010, Marwan and colleagues [151] reported similar findings and conclusions regarding the utility and effectiveness of laparoscopy but questioned the value of laparoscopy in cases with delayed presentation as there was a significant difference in the success rate of laparoscopy between acute and delayed cases. In terms of specific injuries, in 2012, Iqbal and colleagues [152] performed a retrospective review of traumatic pancreatic injuries at 6 large-volume trauma centers and found that the outcomes of those who had a laparoscopic distal pancreatectomy had similar outcomes as those undergoing open resection. Although these studies showed laparoscopy to be useful and effective, there are still disadvantages and areas of concern commonly mentioned when it comes to using laparoscopy in acutely injured pediatric patients. However, the authors reported that in select patients with isolated traumatic pancreatic transection, laparoscopic distal pancreatectomy is very successful in the management of these patients with excellent results (Figs. 14 and 15) [153]. See Table 6 for a list of commonly cited advantages and disadvantages of laparoscopy in trauma.

With regard to thoracic trauma, though there have been a few reports of the use of thoracoscopy in penetrating and blunt thoracic injury, at this point for most pediatric patients, thoracotomy remains the gold standard operative approach [147,154,155]. Although evaluation of the diaphragm is most often accomplished laparoscopically, thoracoscopic evaluation has also been accepted as an approach.

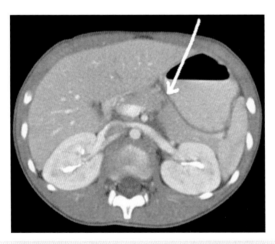

Fig. 14. Traumatic pancreatic laceration (*arrow*). This injury was successfully managed laparoscopically with distal pancreatectomy.

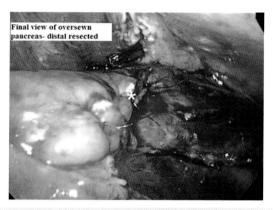

Fig. 15. Intraoperative photograph of pancreatic transection and oversewn proximal pancreatic stump (*star*).

Overall, minimally invasive approaches have diagnostic and therapeutic value in the management of pediatric patients. As advances in technology continue, it is expected that the indications for use in pediatric trauma will continue to expand.

Inflammatory bowel disease

Inflammatory bowel disease (IBD) describes a spectrum of idiopathic and progressive intestinal inflammatory conditions that includes Crohn disease (CD), ulcerative colitis (UC), and indeterminate colitis. Approximately 1 million individuals are affected by IBD in the United States, with 10% to 25% in the pediatric age range [156]. Studies have shown the incidence of pediatric IBD to be

Table 6
Commonly cited advantages and disadvantages of laparoscopy in pediatric trauma patients

	Advantages	Disadvantages
Laparoscopic	• Allows for definitive laparoscopic treatment or conversion to open • Small extensions of umbilical incision (mini-laparotomy) can be used after inspection of abdominal cavity when intracorporeal repair is precluded • Maintenance of bowel in abdomen (less tissue trauma, less temperature and fluid shifts) • Decreased postoperative pain • Shorter hospital stay • Potentially decreased incidence of adhesions/bowel obstructions	• Increased risk of missed injury (false-negative rate approximately 16%–20%) • Trocar site injury • Air embolism • Damage to surrounding structures (omental vessels, splenic capsule) • Increased preoperative setup time in critically injured patients

Data from Refs. [151,218–222]

approximately 7 per 100,000 [157]. The mainstay of management in these patients is primarily medical with immunomodulators and high-dose steroids. Pediatric surgeons typically become involved in the care of children and adolescents with IBD when they become unresponsive to medical therapy, show evidence of developmental delay and nutritional deficiency, or when complications arise. These children often require long-term hyperalimentation, and the chronic nature of the disease may have psychosocial consequences, as they may be unable to attend school or participate in school functions/activities to the level of their similar-aged colleagues.

Because there is no surgical cure for CD (recurrence rates after surgical resection are approximately 25%), surgical therapy is aimed at disease palliation and complication management [158,159]. Despite this, approximately 58% to 92% of patients who have CD will require surgery, depending on the location of the disease [160]. The indications for surgical therapy in patients who have CD are failure of medical therapy or complications of their disease, including stricture, bowel obstruction, hemorrhage, perforation, fistula formation, or abscess. Most patients who undergo surgical therapy for CD have an isolated stricture in the terminal ileum for which an ileocecectomy is required [161]. Laparoscopic-assisted ileocolic resection is an acceptable alternative to traditional open resection in the adult population even in the presence of abscesses and active fistulas, which were initially thought to be contraindications to laparoscopic surgery [162–164]. In 2001, Diamond and Langer [165] published the first report of laparoscopic-assisted ileocecetomy in adolescents. They performed a retrospective review of all adolescents undergoing ileocolic resection for CD. Eleven patients had open resection, and 12 patients had laparoscopic-assisted resection. They found no significant differences in operative time, time to regular diet, or postoperative complications, though the laparoscopic-assisted group was discharged in a significantly shorter time than the patients receiving open resection (2.2 days) [165]. They concluded that lap-assisted ileocecetomy was a safe alternative to open resection in adolescent patients. Shortly after that, von Allmen and colleagues [166] reported similar results from their retrospective review. Their 5-year retrospective review of 12 patients undergoing laparoscopic resection and 16 patients undergoing open resection revealed that the laparoscopic group had significantly shorter hospital stays, decreased days of parenteral narcotics, and a more rapid return to regular diet. They concluded that the laparoscopic approach was more advantageous for patients undergoing initial segmental resection for CD. In these and other studies [167], an extracorporeal anastomosis was performed through a 3- to 5-cm incision. In 2003, Dutta and colleagues [168] published their prospective study of a completely laparoscopic resection in pediatric patients with CD. An intracorporeal anastomosis was performed with no intraoperative complications in 15 patients. Postoperatively, one patient developed a small anastomotic leak on postoperative day 3 and was managed successfully with nonoperative management; another patient developed an anastomotic stricture 9 months postoperatively that was subsequent managed with a laparoscopic resection. They concluded that the completely laparoscopic approach is feasible and safe in pediatric patients with CD.

In contrast to CD, curative therapy is possible with surgery in UC. Operative management of UC is aimed at removing the colon and rectum with preservation of anal sphincter integrity and function. The most commonly performed operation for pediatric UC is total abdominal proctocolectomy with either a direct ileoanal anastomosis or construction of an ileoanal pouch (J pouch) anastomosis. As with many procedures, technological advances have allowed for minimally invasive techniques to be applied to this procedure in pediatric patients. In 2003, Simon and colleagues [169] described their experience performing proctocolectomies with ileoanal anastomosis in 14 patients with UC. Development of a pelvic abscess was the only complication in one patient that was managed with CT-guided drainage, and they concluded that this procedure was a safe alternative in pediatric patients. In 2010, Fraser and colleagues [170] performed a 10-year retrospective review of 27 patients (10 laparoscopic vs 17 open) receiving surgery for UC. They found no significant differences in operative time or complications with the exception of pouchitis. Those patients who underwent a laparoscopic ileal pouch anal anastomosis had a significantly lower incidence of pouchitis when compared with the open group. Mattiolli and colleagues [171] reported similar outcomes and concluded that the laparoscopic approach had become their preferred approach for the management of pediatric patients with IBD.

Overall, in the hands of an experienced laparoscopic surgeon, minimally invasive resection is safe, feasible, and effective for the management of pediatric IBD (Fig. 16). Further studies are needed to assess long-term outcomes moving forward.

Biliary surgery

Choledochal cysts and biliary atresia are the most common indications for biliary reconstruction in pediatric surgery. Surgical management of these conditions involves dissection and resection of bile ducts and reconstruction of biliary drainage using small intestine [172]. The conventional surgical approach for the treatment of biliary atresia or choledochal cysts consists of a generous muscle-cutting laparotomy to expose the critical structures necessary to accomplish the biliary dissection and creation of portoenterostomy in biliary atresia or a choledochojejunostomy/hepaticojejunostomy or hepaticoduodenostomy in the treatment of a choledochal cyst [172–174]. Farello and colleagues [175] reported the first laparoscopic choledochal cyst excision performed in a child in 1995, and Esteves and colleagues [176] reported the first laparoscopic Kasai in 2002. More recently, several cases of laparoscopic Kasai and choledochal cyst repairs have been reported, though very few compare this approach with the open approach. In 2007, Aspelund and colleagues [172] reported their experience comparing open and laparoscopic Kasai and choledochal cyst resection procedures. Over a period of 6 years, 5 laparoscopic and 25 open Kasai procedures were performed along with 4 laparoscopic and 12 open choledochal cyst resections. In

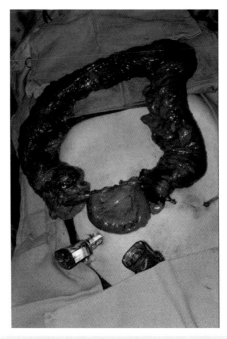

Fig. 16. Laparoscopic total abdominal colectomy for UC in teenaged patient. Notice that the entire colon can be mobilized through relatively small umbilical incision.

their analysis, they found no significant differences in outcomes between the groups and concluded that the laparoscopic approach was feasible and safe in this population. They did report that disadvantages of this approach include the loss of haptic feedback, a 2-dimensional image, and nonarticulating instruments that all lengthen operative time (though not significantly) and may make the learning curve significant. In 2010, Nguyen Thanh and colleagues [177] reported their 12-year experience performing 190 laparoscopic choledochal cyst resections in pediatric patients aged between 2 and 16 years. Of these 190 all of the cyst resections were completed laparoscopically regardless of cyst diameter. Two procedures (1.1%) were converted to open to complete the hepaticojejunostomy. Postoperative leaks occurred in 7 patients (3.7%); however, 6 of these resolved without operative management. Open-approach postoperative leaks have been reported at upwards of 6% (Figs. 17 and 18) [178].

Although the laparoscopic approach has been found to be successful and effective, the disadvantages mentioned earlier have led others to seek out novel approaches to these procedures. In 2006, Woo and colleagues [179] performed the first robotic choledochal cyst resection. In 2007, Meehan and colleagues [180] were the first to present their experience with 2 robotic-assisted Kasai procedures and 2 completely robotic choledochal cyst repairs. The researchers suggested that robotic surgery may provide solutions to some of the difficulties encountered with the laparoscopic approach. They proposed that the

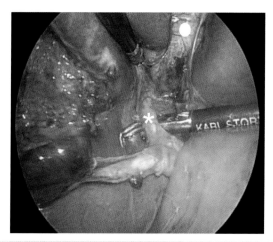

Fig. 17. Laparoscopic choledochal cyst resection. Dissection of biliary structures. Gall-bladder is retracted to screen left (*circle*), and the common hepatic duct is being dissected (*star*). Choledochal cyst is everything below dissector.

articulating robotic instruments offer better dexterity and range of motion than the more rigid laparoscopic tools when it comes to dissecting, suturing, and knot tying, which are most advantageous when it comes to creating the hepaticojejunostomy. In addition, the 3-dimensional camera with high magnification

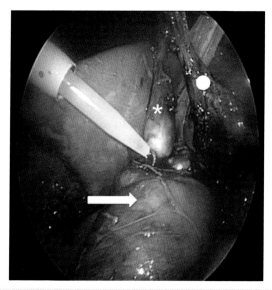

Fig. 18. Laparoscopic choledochal cyst resection with ligation of cyst. Gallbladder is re-tracted to the right (*circle*), and the duodenum is in the foreground of the picture (*arrow*). The distal choledochal cyst (*star*) is held straight up anteriorly and ligated distally with the Endoloop ™ (Ethicon corporation, Cincinnati, OH, USA).

may aid in the dissection of delicate biliary structures. Since these early reports, less than 40 of these procedures have been performed, thus, limiting the ability to perform a meaningful surgical approach comparison. As robotic surgery continues to advance (see "Novel and developing advances in MIS"), the robotic approach to biliary surgery in the pediatric population may become more used.

Endorectal pull-through for anorectal disorders

In 1886, Harold Hirschsprung first described Hirschsprung disease as a cause of constipation in early infancy resulting from the absence of enteric neurons within the myenteric and submucosal plexus of the rectum and colon, which leads to dysmotility. With an incidence of 1 in 5000 live births, early recognition and surgical correction protects affected infants from enterocolitis, obstruction, and debilitating constipation [181]. In 1949, Swenson [182] was the first to report successful surgical correction of Hirschsprung disease in 1948. The basic principles of the repair included resection of the distal aganglionic bowel with reanastomosis of the healthy colon (now neorectum) to the anus while preserving the anal sphincter and avoiding injury to the genitourinary tract [3]. The subsequent modifications of this procedure (specifically the endorectal pull-through) included a diverting ostomy and were aimed at limiting pelvic dissection to minimize the occurrence of urinary incontinence and reproductive organ dysfunction. In 1980, So and colleagues [183] performed the first endorectal pull-through without the placement of a diverting ostomy. This performance was followed in 1995 by the first laparoscopic endorectal pull-through by Georgeson and colleagues [184]. Although a completely transanal approach was also developed and eliminated the need for an intra-abdominal approach, the laparoscopic approach was thought to provide many advantages.

   In 1999, Georgeson and colleagues [185], from 6 pediatric centers, reported on their experience with laparoscopic endorectal pull-through in 80 patients over a 5-year period. Their results revealed average operative times of 2.5 hours, greater than 90% of patients with return of bowel function within 24 hours postoperatively, patient mean discharge time of 3.7 days, and a 28-hour average time to feeding. Early postoperative complications included anastomotic leak (2.5%), recurrent constipation (1%), chronic diarrhea (7%), and enterocolitis (8%). Four patients from the series subsequently required diversion. Two of those patients required diversion for management of anastomotic leaks; one required diversion for severe enterocolitis; and the final patient required diversion for a congenital syndrome. They concluded that overall the laparoscopic endorectal pull-through was characterized by shorter operative and postoperative recovery times as well as fewer perioperative complications [186]. It has been highlighted why the laparoscopic technique provided advantages that would be appealing to pediatric surgeons in contrast to the traditional pull-through techniques [185,186]. First, MIS techniques avoid laparotomy, which minimize peritoneal trauma; secondly, and importantly, using laparoscopy before the transanal endorectal dissection allows the surgeon to more precisely determine the transition zone via biopsy. Finally, laparoscopic mobilization of the rectosigmoid colon minimizes the potential for overdilating the internal anal sphincter, which could compromise fecal continence during the transanal dissection [186]. The laparoscopic approach has also been found to be useful in cases of obstruction secondary to residual aganglionosis when redo operation is necessary [187]. This procedure is now the standard procedure used across many pediatric centers for the management of Hirschsprung with much success. In 2010, Muensterer and colleagues [188] reported on the first single-incision laparoscopic endorectal pull-through with early results that were similar to the conventional laparoscopic approach. More patients and long-term data are needed to make conclusions about the advantages this approach may bring to the management of these patients.

The laparoscopic approach is also useful in repair of high anorectal malformations. Posterior sagittal anorectoplasty (PSARP) first introduced by deVries and Peña [189] is mostly recognized as the standard surgical management of imperforate anus. It requires an incision from the coccyx to the perineal body to provide wide exposure of the external sphincter, levators, rectum, and distal fistula to allow for repair. Before this procedure, patients typically require laparotomy for a diverting colostomy at birth followed by a PSARP after several months of growth. Despite the success of this procedure, only approximately 25% of patients experienced normal continence postoperatively; many require aggressive bowel management [190–192]. In 2000, Georgeson and colleagues [193] proposed the laparoscopic-assisted anorectal pull-through (LAARP) for repair of high imperforate anus. The proposed benefits are that this procedure provides excellent visualization of the deep pelvis and rectal fistula and avoids division of the anal sphincters and levators, which may impact continence. Several studies have shown that the LAARP for high anorectal malformations has equivalent early outcomes when compared with the PSARP as well as a higher incidence of the presence of an anorectal reflex [192,194,195]. The reflex is a manometric expression of the presence of intact perirectal innervation and sphincteric function. Although there are no long-term studies that compare these two procedures, as technology improves and more long-term outcome data are available, this procedure may become the standard of care for the management of these patients.

NOVEL AND DEVELOPING ADVANCES IN MIS

The key to continued success in any field requires a commitment to innovation and to constructively challenging what is considered the standard quo. Although MIS has dramatically changed surgery and patient outcomes over the last several decades, surgeons continue to strive for improvement and advancement of these techniques. In the last 5 years, several new approaches have been developed for use in pediatric patients. Some of these techniques have been briefly mentioned in prior individual sections but deserve further elaboration here.

Single-incision laparoscopic surgery

The advent of single-incision laparoscopic surgery (SILS) began largely in adult surgery. SILS was largely driven by internal and public desire to limit visible scars. Natural orifice transluminal endoscopic surgery (NOTES) was suggested as a potential answer to this dilemma as the entire operation is performed by passing an endoscope through the mouth or vagina [196–198]. An enterotomy is then created in the stomach or vagina to gain access to the abdominal cavity and perform the operation. Challengers of this technique questioned whether obtaining cosmesis was worth the risk of creating an iatrogenic injury to an otherwise normal viscus [199]. Soon after, many of these opponents realized that the same technology of NOTES could be applied through the umbilicus by placing multiple instruments through one single umbilical incision, which resulted in several single-incision procedures, including cholecystectomy and appendectomy, being performed in adults in 2008 and 2009 [199–202]. Shortly after the success of SILS operations, these procedures were attempted in children by Ponsky [199], Dutta [203], and Rothenberg [204] in 2009. In 2010, Muensterer and colleagues [205] first reported single incision procedures in infants. In 2011, Hansen and colleagues [206] reported on the largest series thus far. Over a period of 13 months, 224 pediatric single-incision cases were performed. See Table 7 for the individual procedures performed. They experienced 5 complications, most of which were thermal injury to bowel or traction injuries. All of these except one were managed with conversion to 2 or 3 ports, and none resulted in laparotomy. In addition to their results, the researchers commented on what they considered to be the most challenging aspects of SILS. Trocar and instrument crowding, intra-abdominal exposure, decreased degrees of freedom, suturing, and in-line endoscope viewing were all cited as potential challenges. The researchers suggested techniques like transabdominal

Table 7
Single-incision surgeries performed by Hansen and colleagues [206]

Appendectomy	130
Pyloromyotomy	32
Cholecystectomy	32
Inguinal hernia repairs	11
Nissen fundoplication	6
Laparoscopic-assisted endorectal pull-through	4
Splenectomy	2
Ileocecetomy	2
Total abdominal colectomy	1
Lung biopsy	1
Ovarian cyst aspiration	1
Diagnostic laparoscopy with running of the bowel	1
Peritoneal dialysis catheter revision	1
Total	224

Surgeries performed in largest series to date of single-incision surgery in pediatric patients.
   Data from Gumbs AA, Milone L, Sinha P, et al. Totally transumbilical laparoscopic cholecystectomy. J Gastrointest Surg 2009;13(3):533–4.

retraction sutures, lower profile trocars, angled scopes, and extracorporeal suturing as some of the techniques that can help mitigate these challenges. Although this study and the others discussed speak to the feasibility and safety of these procedures in the pediatric population, further long-term outcome studies are needed as well as further modifications in technology to further mitigate the challenges of this procedure before this technique will have broad application in pediatric surgery.

Endoscopy

The use of endoscopy as an adjunct or alternative to minimally invasive procedures continues to evolve and has shown promise in the adult population [207–209]. These techniques have been reported in children only recently [210,211]. In 2013, Davenport and colleagues [211] reported on their experience performing 30 endoscopic or endoscopic-assisted procedures in children from 2007 to 2010. They defined endoscopy as the successful passage of the endoscope to an area of anatomic abnormality wherein a diagnosis or therapeutic intervention could be achieved. Endoscopy-assisted thoracoscopy was performed in 10 patients (Table 8). For thoracoscopic-assisted esophageal resections, such as diverticulum or duplication cyst resections, the endoscope was used intraoperatively to confirm intact submucosa and the absence of a leak following resection. This confirmation allowed patients to avoid chest tube placement and postoperative upper gastrointestinal contrast studies. For gastroduodenal cases (see Table 8), endoscopy-assisted laparoscopic duodenoduodenostomy was performed in 6 patients (5 for duodenal atresia and 1 for annular pancreas). Intraoperative endoscopy was a useful adjunct for both identifying the atresia and also assessing the anastomosis postlaparoscopic repair. In their 30 cases, no intraoperative complications occurred; the postoperative complications encountered (stricture, postoperative stridor, and esophageal leak) were each managed conservatively. They suggested the use of

Table 8
Endoscopy-assisted procedures performed by Davenport and colleagues [211]

Procedure performed	No. of cases	Indication
Endoscopy-assisted thoracoscopy	10	• Esophageal stricture (5) • Esophageal diverticulum (2) • Esophageal duplication cyst (3)
Endoscopy-assisted laparoscopic duodenoduodenostomy	8	• Duodenal web (5) • Duodenal atresia (3)
Endoscopy + laparoscopic wedge resection	3	• Perforated gastric ulcer (2) • Gastric mass (1)
Endoscopic and percutaneous gastrostomy tube placement	2	• Displaced gastrostomy tube
Endoscopic detorsion and laparoscopic gastropexy	1	• Gastric volvulus
Endoscopic balloon dilation and laparoscopic pyloromyotomy	1	• Pylorospasm

endoscopy in pediatric patients who are not critically ill, have pathology that may be treated by purely endoscopic methods (eg, esophageal stricture dilation) and those that have the potential that endoscopy can assist in identifying alternative pathologies (Figs. 19–22). Although more literature documenting experience with these techniques is needed, the initial results suggest that the use of endoscopy as an adjunctive or alternative surgical approach is safe, effective, and potentially promising.

Robotic surgery

As discussed in the "Biliary surgery" section, robotic surgery is a technology that offers 3-dimensional visualization, instrument articulation, and tremor filtering that has become popular in adult surgery. Pediatric urology was the first division of pediatric surgery to attempt this approach on children with general success [212–215]. In 2008, Meehan and Sandler [216] published the first comprehensive report of robotic surgery in 100 children undergoing general surgery. Twenty-four different procedures were performed (89% abdominal, 11% thoracic) (Box 3). Thirteen percent of the procedures were converted to open, but no conversions or complications occurred as a result of injuries from robotic instruments. In terms of the learning curve, they reported comfort with performing different cases in less than 15 cases per procedure. This finding is less than the learning curve required for some laparoscopic

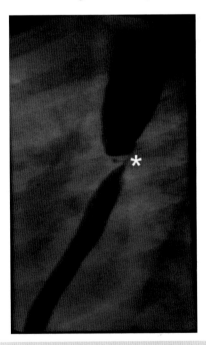

Fig. 19. Upper gastrointestinal series of a 5-year-old patient with a lye stricture (*star*) managed with a gastrostomy tube and was unable to take oral feeds.

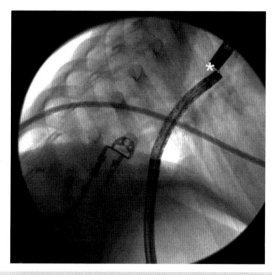

Fig. 20. Two endoscopes are passed through patient's mouth and gastrostomy tube, respectively, to identify strictured area (*star*).

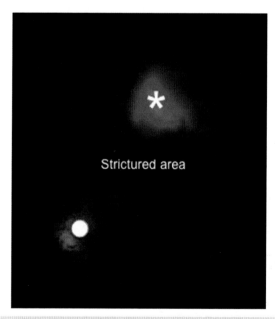

Strictured area

Fig. 21. Right VATS view of endoscopes in upper and lower esophagus at site of stricture. The proximal esophagus (*star*) and distal esophagus (*circle*) are illuminated by the light from the endoscopes. The stricture is the dark area in between the endoscope illuminations; this helps to identify the targeted area of resection.

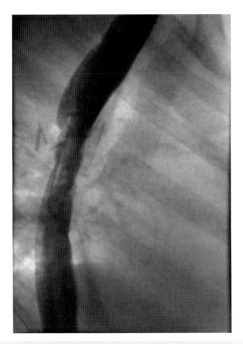

Fig. 22. The patient's normal postoperative esophagram following right VATS resection of the stricture and primary esophageal anastomosis.

Box 3: Partial list of procedures that have been successfully performed via robotic surgery in pediatric patients

Nissen fundoplication

Ladd procedure

Cholecystectomy

Splenectomy

Adrenalectomy

Total proctocolectomy with pull-through

CDH repair (both thoracic and abdominal approaches)

Kasai procedure

Total pyloroplasty

Mediastinal teratoma resection

Meckel diverticulectomy

Pancreatic tumor resection

Heller myotomy

Bronchogenic cyst resection

Congenital cystic adenomatoid malformation resection

procedures [108], and they cited the absence of the fulcrum effect and 3-dimensional magnification as possible reasons for this difference in learning curve. Although significant cost was thought to be the factor that could limit the progress of pediatric robotic surgery, they concluded that with successful team planning, a wide variety of procedures can be performed safely and effectively in pediatric patients. In 2010, Albassam and colleagues [217] reported on 50 children receiving Nissen fundoplications. Twenty-five patients received the laparoscopic approach, whereas the other 25 underwent robotic fundoplication. Their results showed no significant differences in hospital stay, postoperative complications, or postoperative analgesia and agreed with Meehan and Sandler [216] that robotic surgery is feasible in pediatric patients but that the significant cost should limit this approach to only specific procedures.

Overall, robotic surgery is a safe and effective surgical approach in children. Long-term outcome studies as well as cost-reduction strategies are needed in the future to really gage the impact of this technology on the pediatric population.

SUMMARY

Surgery has changed dramatically over the last several decades. The emergence of MIS has allowed pediatric surgeons to manage critically ill neonates, children, and adolescents with improved outcomes in pain, postoperative course, cosmesis, and return to normal activity. Procedures that were once thought to be too difficult to attempt or even contraindicated in pediatric patients in many instances are now the standard of care. New and emerging techniques, such as single-incision laparoscopy, endoscopy-assisted surgery, robotic surgery, and techniques yet to be developed, all hold and reveal the potential for even further advancement in the management of these patients. The future of MIS in pediatrics is exciting; as long as our primary focus remains centered on developing techniques that limit morbidity and maximize positive outcomes for young patients and their families, the possibilities are both promising and infinite.

References

[1] Muhe E. Long-term follow-up after laparoscopic cholecystectomy. Endoscopy 1992;24(9): 754–8.
[2] Dubois F, Berthelot G, Levard H. Cholecystectomy by coelioscopy. Presse Med 1989;18(19):980–2 [in French].
[3] Georgeson KE, Robertson DJ. Minimally invasive surgery in the neonate: review of current evidence. Semin Perinatol 2004;28(3):212–20.
[4] Georgeson KE, Owings E. Advances in minimally invasive surgery in children. Am J Surg 2000;180(5):362–4.
[5] Blatnik JA, Ponsky TA. Advances in minimally invasive surgery in pediatrics. Curr Gastroenterol Rep 2010;12(3):211–4.
[6] Ure BM, Bax NM, van der Zee DC. Laparoscopy in infants and children: a prospective study on feasibility and the impact on routine surgery. J Pediatr Surg 2000;35(8):1170–3.
[7] Bal S, Elshershari H, Celiker R, et al. Thoracic sequels after thoracotomies in children with congenital cardiac disease. Cardiol Young 2003;13(3):264–7.

[8] Bianchi A, Sowande O, Alizai NK, et al. Aesthetics and lateral thoracotomy in the neonate. J Pediatr Surg 1998;33(12):1798–800.

[9] Cherup LL, Siewers RD, Futrell JW. Breast and pectoral muscle maldevelopment after antero-lateral and posterolateral thoracotomies in children. Ann Thorac Surg 1986;41(5):492–7.

[10] Rodgers BM, Talbert JL. Thoracoscopy for diagnosis of intrathoracic lesions in children. J Pediatr Surg 1976;11(5):703–8.

[11] Holcomb GW 3rd, Rothenberg SS, Bax KM, et al. Thoracoscopic repair of esophageal atresia and tracheoesophageal fistula: a multi-institutional analysis. Ann Surg 2005;242(3):422–8 [discussion: 428–30].

[12] Ure BM, Schmidt AI, Jesch NK. Thoracoscopic surgery in infants and children. Eur J Pediatr Surg 2005;15(5):314–8.

[13] Diamond IR, Herrera P, Langer JC, et al. Thoracoscopic versus open resection of congenital lung lesions: a case-matched study. J Pediatr Surg 2007;42(6):1057–61.

[14] Lawal TA, Gosemann JH, Kuebler JF, et al. Thoracoscopy versus thoracotomy improves midterm musculoskeletal status and cosmesis in infants and children. Ann Thorac Surg 2009;87(1):224–8.

[15] Nagahiro I, Andou A, Aoe M, et al. Pulmonary function, postoperative pain, and serum cytokine level after lobectomy: a comparison of VATS and conventional procedure. Ann Thorac Surg 2001;72(2):362–5.

[16] Rothenberg SS. First decade's experience with thoracoscopic lobectomy in infants and children. J Pediatr Surg 2008;43(1):40–4 [discussion: 45].

[17] Lobe TE, Rothenberg SS, Waldschmidt J. Thoracoscopic repair of esophageal atresia in an infant: a surgical first. Journal of Laparoendoscopic and Advanced Surgical Techniques A 1999;3:141–8.

[18] Rothenberg SS. Thoracoscopic repair of tracheoesophageal fistula in a newborn infant. Journal of Laparoendoscopic and Advanced Surgical Techniques A 2000;4:289–94.

[19] Rothenberg SS. Thoracoscopic repair of tracheoesophageal fistula in newborns. J Pediatr Surg 2002;37(6):869–72.

[20] Bax KM, van Der Zee DC. Feasibility of thoracoscopic repair of esophageal atresia with distal fistula. J Pediatr Surg 2002;37(2):192–6.

[21] van der Zee DC, Bax NM. Thoracoscopic repair of esophageal atresia with distal fistula. Surg Endosc 2003;17(7):1065–7.

[22] Burford JM, Dassinger MS, Copeland DR, et al. Repair of esophageal atresia with tracheoesophageal fistula via thoracotomy: a contemporary series. Am J Surg 2011;202(2):203–6.

[23] Rothenberg SS. Thoracoscopic repair of esophageal atresia and tracheoesophageal fistula in neonates, first decade's experience. Dis Esophagus 2013;26(4):359–64.

[24] Nguyen T, Zainabadi K, Bui T, et al. Thoracoscopic repair of esophageal atresia and tracheoesophageal fistula: lessons learned. J Laparoendosc Adv Surg Tech A 2006;16(2):174–8.

[25] Hicks LM, Mansfield PB. Esophageal atresia and tracheoesophageal fistula. Review of thirteen years' experience. J Thorac Cardiovasc Surg 1981;81(3):358–63.

[26] McKinnon LJ, Kosloske AM. Prediction and prevention of anastomotic complications of esophageal atresia and tracheoesophageal fistula. J Pediatr Surg 1990;25(7):778–81.

[27] Colvin J, Bower C, Dickinson JE, et al. Outcomes of congenital diaphragmatic hernia: a population-based study in Western Australia. Pediatrics 2005;116(3):e356–63.

[28] Gallot D, Boda C, Ughetto S, et al. Prenatal detection and outcome of congenital diaphragmatic hernia: a French registry-based study. Ultrasound Obstet Gynecol 2007;29(3):276–83.

[29] Smith NP, Jesudason EC, Featherstone NC, et al. Recent advances in congenital diaphragmatic hernia. Arch Dis Child 2005;90(4):426–8.

[30] van den Hout L, Sluiter I, Gischler S, et al. Can we improve outcome of congenital diaphragmatic hernia? Pediatr Surg Int 2009;25(9):733–43.

[31] Lansdale N, Alam S, Losty PD, et al. Neonatal endosurgical congenital diaphragmatic hernia repair: a systematic review and meta-analysis. Ann Surg 2010;252(1):20–6.

[32] Harrison MR, Adzick NS, Bullard KM, et al. Correction of congenital diaphragmatic hernia in utero VII: a prospective trial. J Pediatr Surg 1997;32(11):1637–42.

[33] Harrison MR, Keller RL, Hawgood SB, et al. A randomized trial of fetal endoscopic tracheal occlusion for severe fetal congenital diaphragmatic hernia. N Engl J Med 2003;349(20):1916–24.

[34] Harrison MR, Sydorak RM, Farrell JA, et al. Fetoscopic temporary tracheal occlusion for congenital diaphragmatic hernia: prelude to a randomized, controlled trial. J Pediatr Surg 2003;38(7):1012–20.

[35] Gomes Ferreira C, Reinberg O, Becmeur F, et al. Neonatal minimally invasive surgery for congenital diaphragmatic hernias: a multicenter study using thoracoscopy or laparoscopy. Surg Endosc 2009;23(7):1650–9.

[36] Kalfa N, Allal H, Raux O, et al. Multicentric assessment of the safety of neonatal videosurgery. Surg Endosc 2007;21(2):303–8.

[37] van der Zee DC, Bax NM. Laparoscopic repair of congenital diaphragmatic hernia in a 6-month-old child. Surg Endosc 1995;9(9):1001–3.

[38] Rothenberg SS, Chang JH, Bealer JF. Experience with minimally invasive surgery in infants. Am J Surg 1998;176(6):654–8.

[39] Becmeur F, Jamali RR, Moog R, et al. Thoracoscopic treatment for delayed presentation of congenital diaphragmatic hernia in the infant. A report of three cases. Surg Endosc 2001;15(10):1163–6.

[40] Yang EY, Allmendinger N, Johnson SM, et al. Neonatal thoracoscopic repair of congenital diaphragmatic hernia: selection criteria for successful outcome. J Pediatr Surg 2005;40(9):1369–75.

[41] Schaarschmidt K, Strauss J, Kolberg-Schwerdt A, et al. Thoracoscopic repair of congenital diaphragmatic hernia by inflation-assisted bowel reduction, in a resuscitated neonate: a better access? Pediatr Surg Int 2005;21(10):806–8.

[42] Cho SD, Krishnaswami S, McKee JC, et al. Analysis of 29 consecutive thoracoscopic repairs of congenital diaphragmatic hernia in neonates compared to historical controls. J Pediatr Surg 2009;44(1):80–6 [discussion: 86].

[43] Kim AC, Bryner BS, Akay B, et al. Thoracoscopic repair of congenital diaphragmatic hernia in neonates: lessons learned. J Laparoendosc Adv Surg Tech A 2009;19(4):575–80.

[44] Gourlay DM, Cassidy LD, Sato TT, et al. Beyond feasibility: a comparison of newborns undergoing thoracoscopic and open repair of congenital diaphragmatic hernias. J Pediatr Surg 2009;44(9):1702–7.

[45] Hamilton BD, Gatti JM, Cartwright PC, et al. Comparison of laparoscopic versus open nephrectomy in the pediatric population. J Urol 2000;163(3):937–9.

[46] Koivusalo AI, Korpela R, Wirtavuori K, et al. A single-blinded, randomized comparison of laparoscopic versus open hernia repair in children. Pediatrics 2009;123(1):332–7.

[47] Rothenberg SS. Experience with 220 consecutive laparoscopic Nissen fundoplications in infants and children. J Pediatr Surg 1998;33(2):274–8.

[48] Shah AV, Shah AA. Laparoscopic approach to surgical management of congenital diaphragmatic hernia in the newborn. J Pediatr Surg 2002;37(3):548–50.

[49] Shah SR, Wishnew J, Barsness K, et al. Minimally invasive congenital diaphragmatic hernia repair: a 7-year review of one institution's experience. Surg Endosc 2009;23(6):1265–71.

[50] Rothenberg SS. Thoracoscopic lung resection in children. J Pediatr Surg 2000;35(2):271–4 [discussion: 274–5].

[51] Merry CM, Bufo AJ, Shah RS, et al. Early definitive intervention by thoracoscopy in pediatric empyema. J Pediatr Surg 1999;34(1):178–80 [discussion: 180–1].

[52] Partrick DA, Rothenberg SS. Thoracoscopic resection of mediastinal masses in infants and children: an evaluation of technique and results. J Pediatr Surg 2001;36(8):1165–7.

[53] Fan LL, Kozinetz CA, Wojtczak HA, et al. Diagnostic value of transbronchial, thoraco-scopic, and open lung biopsy in immunocompetent children with chronic interstitial lung disease. J Pediatr 1997;131(4):565–9.

[54] Rothenberg SS. Thoracoscopic pulmonary surgery. Semin Pediatr Surg 2007;16(4): 231–7.

[55] Rothenberg SS. Experience with thoracoscopic lobectomy in infants and children. J Pediatr Surg 2003;38(1):102–4.

[56] Albanese CT, Sydorak RM, Tsao K, et al. Thoracoscopic lobectomy for prenatally diag-nosed lung lesions. J Pediatr Surg 2003;38(4):553–5.

[57] Albanese CT, Rothenberg SS. Experience with 144 consecutive pediatric thoracoscopic lobectomies. J Laparoendosc Adv Surg Tech A 2007;17(3):339–41.

[58] Vu LT, Farmer DL, Nobuhara KK, et al. Thoracoscopic versus open resection for congenital cystic adenomatoid malformations of the lung. J Pediatr Surg 2008;43(1):35–9.

[59] Panieri E, Rode H, Millar AJ, et al. Oesophageal replacement in the management of cor-rosive strictures: when is surgery indicated? Pediatr Surg Int 1998;13(5–6):336–40.

[60] Luketich JD, Alvelo-Rivera M, Buenaventura PO, et al. Minimally invasive esophagectomy: outcomes in 222 patients. Ann Surg 2003;238(4):486–94 [discussion: 494–5].

[61] Nguyen NT, Gelfand D, Stevens CM, et al. Current status of minimally invasive esophagec-tomy. Minerva Chir 2004;59(5):437–46.

[62] Cury EK, Schraibman V, De Vasconcelos Macedo AL, et al. Thoracoscopic esophagec-tomy in children. J Pediatr Surg 2001;36(9):E17.

[63] Nwomeh BC, Luketich JD, Kane TD. Minimally invasive esophagectomy for caustic esoph-ageal stricture in children. J Pediatr Surg 2004;39(7):e1–6.

[64] Kane TD, Nwomeh BC, Nadler EP. Thoracoscopic-assisted esophagectomy and laparo-scopic gastric pull-up for lye injury. JSLS 2007;11(4):474–80.

[65] Shalaby R, Shams A, Soliman SM, et al. Laparoscopically assisted transhiatal esophagec-tomy with esophagogastroplasty for post-corrosive esophageal stricture treatment in chil-dren. Pediatr Surg Int 2007;23(6):545–9.

[66] van der Zee DC, Bax NM. Thoracoscopic tracheoaortopexia for the treatment of life-threatening events in tracheomalacia. Surg Endosc 2007;21(11):2024–5.

[67] Dave S, Currie BG. The role of aortopexy in severe tracheomalacia. J Pediatr Surg 2006;41(3):533–7.

[68] Weber TR, Keller MS, Fiore A. Aortic suspension (aortopexy) for severe tracheomalacia in infants and children. Am J Surg 2002;184(6):573–7 [discussion: 577].

[69] DeCou JM, Parson DS, Gauderer MW. Thoracoscopic aortopexy for severe tracheomala-cia. Journal of Laparoendoscopic and Advanced Surgical Techniques A 2001;5:205–8.

[70] Schaarschmidt K, Kolberg-Schwerdt A, Pietsch L, et al. Thoracoscopic aortopericardioster-nopexy for severe tracheomalacia in toddlers. J Pediatr Surg 2002;37(10):1476–8.

[71] Perger L, Kim HB, Jaksic T, et al. Thoracoscopic aortopexy for treatment of tracheomalacia in infants and children. J Laparoendosc Adv Surg Tech A 2009;19(Suppl 1):S249–54.

[72] Kane TD, Nadler EP, Potoka DA. Thoracoscopic aortopexy for vascular compression of the trachea: approach from the right. J Laparoendosc Adv Surg Tech A 2008;18(2): 313–6.

[73] Scherer LR, Arn PH, Dressel DA, et al. Surgical management of children and young adults with Marfan syndrome and pectus excavatum. J Pediatr Surg 1988;23(12):1169–72.

[74] Goretsky MJ, Kelly RE Jr, Croitoru D, et al. Chest wall anomalies: pectus excavatum and pectus carinatum. Adolesc Med Clin 2004;15(3):455–71.

[75] Molik KA, Engum SA, Rescorla FJ, et al. Pectus excavatum repair: experience with stan-dard and minimal invasive techniques. J Pediatr Surg 2001;36(2):324–8.

[76] Ravitch MM. The operative treatment of pectus excavatum. Ann Surg 1949;129(4): 429–44.

[77] Nuss D, Kelly RE Jr, Croitoru DP, et al. A 10-year review of a minimally invasive technique for the correction of pectus excavatum. J Pediatr Surg 1998;33(4):545–52.

[78] Nuss D. Minimally invasive surgical repair of pectus excavatum. Semin Pediatr Surg 2008;17(3):209–17.

[79] Croitoru DP, Kelly RE Jr, Goretsky MJ, et al. Experience and modification update for the minimally invasive Nuss technique for pectus excavatum repair in 303 patients. J Pediatr Surg 2002;37(3):437–45.

[80] Petersen C, Leonhardt J, Duderstadt M, et al. Minimally invasive repair of pectus excavatum - shifting the paradigm? Eur J Pediatr Surg 2006;16(2):75–8.

[81] Park HJ, Lee SY, Lee CS. Complications associated with the Nuss procedure: analysis of risk factors and suggested measures for prevention of complications. J Pediatr Surg 2005;39: 391–5.

[82] Ong CC, Choo K, Morreau P, et al. The learning curve in learning the curve: a review of Nuss procedure in teenagers. ANZ J Surg 2005;75(6):421–4.

[83] Nuss D, Croitoru DP, Kelly RE Jr, et al. Review and discussion of the complications of minimally invasive pectus excavatum repair. Eur J Pediatr Surg 2002;12(4):230–4.

[84] Nasr A, Fecteau A, Wales PW. Comparison of the Nuss and the Ravitch procedure for pectus excavatum repair: a meta-analysis. J Pediatr Surg 2010;45(5):880–6.

[85] Chen Z, Amos EB, Luo H, et al. Comparative pulmonary functional recovery after Nuss and Ravitch procedures for pectus excavatum repair: a meta-analysis. J Cardiothorac Surg 2012;7:101.

[86] Gans SL, Berci G. Advances in endoscopy of infants and children. J Pediatr Surg 1971;6(2):199–233.

[87] Esposito C, Montupet P. Complications of laparoscopic minimally invasive surgery. Journal of Laparoendoscopic and Advanced Surgical Techniques A 2003;7(1):13–8.

[88] Chen MK, Schropp KP, Lobe TE. Complications of minimal-access surgery in children. J Pediatr Surg 1996;31(8):1161–5.

[89] Bax NM, van der Zee DC. Complications in laparoscopic surgery in children. In: Bax NM, Najmaldin A, Valla JS, editors. Endoscopic surgery in children. Berlin: Springer-Verlag; 1999. p. 357–68.

[90] Esposito C, Montupet P, Amici G, et al. Complications of laparoscopic antireflux surgery in childhood. Surg Endosc 2000;14(7):622–4.

[91] Esposito C, Mattioli G, Monguzzi GL, et al. Complications and conversions of pediatric videosurgery: the Italian multicentric experience on 1689 procedures. Surg Endosc 2002;16(5):795–8.

[92] Al-Qahtani AR, Almaramhi H. Minimal access surgery in neonates and infants. J Pediatr Surg 2006;41(5):910–3.

[93] Olivares P, Tovar JA. Laparoscopic surgery in children. An Esp Pediatr 1998;48(6):620–4 [in Spanish].

[94] Waldschmidt J, Schier F. Laparoscopic surgery in neonates and infants. Eur J Pediatr Surg 1991;1(3):145–50.

[95] Hegar B, Dewanti NR, Kadim M, et al. Natural evolution of regurgitation in healthy infants. Acta Paediatr 2009;98(7):1189–93.

[96] Ostlie DJ. Gastroesophageal reflux. In: Holcomb GW 3rd, editor. Ashcraft's pediatric surgery. Philadelphia: Saunders; 2010. p. 379–90.

[97] Dranove JE. Focus on diagnosis: new technologies for the diagnosis of gastroesophageal reflux disease. Pediatr Rev 2008;29(9):317–20.

[98] Fonkalsrud EW, Ashcraft KW, Coran AG, et al. Surgical treatment of gastroesophageal reflux in children: a combined hospital study of 7467 patients. Pediatrics 1998;101(3 Pt 1):419–22.

[99] Mattioli G, Esposito C, Lima M, et al. Italian multicenter survey on laparoscopic treatment of gastro-esophageal reflux disease in children. Surg Endosc 2002;16(12): 1666–8.

[100] Mattioli G, Repetto P, Carlini C, et al. Laparoscopic vs open approach for the treatment of gastroesophageal reflux in children. Surg Endosc 2002;16(5):750–2.

[101] International Pediatric Endosurgery Group (IPEG). IPEG guidelines for the surgical treatment of pediatric gastroesophageal reflux disease (GERD). J Laparoendosc Adv Surg Tech A 2009;19(Suppl 1):x–xiii.

[102] Esposito C, Montupet P, Reinberg O. Laparoscopic surgery for gastroesophageal reflux disease during the first year of life. J Pediatr Surg 2001;36(5):715–7.

[103] Esposito C, Montupet P, van Der Zee D, et al. Long-term outcome of laparoscopic Nissen, Toupet, and Thal antireflux procedures for neurologically normal children with gastroesophageal reflux disease. Surg Endosc 2006;20(6):855–8.

[104] Chung DH, Georgeson KE. Fundoplication and gastrostomy. Semin Pediatr Surg 1998;7(4):213–9.

[105] Steyaert H, Al Mohaidly M, Lembo MA, et al. Long-term outcome of laparoscopic Nissen and Toupet fundoplication in normal and neurologically impaired children. Surg Endosc 2003;17(4):543–6.

[106] Subramaniam R, Dickson AP. Long-term outcome of Boix-Ochoa and Nissen fundoplication in normal and neurologically impaired children. J Pediatr Surg 2000;35(8):1214–6.

[107] Kubiak R, Andrews J, Grant HW. Long-term outcome of laparoscopic Nissen fundoplication compared with laparoscopic Thal fundoplication in children: a prospective, randomized study. Ann Surg 2011;253(1):44–9.

[108] Meehan JJ, Georgeson KE. The learning curve associated with laparoscopic antireflux surgery in infants and children. J Pediatr Surg 1997;32(3):426–9.

[109] Mayberry JF, Mayell MJ. Epidemiological study of achalasia in children. Gut 1988;29(1):90–3.

[110] Nurko S. Other motor disorders. In: Walker WA, Durie PH, Hamilton JR, et al, editors. Pediatric gastrointestinal disease. St Louis (MO): Mosby; 2000. p. 322–40.

[111] Hussain SZ, Thomas R, Tolia V. A review of achalasia in 33 children. Dig Dis Sci 2002;47(11):2538–43.

[112] Askegard-Giesmann JR, Grams JM, Hanna AM, et al. Minimally invasive Heller's myotomy in children: safe and effective. J Pediatr Surg 2009;44(5):909–11.

[113] Robertson FM, Jacir NN, Crombleholme TM, et al. Thoracoscopic esophagomyotomy for achalasia in a child. J Pediatr Gastroenterol Nutr 1997;24(2):215–7.

[114] Mehra M, Bahar RJ, Ament ME, et al. Laparoscopic and thoracoscopic esophagomyotomy for children with achalasia. J Pediatr Gastroenterol Nutr 2001;33(4):466–71.

[115] Rothenberg SS, Partrick DA, Bealer JF, et al. Evaluation of minimally invasive approaches to achalasia in children. J Pediatr Surg 2001;36(5):808–10.

[116] Patti MG, Arcerito M, De Pinto M, et al. Comparison of thoracoscopic and laparoscopic Heller myotomy for achalasia. J Gastrointest Surg 1998;2(6):561–6.

[117] Patti MG, Albanese CT, Holcomb GW 3rd, et al. Laparoscopic Heller myotomy and Dor fundoplication for esophageal achalasia in children. J Pediatr Surg 2001;36(8):1248–51.

[118] Khajanchee YS, Kanneganti S, Leatherwood AE, et al. Laparoscopic Heller myotomy with Toupet fundoplication: outcomes predictors in 121 consecutive patients. Arch Surg 2005;140(9):827–33 [discussion: 833–4].

[119] Jara FM, Toledo-Pereyra LH, Lewis JW, et al. Long-term results of esophagomyotomy for achalasia of esophagus. Arch Surg 1979;114(8):935–6.

[120] Katada N, Sakuramoto S, Kobayashi N, et al. Laparoscopic Heller myotomy with Toupet fundoplication for achalasia straightens the esophagus and relieves dysphagia. Am J Surg 2006;192(1):1–8.

[121] Mattioli G, Esposito C, Pini Prato A, et al. Results of the laparoscopic Heller-Dor procedure for pediatric esophageal achalasia. Surg Endosc 2003;17(10):1650–2.

[122] Esposito C, Mendoza-Sagaon M, Roblot-Maigret B, et al. Complications of laparoscopic treatment of esophageal achalasia in children. J Pediatr Surg 2000;35(5):680–3.

[123] Franklin AL, Petrosyan M, Kane TD. Achalasia: a comprehensive review of disease, diagnosis and therapeutic management. World J Gastrointest Endosc 2014;6(4):105–11.

[124] Kobayashi M, Mizuno M, Sasaki A, et al. Single-port laparoscopic Heller myotomy and Dor fundoplication: initial experience with a new approach for the treatment of pediatric achalasia. J Pediatr Surg 2011;46(11):2200–3.

[125] Jaksic T, Yaman M, Thorner P, et al. 20-year review of pediatric pancreatic tumors. J Pediatr Surg 1992;27(10):1315–7.

[126] Perez EA, Gutierrez JC, Koniaris LG, et al. Malignant pancreatic tumors: incidence and outcome in 58 pediatric patients. J Pediatr Surg 2009;44(1):197–203.

[127] Tsukimoto I, Watanabe K, Lin JB, et al. Pancreatic carcinoma in children in Japan. Cancer 1973;31(5):1203–7.

[128] Sohn TA, Yeo CJ, Cameron JL, et al. Resected adenocarcinoma of the pancreas-616 patients: results, outcomes, and prognostic indicators. J Gastrointest Surg 2000;4(6):567–79.

[129] Johnson PR, Spitz L. Cysts and tumors of the pancreas. Semin Pediatr Surg 2000;9(4):209–15.

[130] Sussman LA, Christie R, Whittle DE. Laparoscopic excision of distal pancreas including insulinoma. Aust N Z J Surg 1996;66(6):414–6.

[131] Santoro E, Carlini M, Carboni F. Laparoscopic pancreatic surgery: indications, techniques and preliminary results. Hepatogastroenterology 1999;46(26):1174–80.

[132] Carricaburu E, Enezian G, Bonnard A, et al. Laparoscopic distal pancreatectomy for Frantz's tumor in a child. Surg Endosc 2003;17(12):2028–31.

[133] Melotti G, Cavallini A, Butturini G, et al. Laparoscopic distal pancreatectomy in children: case report and review of the literature. Ann Surg Oncol 2007;14(3):1065–9.

[134] Reynolds EM, Curnow AJ. Laparoscopic distal pancreatectomy for traumatic pancreatic transection. J Pediatr Surg 2003;38(10):E7–9.

[135] Mukherjee K, Morrow SE, Yang EY. Laparoscopic distal pancreatectomy in children: four cases and review of the literature. J Laparoendosc Adv Surg Tech A 2010;20(4):373–7.

[136] Bruzoni M, Sasson AR. Open and laparoscopic spleen-preserving, splenic vessel-preserving distal pancreatectomy: indications and outcomes. J Gastrointest Surg 2008;12(7):1202–6.

[137] Fernandez-Cruz L, Martinez I, Gilabert R, et al. Laparoscopic distal pancreatectomy combined with preservation of the spleen for cystic neoplasms of the pancreas. J Gastrointest Surg 2004;8(4):493–501.

[138] Han HS, Min SK, Lee HK, et al. Laparoscopic distal pancreatectomy with preservation of the spleen and splenic vessels for benign pancreas neoplasm. Surg Endosc 2005;19(10):1367–9.

[139] Aluka KJ, Long C, Rickford MS, et al. Laparoscopic distal pancreatectomy with splenic preservation for serous cystadenoma: a case report and literature review. Surg Innov 2006;13(2):94–101.

[140] Fais PO, Carricaburu E, Sarnacki S, et al. Is laparoscopic management suitable for solid pseudo-papillary tumors of the pancreas? Pediatr Surg Int 2009;25(7):617–21.

[141] Uchida H, Goto C, Kishimoto H, et al. Laparoscopic spleen-preserving distal pancreatectomy for solid pseudopapillary tumor with conservation of splenic vessels in a child. J Pediatr Surg 2010;45(7):1525–9.

[142] Sokolov YY, Stonogin SV, Donskoy DV, et al. Laparoscopic pancreatic resections for solid pseudopapillary tumor in children. Eur J Pediatr Surg 2009;19(6):399–401.

[143] Tsai FJ, Lee JY, Chang YT. Laparoscopic resection of a giant solid pseudopapillary neoplasm of uncinate process of the pancreas in a child. J Laparoendosc Adv Surg Tech A 2011;21(10):979–82.

[144] Kim HH, Yun SK, Kim JC, et al. Clinical features and surgical outcome of solid pseudopapillary tumor of the pancreas: 30 consecutive clinical cases. Hepatogastroenterology 2011;58(107–108):1002–8.

[145] Cavallini A, Butturini G, Daskalaki D, et al. Laparoscopic pancreatectomy for solid pseudopapillary tumors of the pancreas is a suitable technique; our experience with long-term follow-up and review of the literature. Ann Surg Oncol 2011;18(2):352–7.

[146] Gaines BA. Intra-abdominal solid organ injury in children: diagnosis and treatment. J Trauma 2009;67(Suppl 2):S135–9.

[147] Gaines BA, Rutkoski JD. The role of laparoscopy in pediatric trauma. Semin Pediatr Surg 2010;19(4):300–3.

[148] Feliz A, Shultz B, McKenna C, et al. Diagnostic and therapeutic laparoscopy in pediatric abdominal trauma. J Pediatr Surg 2006;41(1):72–7.

[149] Sharp NE, Holcomb GW 3rd. The role of minimally invasive surgery in pediatric trauma: a collective review. Pediatr Surg Int 2013;29(10):1013–8.

[150] Carnevale N, Baron N, Delany HM. Peritoneoscopy as an aid in the diagnosis of abdominal trauma: a preliminary report. J Trauma 1977;17(8):634–41.

[151] Marwan A, Harmon CM, Georgeson KE, et al. Use of laparoscopy in the management of pediatric abdominal trauma. J Trauma 2010;69(4):761–4.

[152] Iqbal CW, Levy SM, Tsao K, et al. Laparoscopic versus open distal pancreatectomy in the management of traumatic pancreatic disruption. J Laparoendosc Adv Surg Tech A 2012;22(6):595–8.

[153] Rutkoski JD, Segura BJ, Kane TD. Experience with totally laparoscopic distal pancreatectomy with splenic preservation for pediatric trauma–2 techniques. J Pediatr Surg 2011;46(3):588–93.

[154] Oak S, Sandesh P, Prakash A, et al. Role of thoracoscopy in blunt thoracic trauma- a case study. Journal of Laparoendoscopic and Advanced Surgical Techniques A 2004;7(3):315–8.

[155] Komatsu T, Neri S, Fuziwara Y, et al. Video-assisted thoracoscopic surgery (VATS) for penetrating chest wound: thoracoscopic exploration and removal of a penetrating foreign body. Can J Surg 2009;52(6):E301–2.

[156] Cuffari C. Inflammatory bowel disease in children: a pediatrician's perspective. Minerva Pediatr 2006;58(2):139–57.

[157] Kugathasan S, Judd RH, Hoffmann RG, et al. Epidemiologic and clinical characteristics of children with newly diagnosed inflammatory bowel disease in Wisconsin: a statewide population-based study. J Pediatr 2003;143(4):525–31.

[158] Lowney JK, Dietz DW, Birnbaum EH, et al. Is there any difference in recurrence rates in laparoscopic ileocolic resection for Crohn's disease compared with conventional surgery? A long-term, follow-up study. Dis Colon Rectum 2006;49(1):58–63.

[159] Fichera A, McCormack R, Rubin MA, et al. Long-term outcome of surgically treated Crohn's colitis: a prospective study. Dis Colon Rectum 2005;48(5):963–9.

[160] Farmer RG, Whelan G, Fazio VW. Long-term follow-up of patients with Crohn's disease. Relationship between the clinical pattern and prognosis. Gastroenterology 1985;88(6): 1818–25.

[161] Ponsky T, Hindle A, Sandler A. Inflammatory bowel disease in the pediatric patient. Surg Clin North Am 2007;87(3):643–58.

[162] Bemelman WA, Slors JF, Dunker MS, et al. Laparoscopic-assisted vs. open ileocolic resection for Crohn's disease. A comparative study. Surg Endosc 2000;14(8):721–5.

[163] Alabaz O, Iroatulam AJ, Nessim A, et al. Comparison of laparoscopically assisted and conventional ileocolic resection for Crohn's disease. Eur J Surg 2000;166(3): 213–7.

[164] Wu JS, Birnbaum EH, Kodner IJ, et al. Laparoscopic-assisted ileocolic resections in patients with Crohn's disease: are abscesses, phlegmons, or recurrent disease contraindications? Surgery 1997;122(4):682–8 [discussion: 688–9].

[165] Diamond IR, Langer JC. Laparoscopic-assisted versus open ileocolic resection for adolescent Crohn disease. J Pediatr Gastroenterol Nutr 2001;33(5):543–7.

[166] von Allmen D, Markowitz JE, York A, et al. Laparoscopic-assisted bowel resection offers advantages over open surgery for treatment of segmental Crohn's disease in children. J Pediatr Surg 2003;38(6):963–5.

[167] Bonnard A, Fouquet V, Berrebi D, et al. Crohn's disease in children. Preliminary experience with a laparoscopic approach. Eur J Pediatr Surg 2006;16(2):90–3.

[168] Dutta S, Rothenberg SS, Chang J, et al. Total intracorporeal laparoscopic resection of Crohn's disease. J Pediatr Surg 2003;38(5):717–9.
[169] Simon T, Orangio G, Ambroze W, et al. Laparoscopic-assisted bowel resection in pediatric/adolescent inflammatory bowel disease: laparoscopic bowel resection in children. Dis Colon Rectum 2003;46(10):1325–31.
[170] Fraser JD, Garey CL, Laituri CA, et al. Outcomes of laparoscopic and open total colectomy in the pediatric population. J Laparoendosc Adv Surg Tech A 2010;20(7):659–60.
[171] Mattioli G, Pini-Prato A, Barabino A, et al. Laparoscopic approach for children with inflammatory bowel diseases. Pediatr Surg Int 2011;27(8):839–46.
[172] Aspelund G, Ling SC, Ng V, et al. A role for laparoscopic approach in the treatment of biliary atresia and choledochal cysts. J Pediatr Surg 2007;42(5):869–72.
[173] Balistreri WF, Grand R, Hoofnagle JH, et al. Biliary atresia: current concepts and research directions. Summary of a symposium. Hepatology 1996;23(6):1682–92.
[174] Ohi R, Yaoita S, Kamiyama T, et al. Surgical treatment of congenital dilatation of the bile duct with special reference to late complications after total excisional operation. J Pediatr Surg 1990;25(6):613–7.
[175] Farello GA, Cerofolini A, Rebonato M, et al. Congenital choledochal cyst: video-guided laparoscopic treatment. Surg Laparosc Endosc 1995;5(5):354–8.
[176] Esteves E, Clemente Neto E, Ottaiano Neto M, et al. Laparoscopic Kasai portoenterostomy for biliary atresia. Pediatr Surg Int 2002;18(8):737–40.
[177] Nguyen Thanh L, Hien PD, Dung le A, et al. Laparoscopic repair for choledochal cyst: lessons learned from 190 cases. J Pediatr Surg 2010;45(3):540–4.
[178] Li MJ, Feng JX, Jin QF. Early complications after excision with hepaticoenterostomy for infants and children with choledochal cysts. Hepatobiliary Pancreat Dis Int 2002;1(2):281–4.
[179] Woo R, Le D, Albanese CT, et al. Robot-assisted laparoscopic resection of a type I choledochal cyst in a child. J Laparoendosc Adv Surg Tech A 2006;16(2):179–83.
[180] Meehan JJ, Elliott S, Sandler A. The robotic approach to complex hepatobiliary anomalies in children: preliminary report. J Pediatr Surg 2007;42(12):2110–4.
[181] Belknap WM. Hirschsprung's disease. Curr Treat Options Gastroenterol 2003;6(3):247–56.
[182] Swenson O, Rheinlander HF, Diamond I. Hirschsprungs disease; a new concept of the etiology; operative results in 34 patients. N Engl J Med 1949;241(15):551–6.
[183] So HB, Schwartz DL, Becker JM, et al. Endorectal "pull-through" without preliminary colostomy in neonates with Hirschsprung's disease. J Pediatr Surg 1980;15(4):470–1.
[184] Georgeson KE, Fuenfer MM, Hardin WD. Primary laparoscopic pull-through for Hirschsprung's disease in infants and children. J Pediatr Surg 1995;30(7):1017–21 [discussion: 1021–2].
[185] Georgeson KE, Cohen RD, Hebra A, et al. Primary laparoscopic-assisted endorectal colon pull-through for Hirschsprung's disease: a new gold standard. Ann Surg 1999;229(5):678–82 [discussion: 682–3].
[186] Kane TD. Endorectal pull-through for Hirschsprung's disease. In: Bax KN, Georgeson KE, Rothenberg SS, et al, editors. Endoscopic surgery in infants and children, vol. XXVII. Berlin: Springer; 2008. p. 367–74.
[187] Coe A, Collins MH, Lawal T, et al. Reoperation for Hirschsprung disease: pathology of the resected problematic distal pull-through. Pediatr Dev Pathol 2012;15(1):30–8.
[188] Muensterer OJ, Chong A, Hansen EN, et al. Single-incision laparoscopic endorectal pull-through (SILEP) for Hirschsprung disease. J Gastrointest Surg 2010;14(12):1950–4.
[189] deVries PA, Pena A. Posterior sagittal anorectoplasty. J Pediatr Surg 1982;17(5):638–43.
[190] Bliss DP Jr, Tapper D, Anderson JM, et al. Does posterior sagittal anorectoplasty in patients with high imperforate anus provide superior fecal continence? J Pediatr Surg 1996;31(1):26–30 [discussion: 30–2].

[191] Langemeijer RA, Molenaar JC. Continence after posterior sagittal anorectoplasty. J Pediatr Surg 1991;26(5):587–90.

[192] Tsuji H, Okada A, Nakai H, et al. Follow-up studies of anorectal malformations after posterior sagittal anorectoplasty. J Pediatr Surg 2002;37(11):1529–33.

[193] Georgeson KE, Inge TH, Albanese CT. Laparoscopically assisted anorectal pull through for high imperforate anus- a new technique. J Pediatr Surg 2000;35(6):927–30 [discussion: 930–1].

[194] Lin CL, Chen CC. The rectoanal relaxation reflex and continence in repaired anorectal malformations with and without an internal sphincter-saving procedure. J Pediatr Surg 1996;31(5):630–3.

[195] Lin CL, Wong KK, Lan LC, et al. Earlier appearance and higher incidence of the rectoanal relaxation reflex in patients with imperforate anus repaired with laparoscopically assisted anorectoplasty. Surg Endosc 2003;17(10):1646–9.

[196] Auyang ED, Hungness ES, Vaziri K, et al. Human NOTES cholecystectomy: transgastric hybrid technique. J Gastrointest Surg 2009;13(6):1149–50.

[197] Mintz Y, Horgan S, Cullen J, et al. NOTES: the hybrid technique. J Laparoendosc Adv Surg Tech A 2007;17(4):402–6.

[198] Pearl JP, Ponsky JL. Natural orifice translumenal endoscopic surgery: a critical review. J Gastrointest Surg 2008;12(7):1293–300.

[199] Ponsky TA, Diluciano J, Chwals W, et al. Early experience with single-port laparoscopic surgery in children. J Laparoendosc Adv Surg Tech A 2009;19(4):551–3.

[200] Podolsky ER, Rottman SJ, Poblete H, et al. Single port access (SPA) cholecystectomy: a completely transumbilical approach. J Laparoendosc Adv Surg Tech A 2009;19(2):219–22.

[201] Canes D, Desai MM, Aron M, et al. Transumbilical single-port surgery: evolution and current status. Eur Urol 2008;54(5):1020–9.

[202] Gumbs AA, Milone L, Sinha P, et al. Totally transumbilical laparoscopic cholecystectomy. J Gastrointest Surg 2009;13(3):533–4.

[203] Dutta S. Early experience with single incision laparoscopic surgery: eliminating the scar from abdominal operations. J Pediatr Surg 2009;44(9):1741–5.

[204] Rothenberg SS, Shipman K, Yoder S. Experience with modified single-port laparoscopic procedures in children. J Laparoendosc Adv Surg Tech A 2009;19(5):695–8.

[205] Muensterer OJ, Adibe OO, Harmon CM, et al. Single-incision laparoscopic pyloromyotomy: initial experience. Surg Endosc 2010;24(7):1589–93.

[206] Hansen EN, Muensterer OJ, Georgeson KE, et al. Single-incision pediatric endosurgery: lessons learned from our first 224 laparoendoscopic single-site procedures in children. Pediatr Surg Int 2011;27(6):643–8.

[207] Alasfar F, Chand B. Intraoperative endoscopy for laparoscopic Roux-en-Y gastric bypass: leak test and beyond. Surg Laparosc Endosc Percutan Tech 2010;20(6):424–7.

[208] Reavis KM, Melvin WS. Advanced endoscopic technologies. Surg Endosc 2008;22(6):1533–46.

[209] Grunhagen DJ, van Ierland MC, Doornebosch PG, et al. Laparoscopic-monitored colonoscopic polypectomy: a multimodality method to avoid segmental colon resection. Colorectal Dis 2011;13(11):1280–4.

[210] Barabino A, Gandullia P, Arrigo S, et al. Successful endoscopic treatment of a double duodenal web in an infant. Gastrointest Endosc 2011;73(2):401–3.

[211] Davenport KP, Mollen KP, Rothenberg SS, et al. Experience with endoscopy and endoscopy-assisted management of pediatric surgical problems: results and lessons. Dis Esophagus 2013;26(1):37–43.

[212] Kutikov A, Nguyen M, Guzzo T, et al. Robot assisted pyeloplasty in the infant-lessons learned. J Urol 2006;176(5):2237–9 [discussion: 2239–40].

[213] Peters CA, Woo R. Intravesical robotically assisted bilateral ureteral reimplantation. J Endourol 2005;19(6):618–21 [discussion: 621–2].

[214] Passerotti C, Peters CA. Robotic-assisted laparoscopy applied to reconstructive surgeries in children. World J Urol 2006;24(2):193–7.
[215] Atug F, Woods M, Burgess SV, et al. Robotic assisted laparoscopic pyeloplasty in children. J Urol 2005;174(4 Pt 1):1440–2.
[216] Meehan JJ, Sandler A. Pediatric robotic surgery: a single-institutional review of the first 100 consecutive cases. Surg Endosc 2008;22(1):177–82.
[217] Albassam AA, Mallick MS, Gado A, et al. Nissen fundoplication, robotic-assisted versus laparoscopic procedure: a comparative study in children. Eur J Pediatr Surg 2009;19(5): 316–9.
[218] Streck CJ, Lobe TE, Pietsch JB, et al. Laparoscopic repair of traumatic bowel injury in children. J Pediatr Surg 2006;41(11):1864–9.
[219] Rossi P, Mullins D, Thal E. Role of laparoscopy in the evaluation of abdominal trauma. Am J Surg 1993;166(6):707–10 [discussion: 710–1].
[220] Ahmed N, Whelan J, Brownlee J, et al. The contribution of laparoscopy in evaluation of penetrating abdominal wounds. J Am Coll Surg 2005;201(2):213–6.
[221] Villavicencio RT, Aucar JA. Analysis of laparoscopy in trauma. J Am Coll Surg 1999;189(1):11–20.
[222] Hasegawa T, Miki Y, Yoshioka Y, et al. Laparoscopic diagnosis of blunt abdominal trauma in children. Pediatr Surg Int 1997;12(2–3):132–6.
[223] Lovorn H, Rothenberg S, Reinberg O, et al. Update on thoracoscopic repair esophageal atresia with and without distal fistula. Journal of Laparoendoscopic and Advanced Surgical Techniques A 2001;5:135–9.
[224] Martinez-Ferro M, Elmo G, Bignon H. Thoracoscopic repair of esophageal atresia with fistula: initial experience. Journal of Laparoendoscopic and Advanced Surgical Techniques A 2002;6:229–37.

Advances in Pediatrics 61 (2014) 197–214

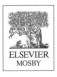

ADVANCES IN PEDIATRICS

ELSEVIER
MOSBY

A Patient/Family-Centered Strategic Plan Can Drive Significant Improvement

Richard J. Brilli, MD[a],*, Wallace V. Crandall, MD[a],
Janet C. Berry, RN, MBA[b],
Linda Stoverock, RN, DNP, MSN, NEA-BC[c],
Kerry Rosen, MD, MBA[a], Lee Budin, MD[a], Kelly J. Kelleher, MD[a],
Sean P. Gleeson, MD, MBA[a], J. Terrance Davis, MD[a]

[a]Quality Improvement Services, Nationwide Children's Hospital, The Ohio State University College of Medicine, 700 Children's Drive, Columbus, OH 43205, USA; [b]Nursing Administration and Perioperative Services, Nationwide Children's Hospital, 700 Children's Drive, Columbus, OH 43205, USA; [c]Nursing Administration, Nationwide Children's Hospital, 700 Children's Drive, Columbus, OH 43205, USA

Keywords
- Strategic plan • Patient/family centered • Employee safety
- Institute of Medicine domains of quality • Preventable harm • Patient satisfaction
- Optimal outcomes • Community health

Key points
- The strategic plan is an essential tool to help an organization achieve its vision. To be fully effective, it must inspire and motivate.
- For most hospitals, the strategic plan is stated from the hospital's viewpoint and is often organized around the Institute of Medicine's (IOM's) domains of quality. As such it often does not inspire or motivate the frontline staff who must operationalize the plan.
- An alternative approach is to reorganize the strategic plan from the patient/family's viewpoint. The Patient/Family-Centered Strategic Plan (PFCSP) consists of 5 domains: (1) Do Not Harm Me (patient safety), (2) Cure Me (disease-specific best outcomes), (3) Treat Me with Respect (patient satisfaction), (4) Navigate My Care (throughput/efficiency), and (5) Keep Us Well (population health/preventive medicine). Our experience with this approach is reported.

Continued

Financial Assistance and Conflicts of Interest: The authors have none to disclose.

*Corresponding author. 7th Floor Administration, Nationwide Children's Hospital, 700 Children's Drive, Columbus, OH 43205. *E-mail address*: rbrilli@nationwidechildrens.org

0065-3101/14/$ – see front matter
http://dx.doi.org/10.1016/j.yapd.2014.03.009 © 2014 Elsevier Inc. All rights reserved.

Continued

- The first pillar developed and implemented was Do Not Harm Me: the Zero Hero Safety Program. After 2 years, efforts were expanded into the other domains. Each was presented as a logical extension of the first, allowing for seamless and integrated programs and avoiding the appearance of isolated short-term initiatives. This article describes each domain and provides detailed examples of relevant initiatives, including results where available.
- The PFCSP is compelling, easily understood by staff at all levels in the organization, and has provided an organizational framework for quality and safety activity. We think it has been a key factor in attaining and sustaining significant improvement results.

INTRODUCTION

Health care organizations generally define themselves and their relationship with others through mission statements, vision statements, value statements, and strategic plans. A mission statement describes an organization's purpose, and therefore provides long-term consistency. Vision statements are complementary to mission statements and describe organizational aspirations over a defined future period often 5 to 10 years. These statements should serve to inspire while describing the art of the possible. Value statements serve as a code of conduct: the moral and ethical principles that guide decision making. Box 1 details the mission, vision, and value statements at Nationwide Children's Hospital (NCH). Finally, strategic plans detail the road map required to achieve the vision.

Formal strategic planning is widely used by health care organizations [1], which are typically updated at 3- to 5-year intervals. The published medical literature generally supports the value of strategic planning and suggests that organizational performance is enhanced by its use [2,3], but rigorous scientific analysis is lacking [4]. Some even suggest that a rigid strategic plan can introduce excessive bureaucracy into decision making and render the organization

---

Box 1: Nationwide Children's Hospital mission, vision, and values statements

- Mission Statement:

    We will provide the highest quality of patient care, advocacy, research, education, and service to our patients and families, without regard to their ability to pay.

- Vision Statement:

    We will create optimal health for every child in our community.

- Values Statement:

    As one team we do the right thing, create a safe day every day, promote health and well-being, are agile and innovative, and get results.

less responsive to changes in the environment [5]. In addition, wide variation exists in the mechanics of strategic planning, including who owns the process (marketing, hospital planning, or an individual within senior management).

For a strategic plan to be effective, the health care professionals who operationalize the road map must have a clear understanding of the plan and feel motivated to do the work. Nurse motivation is in part driven by a desire to help achieve the organization's mission [6], and physician motivation is enhanced by moderately challenging specific performance goals [7,8]. Therefore, a plan with understandable and compelling goals is essential.

Many hospitals have built their strategic plans based on the IOM's domains of quality, as proposed more than a decade ago [9]. The original domains included safety, effectiveness, patient/family centeredness, timeliness, efficiency, and equity. Recently, access and care coordination have been added. Patient/family centeredness is identified as an IOM domain; however, the other domains are not patient or family centered and are more organization centered. As an alternative, our hospital developed a quality and safety strategic plan, organized entirely from the patient's and family's viewpoint. It is a simple, easily understood, compelling, and effective alternative to the IOM domains of quality and transformative strategic thinking.

The PFCSP has 5 domains (Fig. 1): (1) Do Not Harm Me (patient safety), (2) Cure Me (disease-specific outcomes), (3) Treat Me with Respect (patient satisfaction), (4) Navigate My Care (throughput/efficiency), and (5) Keep Us Well (population health/preventive medicine). While the IOM terminology outlines the intellectual content of transformative domains, the PFCSP terminology describes those same concepts from a more compelling point of view—the patient's (Table 1). This article provides implementation details about this novel strategic approach and includes midterm results and progress within each PFCSP domain.

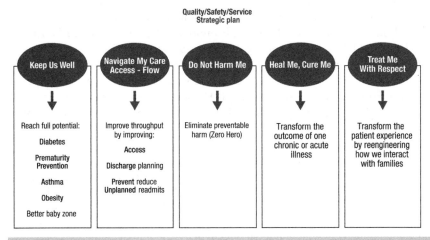

Fig. 1. The 5 domains of PFCSP.

Table 1
NCH patient/family-centered strategic plan compared to the IOM domains of quality

NCH patient/family-centered strategic plan pillar	IOM domain of quality and safety
Do Not Harm Me (patient safety)	Safety
Cure Me (best outcomes)	Effectiveness
Treat Me with Respect (patient satisfaction)	Equity, patient centered
Navigate My Care (throughput/efficiency)	Timeliness, efficiency, coordination
Keep Us Well (population health/preventive medicine)	Access, coordination

DOMAIN 1: DO NOT HARM ME (PATIENT SAFETY)

The first domain developed was patient safety for several reasons. First, safety is the fundamental concern of patients and parents. Even though most come to the hospital seeking diagnosis and cure, any significant patient harm that occurs is likely to obscure an otherwise positive clinical outcome. Also, the quality improvement (QI) infrastructure and culture change needed to significantly address and reduce patient harm is also necessary to support the other strategic plan domains. The dual initiatives to develop a culture of high reliability and to increase the capacity to support numerous robust simultaneous QI projects has been described previously [10,11]. At our institution, establishing a high reliability culture has been a multiyear journey. The mandatory training for the Zero Hero Safety Program taught 8 specific tools to enhance individual reliability. Reinforcement techniques were taught to all managers. More than 300 Safety Coaches provided peer-to-peer coaching on all shifts and all units. Furthermore, in order to provide support so that busy health care providers could fully participate in meaningful QI activities, the Quality Improvement Services Department was quadrupled in size. The new QI support staff was embedded into hospital microsystems and acted as project managers and data analysts, supporting the QI work of clinicians and keeping them on task. A critical mass of health care providers, both physician and nonphysician, were trained in the science of QI. An organizational improvement approach, based on the Institute for Healthcare Improvement Breakthrough Series [12] and the Model for Improvement [13], was selected. A QI Essentials Course was developed, and it is taught twice per year with the goal of training about 300 individuals in QI methodologies. The course is organized around a specific project led by each course participant. Didactic sessions include how to form multidisciplinary microsystem-based teams, the use of rapid improvement Plan-Do-Study-Act cycles, and the interpretation and use of statistical process control charts to drive change.

A useful, easily understood, and motivational metric, the Preventable Harm Index[SM] [14], was developed and is used as the primary outcome metric for harm elimination. By providing real-time, unit level, and specific data about patient harm, the clinical staff can remain engaged in the overall hospital drive toward preventable harm elimination. Other metrics reflecting safety include the Serious Safety Event Rate[SM] (SSER[SM]) [15], the hospital mortality rate, and the cost of preventable harm.

Harm reduction results that derive from the Do Not Harm Me aspect of the strategic plan have been previously described [10,11]. The latest results are as follows: SSER[SM] decreased 88% from peak ($P<.001$), (Fig. 2); Preventable Harm Index[SM] (PHI) decreased 50% from peak ($P<.001$) (Fig. 3); annual hospital severity-adjusted mortality decreased by 25% ($P<.001$); and harm-related hospital costs decreased by 22.0%. Furthermore, hospital-wide safety climate scores have significantly improved. Results have been sustained since the completion of previous publications.

Approximately 4 years after the patient safety program was launched, it was expanded to include employee safety. Two patient safety metrics, the SSER[SM] and PHI, were modified for use as employee safety outcome metrics. These are the employee SSER (eSSER) (Fig. 4) and the employee PHI (ePHI) (Table 2) and parallel the patient safety metrics. Using these 2 metrics allowed for the straightforward addition of employee safety to the patient safety work because the metrics' fundamentals were already widely understood. It is still early in the program, but Fig. 5 shows an 18-month downward trend in the eSSER. This trend predates any specific employee safety improvement efforts and may reflect the maturing influence of the patient safety program (Zero Hero). No improvement in ePHI has yet occurred.

DOMAIN 2: CURE ME (DISEASE-SPECIFIC BEST OUTCOMES)

Approximately 2 years after the Zero Hero program (Do Not Harm Me) began, attention turned to the other PFCSP domains, beginning with Cure Me. The premise of this domain is to optimize care by reducing variation in clinical practice and achieve transformative outcomes for specific diseases. Clinical divisions chose one chronic illness that is an important component of their

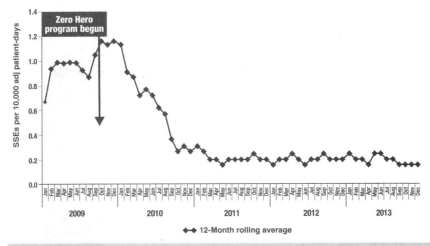

Fig. 2. Rolling 12-month average of serious safety events per 10,000 adjusted patient-days, 2009 to 2013. Decrease from peak = 88% (P<.001). Adj, adjusted; SSE, serious safety events.

Number of harm events
600
500
400
300
200
100
0
446
530
426
342
266
2009
2010
2011
2012
2013

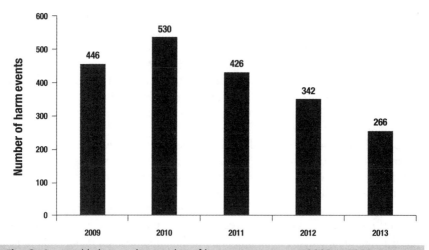

Fig. 3. Preventable harm index: number of harm events per year, 2009 to 2013. Decrease from peak = 50% (P<.001).

clinical population. Transformative outcome metrics such as remission rate, mortality, or total hospital days are identified for each disease being targeted. Standardized QI methodology is used to drive change and is aimed at achieving transformative and clinically important outcomes.

For example, the Gastroenterology Section selected remission rates in children and adolescents with inflammatory bowel disease (IBD) as the outcome metric. Multiple interventions (Box 2), targeting remission rate improvement, were implemented locally and also as part of a national collaborative [16,17].

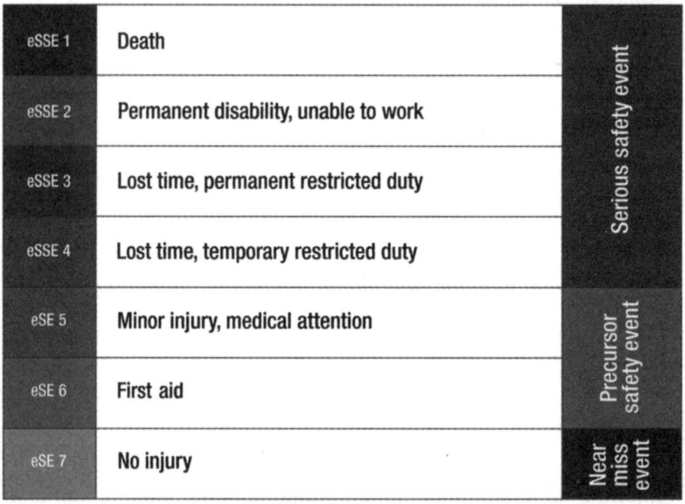

eSSE 1
Death
eSSE 2
Permanent disability, unable to work
eSSE 3
Lost time, permanent restricted duty
eSSE 4
Lost time, temporary restricted duty
eSE 5
Minor injury, medical attention
eSE 6
First aid
eSE 7
No injury
Serious safety event
Precursor safety event
Near miss event

Fig. 4. Taxonomy of employee safety events.

Table 2
Employee preventable harm index

Employee safety domain	n
Needle sticks or sharps injuries	n1
Serious falls	n2
Back injuries	n3
Miscellaneous injuries	n4
ePHI	Sum of n1–n4

All injuries are occupational safety and health administration reportable. For a given time frame, the ePHI is the sum of all reportable injuries in 4 categories.

Remission rates increased from approximately 50% to more than 85% (Fig. 6). These results were achieved by reliably implementing best practices and without introducing new therapies—an important concept in driving better outcomes for many chronic illnesses.

Because many important illnesses selected for Cure Me are chronic illnesses for which a total cure is not currently available, we continue to develop unique metrics intended to reflect success in maximizing the overall well-being of patients. Some metrics in use include total annual hospital days and the Cancer Care Index, developed by Hematology/Oncology. This metric sums the total number of undesirable events occurring in their population of patients with cancer each month. Examples include any preventable harm episode, missing specific consultations (Nutrition, Social Work, etc), or central venous line malposition. The index facilitates tracking of outcomes for all patients with cancer, regardless of the specific type, and therefore reflects the system of cancer care provided. In keeping with QI practice, balancing measures are included

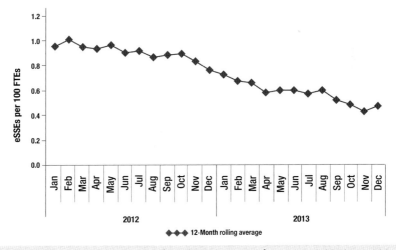

Fig. 5. Rolling 12-month average of employee serious safety events (eSSEs) per 100 employees, June 2012 to July 2012. FTE, full time equivalent employees.

Box 2: Interventions for patients with IBD

• Systematic previsit planning for all routine IBD clinic visits was done
  ○ Review medication dosing
  ○ Laboratory monitoring
  ○ Review clinical history
  ○ Recommendations based on disease activity
• A weekly population management program was instituted
  ○ Review of groups of patients outside of the clinic setting
    ▪ Patients not seen in 6 months
    ▪ Patients being treated with corticosteroids
    ▪ Patients with the highest risk scores
  ○ Recommendations are provided to the treating physician that can be instituted before the patients next clinic visit
• Self-management tools and techniques were developed and implemented

---

in each effort so that, for example, programs that reduce hospital days do not increase hospital readmissions.

Cure Me efforts are now underway in 20 clinical divisions. Interval progress reports are tracked by the QI team, the Associate Medical Director for Quality, and the Chief Medical Officer. Table 3 lists a few examples of other Cure Me projects underway, salient details about methods and metrics used, and results to date.

DOMAIN 3: TREAT ME WITH RESPECT (PATIENT SATISFACTION)

The third domain reflects the patient's and family's desire to be treated as a colleague and partner in the journey to wellness. The QI initiatives in this

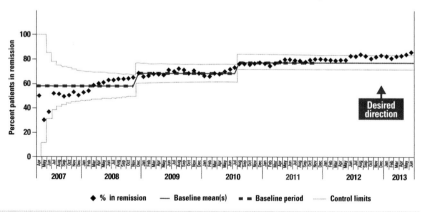

Fig. 6. Percentage of NCH patients with IBD in remission by month.

Table 3
Cure Me sample projects in selected divisions/departments

Section or department	Disease entity	Problem selected	Metric	Method(s)	Results to date
Neonatology	Prematurity	BPD rate	Incidence of BPD on day of life 28 and 36-wk corrected gestational age	Improved nutrition; respiratory management protocols; small baby unit/team established	20% reduction in incidence
The Heart Center	HLHS	Improving interstage quality of life	Percentage of patients with fewer than 60 hospital days in year 1	Care Journey; with standardized management protocols	100% compliance in 3 of 5 components for the Care Journey
Hematology, Oncology	Quality of cancer care	Reliability of delivery of evidence-based care	Cancer Care Index	Appropriate bundles and guidelines	25% reduction in Cancer Care Index (2013 vs 2012)
Neurology	Epilepsy	Decreasing total hospital days	Total annual days in hospital; reduction in unplanned admissions and ED visits	Clinical Guidelines for infantile spasms; seizure action plan; case management checklist	49% decrease in LOS for patients with infantile spasms

Abbreviations: BPD, bronchopulmonary dysplasia; ED, Emergency Department; HLHS, hypoplastic left heart syndrome; LOS, length of stay.

domain are based on the Principles of Patient- and Family-Centered Care as articulated by the Institute for Patient- and Family-Centered Care. These are (1) respect and dignity, (2) information sharing, (3) family participation at a level they choose, and (4) collaboration in all aspects of care [18]. Two metrics are used to gauge success. The first is the percentage of questions on the inpatient Press Ganey patient satisfaction survey [19] that are rated at the top (a score of 5/5—very good). The second is the number of grievances as defined by the center for medicaid and medicare services, filed by families against our organization.

This article highlights 3 of the 31 interventions underway in this domain: (1) hospital-wide training in Treat-Me-with-Respect techniques, (2) family-centered rounds (FCRs), and (3) managers rounding with families on inpatient units.

Hospital-wide satisfaction/service training for all employees extends the Zero Hero high reliability principles and tools to the arena of interactions and respect for patients and family as well as between coworkers. The 1.5-hour training program for all staff makes the case for clinician-family partnership and provides specific tools for clinical and administrative staff to resolve family concerns before dissatisfaction escalates. This training began QI 2014.

A second work stream is a multifaceted campaign to increase FCR. This campaign includes conducting daily clinical rounds in the patient's room and fully involving the family in the rounding process. To generate enthusiasm for this process change, considerable education was provided about the proven benefits of this rounding format. These benefits include improved family satisfaction and enhanced intrateam communication [20,21]. Hotel-room-like hang tags (like hotels' do not disturb tags) have been used to let the clinical rounding team know that the family wants to participate when the team arrives at the patient's room. Overall hospital compliance has increased substantially (Fig. 7), and our experience has been positive and does not reflect the few negative reports about FCR found in the literature [22].

The third work stream relates to managers conducting routine rounds in the inpatient units. The manager is expected to engage with the family regularly and simply ask "do you have any concerns?" with scripted responses for positive, negative, or neutral responses. The expectation is that managers will do at least 10 such rounds per week. A positive correlation has been observed between the percentage of time managers achieve the rounding expectation and the Press Ganey mean patient satisfaction scores for that unit (Fig. 8).

In order to fully operationalize a PFCSP, families must be fully integrated into the system. Families are involved at every level of the organization, from the traditional Family Advisory Council to membership on the hospital Board of Directors Quality Committee. The Family Advisory Committee is an active group of volunteers, many of whom have chronically ill children and therefore can speak to system issues that represent opportunities for improvement. Family members serve on many hospital committees. Children's Family as Faculty is another family member group that meets all new hires and physician house staff. This group describes the family- clinician partnership

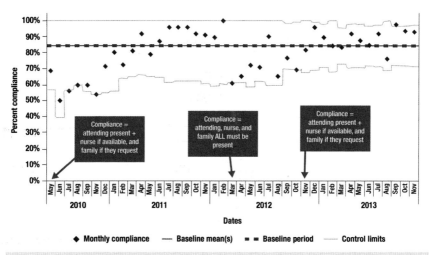

Fig. 7. Hospital-wide compliance with family-centered rounds. Note changes in compliance definition over time.

through its personal stories. Furthermore, many QI teams include family members. The parent's perspective has been exceedingly valuable in helping us achieve improved partnerships between clinician and family.

Fig. 9 demonstrates a slow increase in the percentage of questions answered as a "5" (Very Good). The current rate is 72% with a short-term goal of at least 75%. To date, no progress has been made toward the goal of decreasing filed grievances.

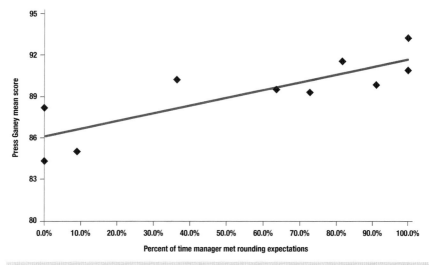

Fig. 8. Percentage of time manager meets rounding expectations compared to Press Ganey in-patient satisfaction mean scores. $Y = 5.6391$; $x = 86.068$; $R^2 = 0.6959$.

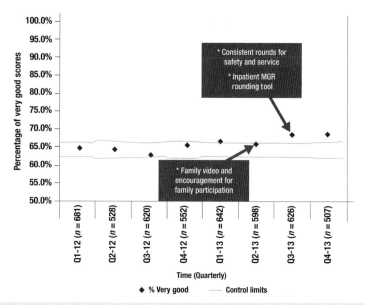

Fig. 9. Percentage of 5's on in-patient Press Ganey survey over time. MGR, manager.

DOMAIN 4: NAVIGATE MY CARE (THROUGHPUT/EFFICIENCY)

Efforts in this domain, although applicable to all patients, have concentrated on the care of complex, chronically ill children. Specifically, efforts have centered on standardizing and facilitating care for patients with cerebral palsy (CP). Because of frequent inpatient and outpatient care, and multiple medical needs, these patients may benefit the most from integrated care coordination. A multidisciplinary and multifaceted approach was developed including a specialized complex care team providing outpatient management, as well as inpatient and outpatient care coordination.

As an example, feeding tube difficulties in the CP population are a major source of dissatisfaction for families. Inconsistent recommendations and management of feeding tubes for patients with CP had led to confusion for families and even staff resulting in unnecessary clinic visits, emergency department visits, and sometimes hospital admissions. In response, activities on many fronts have standardized care and reduced variation (Box 3). These initiatives have served to empower patients and their families with the ability to better care for their children and their feeding tube after hospital discharge. As a result, we have seen a 14% decrease in the number of hospital admissions per 100 patients with feeding tubes and a 16% decrease in the average length of stay for patients with feeding tubes. The methods and interventions that prove most effective in the CP population will be spread to other chronic conditions.

Table 4 lists a sample of other initiatives in the Navigate My Care domain. The use of care bundles in some initiatives have proven effective and important.

Box 3: Management tools for patients with feeding tubes

- Standardize feeding tube procedures:
  - Postinsertion feeding tube care
  - Feeding-tube-related documentation procedures in the electronic medical record
  - Nutrition management for children with feeding tubes
- Develop tools within the electronic medical record that ensure the patient's feeding tube care team is identified before a tube insertion. Clearly identify:
  - The provider responsible for insertion
  - Those providing ongoing care of the tube and the surrounding skin
  - The outpatient nutrition manager
  - The provider responsible for reassessing the initial and ongoing need for the tube
- Streamline and centralize the process by which families of children with new feeding tubes are educated before leaving the hospital.
  - A care journey that identifies educational milestones families must achieve before leaving
  - Referral to the FRC for first-line, one-on-one teaching with a nurse educator
  - A tablet-based competency assessment kiosk to evaluate knowledge pre and post teaching in the FRC
  - A new educational workbook available in print and online and how-to videos to accompany the online version of the workbook

Abbreviation: FRC, Family Resource Center.

DOMAIN 5: KEEP US WELL (POPULATION HEALTH/ PREVENTIVE MEDICINE)

Keep Us Well expands the focus to all children in our region with the ambitious goal to ensure that all children can reach their full potential. This effort is facilitated by our Physician Hospital Organization, Partners for Kids (PFK), that accepts full risk capitation from Medicaid managed care plans for the hospital's primary and secondary service areas. This entry into managed care provided both the motive and the method to enable our population health decisions. Specifically, NCH is responsible for the full cost of care for a population approaching 300,000 children. Maximizing and maintaining the health and wellness of this population has direct financial benefits, reinforcing the mission-based motive to work toward positive health outcomes. PFK also supplies the method because, as the ultimate payer, PFK has access to health insurance records and the claims history for all children. This administrative database provides a way to measure the health of the population through its interactions (or lack thereof) with the health care system. The hospital considered many clinical areas as potential targets for the population health efforts, and ultimately 6 areas were selected: asthma, diabetes, health supervision, obesity, prematurity prevention, and the creation of a "better babies zone."

Table 4
Navigate My Care sample projects

Initiative	Interventions	Metric	Results to date
Improve care coordination	Increase CC; standardize CC job description; focus on complex patients	Compliance with various regulatory and state Medicaid care coordination standards; total hospital days; preventable harm; total cost of care	Developed EHR tools for identifying, tracking and documenting care coordination efforts
Reduce unplanned readmissions	Discharge bundle; predictive modeling for risk and interventions for readmission; define preventable readmission	Compliance with discharge bundle	Bundle elements have been tested; spreading house-wide
Reduce variability in tracheostomy care	Preinsertion checklist; development of tracheostomy care bundle; tracheostomy care Journey Board	Inpatient hospital days per cohort patient per month	Baseline = 1.3 hospital days per patient per month. Goal to reduce to 1.1

Abbreviations: CC, care coordinators; EHR, electronic Health Record.

As an example, efforts in obesity addressed the issue through 4 key drivers: energy imbalance, detection/intervention, coordination efforts, and measurement/accountability. A local team led the charge to pursue policy change through the Ohio legislature to pass laws requiring healthy food choices and minimum physical activity levels in schools. Increases in availability of nutritious food choices were pursued through community gardens, teaching preschools better menu and food preparation choices, and starting farmer's markets in areas previously described as a "food desert." Exercise was increased through after-school programs, community-sponsored walks in the park, and engaging with the First Lady of Ohio to develop an exercise digital video disc for schools. Partnering with the local school district, analytic and information technology support for the biometric screening program for all students was provided. External grant funding was obtained to support training physicians on early identification and counseling high-risk families. Finally, the hospital led by example through employee health activities such as fitness challenges and removing sugar-sweetened drinks from all hospital concessions. Although reasons for improvement are multifactorial and the NCH cannot take full credit for changes, there had been an average 24% decrease in body mass index for children in those Columbus City schools that enrolled the entering kindergarten cohort. Table 5 summarizes some of the other initiatives underway in the Keep Us Well domain of the strategic plan.

Table 5
Select examples of Keep Us Well initiatives

Section/department	Disease entity	Problem selected	Metric	Method(s)	Results to date
Infectious disease	Influenza	Low immunization rates	Hospital-wide immunization rate: patients seen during flu season and patients with chronic disease	Computer alerts; reminder lists; nurse-initiated protocols; overall hospital flu vaccine campaign	37% increase in all clinic patients (2010–2011 vs current); 8% increase in long-term patients
Ambulatory pediatrics	Childhood immunizations	Low childhood immunization rates	Immunization rate of population	EMR and POC alerts; immunize during any clinic visit	23% increase for patients in ambulatory care clinic; (2005 vs current)
Pulmonary	Asthma	Poorly controlled asthma in patients receiving managed care in Franklin County, OH, USA	ED visit rate/1000 member months	QI programs for PCPs; patient education; increased asthma action plan use, early ED steroid use; school-based asthma program	10.2% decrease in ED visit rate compared to previous year
Healthy neighborhoods healthy families	Community-based risk factors to optimal health	High number of vacant—abandoned—houses	OOR	Partner with city and state to rehab homes	OOR = 39.7%; 104 homes rehabbed or remodeled

Abbreviations: ED, Emergency Department; EMR, electronic medical record; OOR, owner occupancy rate; PCP, primary care physician; POC, point of care.

DISCUSSION

Motivation is a mental state or condition that determines the form, direction, intensity, and duration of behavior [23]. There are 24 separate theories about what motivates individuals [6,7], but most involve the relationship of the individual to the perceived goal. Goal setting theory holds that professionals are motivated to improve their performance when they accept moderately challenging and specific performance goals to which they feel committed [7]. Because strategic planning is viewed by hospital leadership as a key value-added function for health care organizations [1], the optimal plan should be one that engenders commitment. Creating a strategic plan from the patient's and family's viewpoint is a way to engage individuals whose professional lives are dedicated to improving the lives of patients—hence the reason for the PFCSP.

The 5 PFCSP domains presented here subsume all the IOM domains of quality (see Fig. 1, Table 1). The IOM domains, although comprehensive and succinct, clearly represent the perspective of the health care system. Conversely, the PFCSP covers the same conceptual domains, but does so from the patient and family perspective—a perspective that resonates with clinicians, hospital staff, and board members. Indeed, some NCH Board Members were the most enthusiastic supporters of this quality and safety organizational framework. Finally, the simplicity and focus of the PFCSP has been particularly valuable in helping nonclinical staff link the strategic plan and organizational vision.

The use of this paradigm has supported the sequential rollout of multiple initiatives over a period of years in a logical manner, without a shift in focus, and within the same framework. Beginning with Do Not Harm Me, the principles of highly reliable organizations, increased QI infrastructure, and institutional application of the Model for Improvement methods were established as the way our hospital approaches improvement work. Subsequent initiatives in the other domains used these same principles and techniques to achieve change. For example, every project is organized around a Specific Aim and has a Key Driver Diagram guiding the activities. The PFCSP has provided a unified conceptual framework for quality, safety, outcomes, and service initiatives, while avoiding the potentially distracting appearance of multiple disjointed efforts.

As the road map to the vision, the PFCSP forms the basis of operational decisions and prioritization for programs or initiatives pertaining to outcomes, quality, and safety. As such, it is widely used throughout the organization. Furthermore, unwavering, enthusiastic, and visible support by senior hospital leadership is essential to executing any strategic plan—even one organized with the patient and family as the priority. The most remarkable evolution has been the gradual engagement of families through Treat Me with Respect and Navigate My Care where patients are seen more fully as partners in their services. We expect this locus of participation to shift even further as we engage multiple neighborhoods, agencies, and community partners in the Keep Us Well programs focused on population health. The PFCSP has moved engagement in the plan from hospital centric to family centric and now community centric.

Five years after initiating the PFCSP, all early gains previously reported in the Do Not Harm Me domain have been sustained. In addition, substantial activity has been initiated and progress obtained in the other 4 domains. Currently, approximately 150 individual QI projects are underway supporting all 5 strategic plan domains. The initial declaration of zero as the goal for preventable harm once seemed outrageous, but in time has come to be widely accepted. Even though true zero has not been attained, major improvements have been made, and we think that the PFCSP has been an essential contributing factor.

SUMMARY

The use of a PFCSP, as a road map to operationalize the hospital's vision, has been a compelling paradigm to achieve significant QI results. The framework is simple yet directly aligns with the IOM domains of quality. It has inspired and helped actively engage hospital personnel in the work required to achieve the goals and vision of the hospital system. Five years after initiating this type of plan, activity is flourishing in each of the domains and midterm results are substantial. We think that the nature of this strategic plan has been an important aspect of our success to date.

References

[1] Begun JW, Kaissi AA. An exploratory study of healthcare strategic planning in two metropolitan areas. J Healthc Manag 2005;50(4):264–74.
[2] Begun J, Heatwole KB. Strategic cycling: shaking complacency in healthcare strategic planning. In: Kovner AR, Neuhauser D, editors. Health services management: readings, cases, and commentary. Chicago: Health Administration Press; 2004. p. 263–76.
[3] Zuckerman AM. Healthcare strategic planning. 2nd edition. Chicago: Health Administration Press; 2005.
[4] Kovner AR, Elton JJ, Billings J. Evidence based management. Front Health Serv Manage 2000;16(4):3–24.
[5] Begun JW, Zimmerman B, Dooley KJ. Healthcare organizations as complex adaptive systems. In: Mick SS, Wyttenback ME, editors. Advances in healthcare organization theory. San Francisco (CA): Josse-Bass; 2003. p. 253–88.
[6] Toode K, Routasalo P, Suominen T. Work motivation of nurses: a literature review. Int J Nurs Stud 2011;48:246–57.
[7] Buetow S. What motivates health professionals? Opportunities to gain greater insight from theory. J Health Serv Res Policy 2007;12(3):183–5.
[8] Wright SM, Beasley BW. Motivating factors for academic physicians within departments of medicine. Mayo Clin Proc 2004;79(9):1145–50.
[9] Crossing the quality chasm. A new health system for the 21st century. Washington, DC: Institute of Medicine, National Academy Press; 2001.
[10] Crandall W, Davis JT, McClead R, et al. Preventable harm: the right metric? Pediatr Clin North Am 2012;59:1279–92.
[11] Brilli RJ, McClead RM, Crandall WV, et al. A comprehensive patient safety program can reduce significantly preventable harm, associated costs, and hospital mortality. J Pediatr 2013;163(6):1638–45.
[12] Kilo CM. A framework for collaborative improvement: lessons from the institute for healthcare improvement's breakthrough series. Qual Manag Health Care 1998;6:1–14.

[13] Langley GJ, Moen R, Nolan KM, et al. The improvement guide: a practical approach to enhancing organizational performance. San Francisco (CA): Jossey-Bass; 2009.

[14] Brilli R, McClead R, Davis T, et al. The Preventable Harm Index: an effective motivator to facilitate the drive to zero. J Pediatr 2010;157:681–3.

[15] Healthcare performance improvement, LLC: innovative solutions in healthcare performance. Available at: http://hpiresults.com. Accessed September 28, 2012.

[16] Crandall W, Kappelman MD, Colletti RB, et al. ImproveCareNow: the development of a pediatric inflammatory bowel disease improvement network. Inflamm Bowel Dis 2011;17(1): 450–7.

[17] Crandall WC, Margolis PA, Kappelman MD, et al. Improved outcomes in a quality improvement collaborative for pediatric inflammatory bowel disease. Pediatrics 2012;129: e1030–41.

[18] Strategies for leadership: patient- and family-centered care, a hospital self-assessment inventory. Available at: http://www.aha.org/content/00-10/assessment.pdf. Accessed January 6, 2014.

[19] Press Ganey Associates. South Bend (IN). Available at: http://www.pressganey.com. Accessed January 6, 2014.

[20] Muething SE, Kotagal UR, Schoettker PJ, et al. Family-centered bedside rounds: a new approach to patient care and teaching. Pediatrics 2007;119:829–32.

[21] Kuo DZ, Sisterhen LL, Sigrest TE, et al. Family experiences and pediatrics health services use associated with family-centered rounds. Pediatrics 2012;130(2):1–7.

[22] Fenton JJ, Jerant AF, Bertakis KD, et al. The cost of satisfaction: a national study of patient satisfaction, health care utilization, expenditures, and mortality. Arch Intern Med 2012;172(5):405–11.

[23] Latham G, Pinder C. Work motivation theory and research at the dawn of the 21st century. Annu Rev Psychol 2005;56:485–516.

Advances in Pediatrics 61 (2014) 215–223

ADVANCES IN PEDIATRICS

ELSEVIER
MOSBY

Hypothermia in Hypoxic Ischemic Encephalopathy
A 5-Year Experience at Phoenix Children's Hospital Neuro NICU

Jorge I. Arango, MD, Kimberlee Allred, RN, NNP-BC,
P. David Adelson, MD, Parita Soni, MD, Ryan Stradleigh, BS,
Remy Wahnoun, PhD, Cristina Carballo, MD*

Barrow Neurological Institute at Phoenix Children's Hospital, 1919 East Thomas Road, Phoenix, AZ 85016, USA

Keywords
- Hypoxic ischemic encephalopathy • Therapeutic hypothermia
- Neurodevelopmental • NICU

Key points
- TH is safe and effective at improving survival and neurodevelopmental outcomes following HIE in term children.
- A properly staffed and equipped environment ensuring optimal monitoring and timely intervention is essential for the adequate management of these patients.
- The retrospective character of our study limited our capacity to identify the specific sources for our improved outcomes, further prospective efforts are necessary to define them.

INTRODUCTION

Perinatal cerebral hypoxia remains a significant cause of death and disability affecting approximately 1 to 2 per 1000 full-term newborns and up to 9 per 1000 preterm live births in developed countries [1–4]. These numbers are substantially higher in developing countries where its incidence can reach up to 75 per 1000 live births [5]. More than 15% of infants experiencing cerebral hypoxia die during the newborn period and from those who survive, a quarter develop permanent neurodevelopmental conditions ranging from cerebral palsy to area-specific learning disabilities and epilepsy [6].

*Corresponding author. E-mail address: ccperelman@me.com

0065-3101/14/$ – see front matter
http://dx.doi.org/10.1016/j.yapd.2014.03.004 © 2014 Elsevier Inc. All rights reserved.

   Limited therapeutic alternatives and a relative increment in the incidence of hypoxic ischemic encephalopathy (HIE) secondary to the constantly improving survival of preterm babies led to the identification and re-evaluation of new and former therapies [7–9]. Several studies focused on the evaluation of hypothermia as a potential neuroprotective alternative following brain insult in animal models [10–17]. During the past decade, several investigators have been working on the evaluation of the safety and effectiveness of therapeutic hypothermia (TH) in term babies with moderate to severe HIE; their results have been consistent at demonstrating improved survival and decreasing short-term disability [18–24].

   In 2006, the National Institute of Child Health and Human Development invited a panel of experts to review the available evidence on TH in HIE. The panel concluded that TH was an evolving therapy and that given this condition, institutions providing TH in patients with HIE must develop appropriate cooling protocols and standardized testing mechanisms while gathering short- and long-term evidence about the safety and effectiveness of the therapy [25].

   The administration of TH to term babies with HIE at Phoenix Children's Hospital (PCH) was strategically planned and instituted only after establishing a dedicated neurologic neonatal intensive care unit (Neuro NICU) that includes a multidisciplinary approach to care combining neonatology and neurocritical care rounds, pediatric neuroradiology support with prioritized neonatal magnetic resonance imaging (MRI) and MRI spectroscopy, bedside electroencephalographic monitoring, and cerebral near-infrared spectroscopy. A Neuro NICU provides patients with the necessary elements for TH treatment and continuous cerebral function monitoring to ensure optimum care during treatment.

METHODS

The PCH Neuro NICU database was queried to perform a systematic evaluation of the information from patients referred for and/or treated with TH at PCH for the management of HIE during the 5-year period between April 1, 2008 and March 31, 2013. This review was made under PCH Institutional Review Board (IRB) exempt determination #13-135.

COOLING PROTOCOLS

In 2008, the TH program was established at PCH based on previously established models using selective head cooling with the Olympic Cool-Cap from Tiara Medical Systems (Lakewood, OH) [21,26,27]. TH was initiated in infants greater than or equal to 36 weeks of gestational age and greater than or equal to 1800 g of weight who met specific inclusion criteria evaluated in two steps: presentation and neurologic examination (Table 1). Once enrolled, patients were cooled to a rectal temperature of $34.5 \pm 0.5°C$ and maintained in such range for 72 hours. The rewarming period was aimed to an incremental rate of $0.5°C$ per hour. After our first year using selective head cooling and despite the potential complications of whole-body hypothermia [22], it was decided through a consensus to change to whole-body hypothermia because scalp

Table 1
Eligibility criteria for modest hypothermia therapy

Step A (presentation)

1. History of an acute perinatal event
2. Apgar score ≤ 5 at 10 min
3. Cord or first postnatal blood pH ≤ 7.0
4. Cord or first postnatal blood gas base deficit ≥ 16 mEq/L
5. Continued need for ventilation for >10 min after birth
A1: If blood gas is available
Infant should meet items 3 OR 4
A2: If blood gas is not available or pH between 7.0 and 7.15 or base deficit between 10 and 15.9
Infant should meet items 1 AND 2 OR 5

| | Step B (neurologic examination) | | |
	Category	Moderate encephalopathy	Severe encephalopathy
1	Level of consciousness	Lethargic	Stupor/coma
2	Spontaneous activity	Decreased	No activity
3	Posture	Distal flexion	Decerebrate
4	Tone	Hypotonia	Flaccid
5	Primitive reflexes		
	Suck	Weak	Absent
	Moro	Incomplete	Absent
6	Autonomic function		
	Pupils	Constricted	Deviation/dilation/nonreact
	Respiration	Periodic breathing	Apnea

Presence of seizures OR symptoms on three of the six categories.

edema caused by the cooling cap limited proper electroencephalographic monitoring. This decision to change was also supported by the results obtained from the TOBY and ICE trials reported by Azzopardi and coworkers [28] and Jacobs and coworkers [29], respectively.

AGGRESSIVE CARE AND BRAIN FUNCTION MONITORING
Early in the process, electroencephalography (EEG) involved an amplitude integrated EEG to define criteria for cooling, followed by conventional EEG before cooling was initiated, and a subsequent conventional EEG after cooling to evaluate postinterventional function. This pattern was shown to provide limited information and not enough accuracy for proactive care and time-dependent decisions. The transition from head cooling to whole-body cooling permitted the use of continuous conventional EEG during the whole cooling and rewarming periods. The new model offered a more timely and comprehensive overview of the patients' brain activity in addition to allowing for more efficient and flexible monitoring of cerebral perfusion through near-infrared spectroscopy. The up-to-the-minute capacity to evaluate brain function and perfusion allowed us to make time-sensitive decisions while TH was ongoing.

QUALITY ASSESSMENT

In response to the National Institute of Child Health and Human Development request to use standardized protocols for the delivery of TH and the evaluation of patients receiving it, PCH developed a registry to track patients' characteristics and presentation along with their management, evaluations, and outcomes. This registry was initially established as a research initiative under PCH IRB #09-026. The registry system was improved and transformed into a quality tool including all individuals who received or were referred for TH at PCH. This transition took place with the development of a Web–based database connected to the hospital medical record system and it allowed for the reliable recollection of data that made for the body of this report.

OUTCOMES ANALYSIS

The information reviewed included patients' demographic information; clinical presentation (gestational age, Apgar scores [30], and Modified Sarnat staging scores [31]); radiologic evaluation reports; electroencephalographic reports; laboratory results; and outcome markers including survival, hospital stay, disposition, and neurologic development as assessed during neurologic follow-up evaluation or by neuropsychological application of Bayley Infant Scale of Development III [32]. Patients were stratified and their information analyzed based on their encephalopathy stage at admission. Patients with stage 2 in the Sarnat grading scale were considered as having moderate encephalopathy and those with stage 3 were considered as having severe encephalopathy. A subanalysis was performed on patients receiving extracorporeal membrane oxygenation (ECMO) and TH concomitantly.

STATISTICAL ANALYSIS

Analysis was performed using SPSS (Chicago, IL) and Matlab Math Works (Natick, MA). Descriptive statistics were calculated for all categorical and dichotomous variables. Mean, median, standard deviation, and 10th and 90th percentiles were calculated for continuous variables as appropriate. Fisher exact test or Pearson chi-square were used when appropriate to identify potential associations between independent fields. Statistical significance was defined as α less than or equal to 0.05 with two-tail hypotheses.

RESULTS

From the 195 babies referred to PCH with diagnosis of HIE during the 5-year period between April 2008 and March 2013, 157 (80.5%) met criteria for TH. Thirty-seven (23.6%) of these patients received head selective cooling and the rest received whole-body cooling. TH was initiated in less than 6 hours from birth in 124 (79.0%) patients and between 6 and 12 hours in 20 (12.7%) patients. Two (1.3%) patients were placed on TH after 12 hours; these patients were not candidates for TH at time of birth but one developed fetal thrombotic vasculopathy and the other developed hypoxia while in ECMO. No information is available about the time at which TH was initiated in the remaining 11 patients.

A total of 102 (65.0%) patients were diagnosed with moderate encephalopathy and 55 (35.0%) with severe encephalopathy. Patients' demographic characteristics were similar among groups (moderate and severe encephalopathy) and were in accordance with regional racial and ethnic distribution (Table 2).

A total of 23 (14.6%) patients died during their initial hospitalization and one (0.6%) patient died 9 weeks after birth for reasons unrelated to HIE or its treatment. Survival was 99% for patients with moderate encephalopathy and 60% for those with severe encephalopathy. Three patients presented with chromosomal abnormalities and were excluded from analysis.

Patients' clinical appearance at birth (as determined by Apgar score) and laboratory findings at presentation were consistent among groups (Table 3).

The mean Neuro NICU length of stay was 18.3 (standard deviation, 11.3) days and the median was 15 days with 10th and 90th percentiles at 10 and 31 days, respectively, for the patients who survived past the initial admission period. No significant difference was observed between patients with moderate and severe encephalopathy in terms of length of stay.

Table 2
Population characteristics

	All patients	Patients with moderate encephalopathy	Patients with severe encephalopathy
Number of patients	157	102	55
Gender			
Female	77 (49%)	51 (50.0%)	26 (47.3%)
Male	80 (51%)	51 (50.0%)	29 (52.7%)
Race/ethnicity			
Asian	5 (3.2%)	2 (2.0%)	3 (5.5%)
African American	11 (7.0%)	8 (7.8%)	3 (5.5%)
Hispanic	56 (35.7%)	39 (38.2%)	17 (30.9%)
Native American	14 (8.9%)	8 (7.8%)	6 (10.9%)
White	66 (42.0%)	41 (39.0%)	25 (45.5%)
Other	5 (3.2%)	4 (40.2%)	1 (1.8%)
Gestational age			
≤34 wk	4 (2.6%)	2 (2.0%)	2 (3.2%)
35 wk	2 (1.3%)	1 (1.0%)	1 (1.8%)
36 wk	23 (14.6%)	12 (11.8%)	11 (20.0%)
37 wk	16 (10.2%)	9 (8.8%)	7 (12.7%)
38 wk	22 (14.0%)	17 (16.7%)	5 (9.1%)
39 wk	41 (26.1%)	29 (28.4%)	12 (21.8%)
40 wk	35 (22.3%)	23 (22.5%)	12 (21.8%)
≥41 wk	13 (6.4%)	8 (7.9%)	5 (9.1%)
Unknown	1 (1.3%)	1 (1.0%)	0 (0.0%)
Disposition			
Discharged home	131 (83.4%)	100 (98.0%)	31 (56.4%)
Transferred to lower level of care	3 (1.9%)	1 (1.0%)	2 (3.6%)
Died during initial hospitalization	23 (14.6%)	1 (1.0%)	22 (40.0%)

Table 3
Clinical presentation at birth and initial laboratory findings

Sarnat		Apgar 1 min	Apgar 5 min	Apgar 10 min	LA	PCO₂	pH
Stage 2	Mean (SD)	2.3 (1.9)	4.6 (2.2)	5.8 (1.9)	6.9 (4.9)	43.4 (20.2)	7.05 (0.2)
	Median	2.00	4.00	6.00	5.00	39.00	7.05
Stage 3	Mean	1.9 (1.9)	4.2 (2.2)	5.2 (2.0)	8.7 (6.3)	42.8 (21.8)	7.02 (0.2)
	Median	1.00	4.00	6.00	8.00	40.00	7.02
Total	Mean	2.2 (1.9)	4.5 (2.2)	5.7 (2.0)	7.4 (5.3)	43.3 (20.5)	7.04 (0.2)
	Median	2.00	4.00	6.00	6.00	39.00	7.04

Abbreviations: LA, lactic acid; SD, standard deviation.

Neurodevelopmental follow-up information was available for 81 (61.8%) patients; 59 (72.8%) out of the 81 had moderate encephalopathy and 22 (27.2%) had severe encephalopathy. Thirty-one (38.3%) patients were evaluated once and the rest had two or more evaluations, with a median of two evaluations per patient and a maximum of 11. The mean follow-up period was 10 months.

From the patients with moderate encephalopathy who were evaluated once, 20 (91%) were found developing normally without deficits, one (4.5%) was found having motor delay, and one (4.5%) was found having combined motor and speech delays. Thirty-seven patients were evaluated two or more times, 23 (85.2%) of them were found normal without deficits at the first evaluation and 21 (56.8%) remained as such on all subsequent evaluations, and two (5.4%) were found developing deficits in subsequent evaluations. Fourteen patients were found with deficits during the first evaluation but these deficits improved to normality in six (42.6%) of the patients.

From the patients with severe encephalopathy, nine were evaluated only once and seven (77.8%) out of those nine were found developing normally without deficits; one (11.1%) was found having motor delay; and one (11.1%) was found with combined motor, speech, and cognitive delay. Thirteen patients were evaluated two or more times; eight (61.5%) were found developing normally without deficits during the first visit and remained as such on any subsequent visits. Five (38.5%) patients were found with deficits during their initial neurodevelopmental evaluations but these deficits improved to normal limits in four (80%) of the patients.

The overall incidence of cerebral palsy among our population was 18.5% with 1.8 (odds ratio, 2.08) times higher risk for patients with severe encephalopathy than for those with moderate encephalopathy.

Concomitant ECMO therapy failed to suggest any additional risk for developmental delay but the number of patients receiving both therapies was too low to discard any potential correlation or lack of it.

Early seizures were present in 17 (10.8%) out of 157 patients; six (3.8%) of them presented continued seizure activity in subsequent EEG monitoring and required chronic pharmacologic management.

Imaging was available for 149 patients and abnormalities were observed in 72 (48.3%) of the patients, with the most common being diffusion restriction (41.6%) and ischemic changes (20.8). Fifteen patients had a single MRI and from those nine (60%) were found to be abnormal. A total of 134 patients had two or more MRI studies and from those 71 (53%) were found to be normal during their initial evaluation. Ten (14.1%) out of these 71 patients were found to develop radiologic abnormalities in subsequent studies. MRI abnormalities were observed in 63 (47%) patients but these resolved in 37 (58.7%) of the patients.

Modified Barium Swallowing (MBS) evaluations were performed in 115 (73.2%) patients. Initial evaluations revealed swallowing issues in 96 (83.5%) patients. Normalization was observed in most patients but it was only evidenced with further swallowing studies in a fraction of the patients.

DISCUSSION

TH is a safe and efficacious therapy for patients with perinatal cerebral hypoxia. A multidisciplinary environment with appropriate technologic resources is ideal to improve patient survival and to limit the magnitude of the insult. Our evaluation identified an overall mortality and incidence of cerebral palsy reduction of 44% and 29%, respectively, when compared with the recent meta-analytic results reported by Tagin and colleagues [33].

No difference was observed in terms of survival or neurodevelopmental outcomes between the use of head selective and whole-body TH. However, whole-body cooling allowed for improved monitoring of brain activity and perfusion. We believe that aggressive monitoring in association with comprehensive neurologic care while HT is ongoing facilitates the delivery of appropriate and well-timed strategies to improve cerebral perfusion and/or eliminate further insult, allowing for overall improvement of neurodevelopmental outcomes.

Continuous EEG monitoring during the acute and subacute phases of injury is necessary for the early identification of seizures, their intervention, and the reduction of their subacute prevalence. Our experience is however limited in terms of length of follow-up and as such inappropriate to draw conclusions about the development of epilepsy secondary to HIE during the preschool and school periods as described by Robertson and Finer [34]. Initial EEG abnormalities showed strong association with mortality and developmental delay also associated with abnormal findings on initial EEG and MRI. These results were not explored further because they deviate from the goal of presenting our experience. Further studies may be useful to define the predictive value these may have on the outcomes of patients with HIE.

A recurring issue observed with the use of TH was the development of feeding abnormalities. The identification of this issue created the need for its evaluation and MBS was added to the cooling protocol. The high incidence of swallowing abnormalities observed with the use of cooling makes its evaluation an important factor in the care of these patients.

SUMMARY

We found TH to be safe and effective in improving survival and neurodevelopmental outcomes following HIE in term children. Additionally, the use of a multidisciplinary team involved with these complex patients and the use of advanced monitoring techniques will likely assist in identifying second insults (ie, seizures), leading to more rapidly instituted treatments. Our study, however, had the limitation of including only retrospective data from patients in whom TH was provided. This makes it difficult to identify the specific sources for the improved outcomes and/or the presence of complications.

Acknowledgments

This project was possible because of the support of United Cerebral Palsy of Central Arizona and the collaboration of Bryan Brannon from Bluefish Systems.

References

[1] Palsdottir K, Thorkelsson T, Hardardottir H, et al. Birth asphyxia, neonatal risk factors for hypoxic ischemic encephalopathy. Laeknabladid 2007;93(10):669–73 [in Icelandic].

[2] Jacobs S, Hunt R, Tarnow-Mordi W, et al. Cooling for newborns with hypoxic ischaemic encephalopathy. Cochrane Database Syst Rev 2007;(4) CD003311.

[3] Gunn AJ. Cerebral hypothermia for prevention of brain injury following perinatal asphyxia. Curr Opin Pediatr 2000;12(2):111–5.

[4] Costello AM, Manandhar DS. Perinatal asphyxia in less developed countries. Arch Dis Child Fetal Neonatal Ed 1994;71(1):F1–3.

[5] Schmidt JW, Walsh WF. Hypoxic-ischemic encephalopathy in preterm infants. J Neonatal Perinatal Med 2010;3(4):277–84.

[6] Vannucci RC, Perlman JM. Interventions for perinatal hypoxic-ischemic encephalopathy. Pediatrics 1997;100(6):1004–14.

[7] Westin B, Enhorning G. An experimental study of the human fetus with special reference to asphyxia neonatorum. Acta Paediatr Suppl 1955;44(Suppl 103):79–81.

[8] Vannucci RC. Current and potentially new management strategies for perinatal hypoxic-ischemic encephalopathy. Pediatrics 1990;85(6):961–8.

[9] Clark SL, Hankins GD. Temporal and demographic trends in cerebral palsy: fact and fiction. Am J Obstet Gynecol 2003;188(3):628–33.

[10] Thoresen M, Penrice J, Lorek A, et al. Mild hypothermia after severe transient hypoxia-ischemia ameliorates delayed cerebral energy failure in the newborn piglet. Pediatr Res 1995;37(5):667–70.

[11] Edwards AD, Yue X, Squier MV, et al. Specific inhibition of apoptosis after cerebral hypoxia-ischaemia by moderate post-insult hypothermia. Biochem Biophys Res Commun 1995;217(3):1193–9.

[12] Laptook AR, Corbett RJ, Sterett R, et al. Modest hypothermia provides partial neuroprotection for ischemic neonatal brain. Pediatr Res 1994;35(4 Pt 1):436–42.

[13] Gunn AJ, Gunn TR, de Haan HH, et al. Dramatic neuronal rescue with prolonged selective head cooling after ischemia in fetal lambs. J Clin Invest 1997;99(2):248–56.

[14] Bona E, Hagberg H, Loberg EM, et al. Protective effects of moderate hypothermia after neonatal hypoxia-ischemia: short- and long-term outcome. Pediatr Res 1998;43(6):738–45.

[15] Gunn AJ, Gunn TR, Gunning MI, et al. Neuroprotection with prolonged head cooling started before postischemic seizures in fetal sheep. Pediatrics 1998;102(5):1098–106.

[16] Laptook AR, Shalak L, Corbett RJ. Differences in brain temperature and cerebral blood flow during selective head versus whole-body cooling. Pediatrics 2001;108(5):1103–10.

[17] Wagner BP, Nedelcu J, Martin E. Delayed postischemic hypothermia improves long-term behavioral outcome after cerebral hypoxia-ischemia in neonatal rats. Pediatr Res 2002;51(3):354–60.

[18] Gunn AJ, Gluckman PD, Gunn TR. Selective head cooling in newborn infants after perinatal asphyxia: a safety study. Pediatrics 1998;102(4 Pt 1):885–92.

[19] Azzopardi D, Robertson NJ, Cowan FM, et al. Pilot study of treatment with whole body hypothermia for neonatal encephalopathy. Pediatrics 2000;106(4):684–94.

[20] Shankaran S, Laptook A, Wright LL, et al. Whole-body hypothermia for neonatal encephalopathy: animal observations as a basis for a randomized, controlled pilot study in term infants. Pediatrics 2002;110(2 Pt 1):377–85.

[21] Gluckman PD, Wyatt JS, Azzopardi D, et al. Selective head cooling with mild systemic hypothermia after neonatal encephalopathy: multicentre randomised trial. Lancet 2005;365(9460):663–70.

[22] Eicher DJ, Wagner CL, Katikaneni LP, et al. Moderate hypothermia in neonatal encephalopathy: safety outcomes. Pediatr Neurol 2005;32(1):18–24.

[23] Eicher DJ, Wagner CL, Katikaneni LP, et al. Moderate hypothermia in neonatal encephalopathy: efficacy outcomes. Pediatr Neurol 2005;32(1):11–7.

[24] Edwards AD, Brocklehurst P, Gunn AJ, et al. Neurological outcomes at 18 months of age after moderate hypothermia for perinatal hypoxic ischaemic encephalopathy: synthesis and meta-analysis of trial data. BMJ 2010;340:c363.

[25] Higgins RD, Raju TN, Perlman J, et al. Hypothermia and perinatal asphyxia: executive summary of the National Institute of Child Health and Human Development workshop. J Pediatr 2006;148(2):170–5.

[26] Gunn AG, Gluckman PD, Wyatt JS, et al. Selective head cooling after neonatal encephalopathy. Lancet 2005;365:1619–20.

[27] Department of Health and Human Services. FDA approval order P040025. T.C.f.D.a.R. Health, editor. 2006. U.S. Food and Drug Administration. Available at: http://www.accessdata.fda.gov/cdrh_docs/pdf4/P040025a.pdf.

[28] Azzopardi DV, Strohm B, Edwards AD, et al. Moderate hypothermia to treat perinatal asphyxial encephalopathy. N Engl J Med 2009;361(14):1349–58.

[29] Jacobs SE, Morley CJ, Inder TE, et al. Whole-body hypothermia for term and near-term newborns with hypoxic-ischemic encephalopathy: a randomized controlled trial. Arch Pediatr Adolesc Med 2011;165(8):692–700.

[30] Apgar V. The newborn (Apgar) scoring system. Reflections and advice. Pediatr Clin North Am 1966;13(3):645–50.

[31] Sarnat HB, Sarnat MS. Neonatal encephalopathy following fetal distress. A clinical and electroencephalographic study. Arch Neurol 1976;33(10):696–705.

[32] Bayley N. Bayley Scales of Infant and Toddler Development®. 3rd Edition (Bayley-III®). (2006).

[33] Tagin MA, Woolcott CG, Vincer MJ, et al. Hypothermia for neonatal hypoxic ischemic encephalopathy: an updated systematic review and meta-analysis. Arch Pediatr Adolesc Med 2012;166(6):558–66.

[34] Robertson C, Finer N. Term infants with hypoxic-ischemic encephalopathy: outcome at 3.5 years. Dev Med Child Neurol 1985;27(4):473–84.

Advances in Pediatrics 61 (2014) 225–243

ADVANCES IN PEDIATRICS

ELSEVIER
MOSBY

Advances in the Diagnosis and Treatment of Cystic Fibrosis

Stacey L. Martiniano, MD*, Jordana E. Hoppe, MD,
Scott D. Sagel, MD, PhD, Edith T. Zemanick, MD, MSCS

Department of Pediatrics, Children's Hospital Colorado, University of Colorado Denver, 13123
East 16th Avenue, B-395, Aurora, CO 80045, USA

Keywords
- Cystic fibrosis • CFTR • Newborn screen • Bronchiectasis • CFTR modulators
- Ivacaftor

Key points
- Cystic fibrosis (CF) is an autosomal recessive disorder that leads to chronic multisystem disease consisting of chronic sinopulmonary infections, malabsorption, and nutritional abnormalities.
- Current therapies for CF lung disease primarily target the progressive cycle of mucus obstruction; chronic, persistent infections; and excessive inflammatory response to reduce progressive airway damage and dilatation, known as bronchiectasis.
- CF care is provided with a multidisciplinary approach. Team members commonly include a CF provider, nurse, respiratory therapist, dietician, social worker, and a primary care physician.
- CF transmembrane conductance regulator modulators, small molecule pharmaceuticals that target the basic defect in CF, are available for a limited group of people with CF, and offer the hope of improved treatment options for many more people with CF over the next decade.

INTRODUCTION

Cystic fibrosis (CF) is a genetic disorder that leads to chronic multisystem disease consisting of chronic sinopulmonary infections, malabsorption, and nutritional abnormalities. It is the most common autosomal recessive life-shortening disease among white people in the United States. Although multiple organ

Disclosure: The authors have no relationships to disclose.

*Corresponding author. E-mail address: stacey.martiniano@childrenscolorado.org

0065-3101/14/$ – see front matter
http://dx.doi.org/10.1016/j.yapd.2014.03.002 © 2014 Elsevier Inc. All rights reserved.

systems are affected in this disease, lung involvement is the major cause of morbidity and mortality. From a pulmonary perspective, a cycle of chronic, persistent infections with CF-related pathogens and an excessive inflammatory response progressively damages the airways and lung parenchyma, resulting in widespread bronchiectasis and early death from respiratory failure [1,2].

CF is caused by mutations in a gene on chromosome 7 that encodes the CF transmembrane conductance regulator (CFTR) protein, a cyclic adenosine monophosphate–regulated ion channel. CFTR functions primarily as a chloride channel and controls the movement of salt and water into and out of epithelial cells lining the respiratory tract, biliary tree, intestines, vas deferens, sweat ducts, and pancreatic ducts. More than 1500 mutations in CFTR have been identified. The most common mutation in the United States, F508del, is a deletion of 3 base pairs encoding for phenylalanine at amino acid position 508 in the normal protein. This gene mutation as well as others leads to defects or deficiencies in CFTR, causing problems in salt and water movement across cell membranes, resulting in abnormally thick secretions in various organ systems and critically altering host defense in the lung.

Since its initial pathologic description 75 years ago [3], life expectancy in CF has improved, with a median predicted survival now approaching 40 years [4]. The improved survival in CF is one of the great success stories in pediatrics. Over these 75 years, CF has changed from an early fatal childhood disease, in which most afflicted infants died at a young age, to a chronic disorder in which most patients with CF are expected to live well into adulthood. There are myriad reasons for this improved survival, summarized in recent reviews (Fig. 1) [5,6], which include pancreatic enzyme replacement therapy; advancements in airway clearance techniques/devices; development of antimicrobial agents, including inhaled antibiotics targeting CF-specific pathogens; and

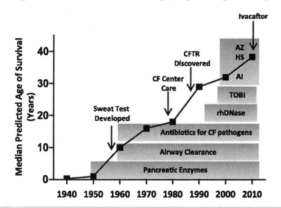

Fig. 1. Survival in CF since 1940. CF survival over time (line), associated CF therapies (bars), and milestones (arrows). AI, inhaled aztreonam; AZ, azithromycin; HS, hypertonic saline. (Reprinted with permission of the American Thoracic Society. Copyright © 2014 American Thoracic Society. Clancy JP, Jain M. Personalized medicine in cystic fibrosis: dawning of a new era. Am J Respir Crit Care Med 2012;186:594. Official Journal of the American Thoracic Society.)

inhaled mucolytic agents. Along with these therapeutic approaches, other developments that have had a positive impact on health outcomes and survival in CF include a network of accredited CF care centers with multidisciplinary specialized teams, dedicated quality improvement efforts, and early diagnosis through the nationwide implementation of newborn screening for CF.

This article reviews advances in both the diagnosis and treatment of CF. Based on recommendations from the Centers for Disease Control and Prevention [7] and the CF Foundation (CFF) [8], all states are now performing newborn screening for CF, which provides the opportunity for early intervention and improved outcomes. As a result, most individuals with CF are diagnosed through newborn screening. From a therapeutic perspective, the CF community has historically focused on treatments that counteract downstream manifestations of CF lung disease including mucus obstruction, infection, and inflammation. In an effort to address the root cause of CF, defective CFTR, the CFF established collaborations with biopharmaceutical companies to develop novel drugs targeting mutant CFTR. These efforts have led to the recent approval of one compound, ivacaftor (Kalydeco), for patients with CF with the G551D gating mutation. Drugs targeting F508del and other mutations are currently undergoing clinical trials. Development of CFTR-targeted drugs represents a new era in CF treatment, one that is expected to revolutionize the care of patients with CF.

DIAGNOSIS OF CF

A diagnosis of CF has historically required clinical evidence of typical phenotypic features in combination with laboratory confirmation. In 1996, a CFF consensus panel recommended that the diagnosis of CF should be based on the presence of one or more characteristic clinical features (Box 1), a history of CF in a sibling, or a positive newborn screening test, plus laboratory evidence of an abnormality in the CFTR gene or protein [9]. Acceptable evidence of a CFTR abnormality includes biological evidence of protein dysfunction (ie, abnormal sweat chloride concentration or nasal potential difference) and/or identification of 2 disease-causing CFTR mutations. Widespread implementation of newborn screening has now changed the diagnostic paradigm from one in which individuals are diagnosed from clinical features suggesting CF, to one in which most infants are referred for diagnostic testing after a positive newborn screen, many of whom do not have overt clinical manifestations. To this end, the CFF convened another meeting of experts in CF diagnosis in 2007 and a consensus report on updated CF diagnostic criteria was issued [10]. The recommendations involve a combination of clinical presentation, laboratory testing, and genetics to confirm a diagnosis of CF. The various laboratory methods to diagnose CF are discussed in this article.

Newborn screening for CF

Colorado was the first state to implement newborn screening for CF in 1982 [11]. Because of the published benefits of earlier detection afforded by newborn screening, many of which came from the Colorado and Wisconsin newborn

Box 1: Phenotypic features consistent with a diagnosis of CF

1. Chronic sinopulmonary disease, manifested by:
   - Airway infection with typical CF pathogens, including *Staphylococcus aureus*, nontypeable *Haemophilus influenzae*, mucoid and nonmucoid *Pseudomonas aeruginosa*, *Stenotrophomonas maltophilia*, and *Burkholderia cepacia*
   - Chronic cough and sputum production
   - Persistent chest radiograph abnormalities (eg, bronchiectasis, atelectasis, infiltrates, or hyperinflation)
   - Airway obstruction, manifested by wheezing and air-trapping
   - Nasal polyps; radiographic or computed tomography abnormalities of the paranasal sinuses
   - Digital clubbing
2. Gastrointestinal and nutritional abnormalities, including:
   - Intestinal: meconium ileus, distal intestinal obstruction syndrome, rectal prolapse
   - Pancreatic: pancreatic insufficiency, recurrent acute pancreatitis, chronic pancreatitis, pancreatic abnormalities on imaging
   - Hepatic: prolonged neonatal jaundice, chronic hepatic disease manifested by clinical or histologic evidence of focal biliary cirrhosis or multilobular cirrhosis
   - Nutritional: failure to thrive (protein-calorie malnutrition), hypoproteinemia and edema, complications secondary to fat-soluble vitamin deficiencies
3. Salt loss syndromes: acute salt depletion, chronic metabolic alkalosis
4. Genital abnormalities in male patients, resulting in obstructive azoospermia

Adapted from Rosenstein BJ, Cutting GR. The diagnosis of cystic fibrosis: a consensus statement. Cystic Fibrosis Foundation Consensus Panel. J Pediatr 1998;132:590; with permission.

screening programs, the Centers for Disease Control and Prevention and the CFF issued guidelines in 2004 supporting the clinical usefulness of newborn screening for CF [7]. As of 2010, all 50 states are performing newborn screening for CF and most new diagnoses are now made through this diagnostic approach [4].

All newborn screening methods for CF begin with the measurement of immunoreactive trypsinogen (IRT) in dried blood spots collected from newborn infants. IRT is a pancreatic enzyme precursor that serves as a biomarker of pancreatic injury. IRT is increased in most newborns with CF because of in utero blockage of pancreatic ducts. Newborn screening protocols vary by state and individual states set the specific cutoff value that defines an increased IRT. After a high IRT value is identified, the next step involves either DNA mutation analysis (IRT/DNA) or obtaining a second IRT (IRT/IRT) to assess for persistent increase. Those infants with a positive IRT who have at least one CFTR mutation and those with persistently increased IRT values are referred for a confirmatory sweat test. Thus, the sweat chloride test remains the fundamental test for diagnosing CF and completing the newborn screen process. An algorithm published by the CFF Consensus Committee provides a detailed, time-based description of the process from newborn screen to diagnosis, including the expectation that the initial sweat chloride test will be performed at 2 to 4 weeks of age (Fig. 2) [10].

Sweat testing for CF

The quantitative measurement of chloride in sweat (commonly called the sweat test) is the standard procedure for diagnosing CF. Despite more than 5 decades of experience with sweat testing, technical and interpretative challenges remain. Therefore, the CFF requires that sweat testing conducted at accredited CF care centers adheres to specific standards and requirements [12]. The sweat test involves transdermal administration of pilocarpine by iontophoresis to stimulate sweat gland secretion, followed by collection and quantitation of sweat onto gauze or filter paper or into a Macroduct coil (Wescor Inc, Logan, UT) and

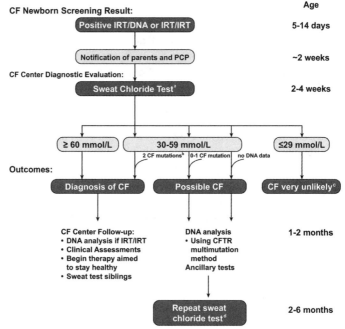

a If the baby is at least 2kg and more than 36 weeks gestation at birth, perform bilateral sweat sampling/analysis with either Gibson-Cooke or Macroduct® method; repeat as soon as possible if sweat quantity is less than 75 mg or 15 μl, respectively.

b CF mutation refers to a CFTR mutant allele known to cause CF disease.

c The disease is very unlikely; however, if there are 2 CF mutations in trans, CF may be diagnosed.

d After a repeat sweat test, further evaluation depends on the results as implied above.

Fig. 2. The CF diagnostic process for screened newborns. IRT, immunoreactive trypsinogen; PCP, primary care provider. (*Reprinted from* Farrell PM, Rosenstein BJ, White TB, et al. Guidelines for diagnosis of cystic fibrosis in newborns through older adults: Cystic Fibrosis Foundation consensus report. J Pediatr 2008;153:S6; with permission.)

analysis of chloride concentration, as described by the Clinical and Laboratory Standards Institute [12].

A sweat chloride value greater than 60 mmol/L has traditionally been considered diagnostic of CF. However, there have been instances in which individuals diagnosed with CF had lower sweat chloride values, and data emerging from newborn screening programs suggest that some infants eventually diagnosed with CF have initial sweat chloride values less than 60 mmol/L. This finding has led to recently revised reference values [10]. CF is now deemed to be very unlikely when the sweat chloride value is less than or equal to 29 mmol/L in infants up to age 6 months old or when the sweat chloride value is less than or equal to 39 mmol/L in individuals more than 6 months old (see Fig. 2). Individuals with intermediate results (30–59 mmol/L in infants up to age 6 months or 40–59 mmol/L in individuals more than 6 months of age) should undergo additional evaluation and be referred to a CF care center with expertise in diagnosing CF.

CF genotyping

DNA analysis for detection of CFTR mutations is recommended for all individuals with a sweat chloride in the positive or intermediate range [10]. Individuals with normal sweat chloride but features strongly suggesting CF should also have genetic testing performed, because, rarely, CF may still be diagnosed [13]. The most common mutation, F508del, is detected in up to 80% of people with CF in the Unites States. The detection rate of CFTR mutations varies based on mutation panel, testing method, and ethnic background. For example, targeted mutation analysis with a 23-mutation panel detects 2 CFTR mutations in more than 90% of Ashkenazi Jewish individuals, ~70% of white people, and only ~25% of Hispanic individuals [14]. The 23-mutation screening panel recommended by the American College of Medical Genetics is used for prenatal CF carrier screening and in newborn screening programs that rely on DNA analysis. Some states have implemented the use of expanded mutation panels or gene sequencing approaches in their newborn screening algorithms in order to capture individuals of more diverse ethnic backgrounds. DNA analyses that are commercially available typically include an initial panel of ~100 mutations. If no or only 1 CFTR mutation is detected, then extended full-gene sequencing and deletion/duplication testing is indicated; full-gene testing detects 2 mutations in ~97% of people with CF. In the era of CFTR modulator therapy, every effort should be made to identify 2 CFTR mutations in all persons with CF.

Genotype/phenotype correlations

Each of the CFTR mutations identified results in different functional protein consequences, ranging from complete protein absence to defective protein activity at the plasma membrane. CFTR mutations are broadly categorized into 5 classes based on the effect of the gene mutation on the CFTR protein function (Fig. 3) [15]. Class I (nonsense mutations) includes premature termination codons and frameshift mutations that result in either no significant protein

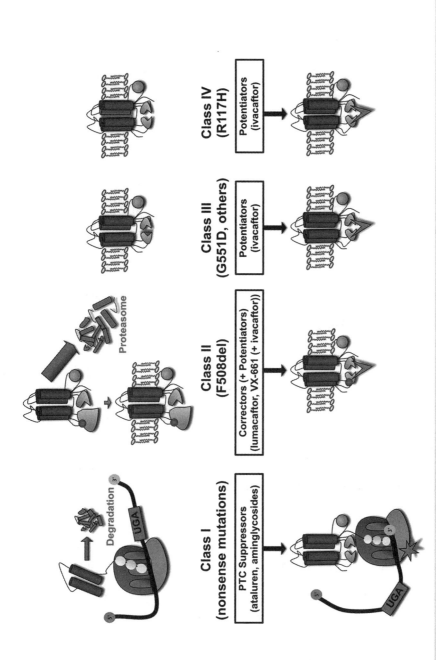

Fig. 3. CFTR gene mutation classes and therapeutic approaches. PTC, post-transcriptional control; UGA, stop codon genetic code. *(From Rowe SM, Borowitz DS, Burns JL, et al. Progress in cystic fibrosis and the CF Therapeutics Development Network. Thorax 2012;67:883; with permission.)*

synthesis or low levels of truncated CFTR proteins. Class II mutations, which include the most common F508del mutant, cause folding or maturation defects, and little detectable CFTR at the plasma membrane. Class III mutations (eg, G551D) lead to the formation of CFTR proteins that reach the plasma membrane but are nonfunctional secondary to gating defects that limit channel opening. As such, classes I to III mutations typically have minimal protein function and are associated with a classic CF phenotype including pancreatic insufficiency. Class IV and V mutations are associated with either reduced chloride conductance through the CFTR protein or reduced levels of the CFTR protein at the plasma membrane, respectively. Individuals with 1 class IV or V mutation typically have residual CFTR function (ie, partial function mutations), often have sufficient pancreatic function to absorb nutrients without supplemental pancreatic enzymes (ie, pancreatic sufficiency), and may have sweat chloride values in the CF diagnostic or intermediate ranges [16]. The most commonly detected class IV mutation is R117H, which has an additional layer of clinical phenotype variability based on polymorphisms in the poly T tract in intron 8 of the CFTR gene [17]. Individuals with the R117H mutation, particularly with a 7T poly T tract, are generally expected to do well with low risk of disease progression, whereas those with a 5T poly T tract are at higher risk of developing lung disease. Although underlying CFTR mutations are strong predictors of pancreatic status, mutation class is a poor predictor of lung disease phenotype. It is thought that, in addition to the CFTR genotype, both CF modifier genes and environmental factors influence the variability of CF symptoms and comorbidities [18–20].

Although more than 1500 CFTR mutations have been identified, the functional consequence of many mutations remain unclear. The Clinical and Functional Translation of CFTR (CFTR2) is a joint venture between international researchers and the CFF [21]. The CFTR2 Web site (www.cftr2.org) provides information about specific CF mutations to patients, researchers, and the general public from a database of almost 40,000 people with CF worldwide. Because clinical phenotypes can vary, individuals with abnormal genetic testing and unclear diagnoses should be referred to an accredited CF care center for evaluation.

CFTR-related metabolic syndrome
CFTR-related metabolic syndrome (CRMS) is the diagnostic term used for infants with a positive newborn screen, sweat chloride less than 60 mmol/L, and up to 2 CFTR mutations, at least one of which is not clearly CF disease causing [22]. Infants with CRMS differ from individuals diagnosed later in life with nonclassic CF or CFTR-related disorders (eg, congenital absence of the vas deferens, recurrent pancreatitis, and bronchiectasis) because infants with CRMS are typically asymptomatic, whereas evaluation in older individuals is initiated by clinical symptoms. There is a paucity of data on the clinical course and outcomes of infants with CRMS; however, population data suggest that most

people with CRMS remain healthy. The CFF issued guidelines in 2009 for the management of infants with CRMS [22].

Nasal potential difference

Transepithelial nasal potential difference (NPD) is a method of testing for CFTR activity by measuring the electrical potential difference across respiratory epithelia lining the nasal mucosa [14]. The electrical potential difference relies on active ion transport, which is abnormal in individuals with absent or decreased CFTR function. Changes in the NPD are measured by a small catheter placed in the nostril while amiloride, low ion, and beta-agonist solutions are used to bathe the nasal mucosa. NPD can be performed reliably in children as young as 6 to 8 years of age in specialized CF centers. NPD measurements are most useful in patients with inconclusive sweat chloride values and as outcome measures in clinical trials of CFTR modulators [23].

Conventional diagnosis

Before newborn screening, individuals with CF were diagnosed based on clinical presentation (including 15%–20% presenting at birth with meconium ileus) or a known family history of CF. Over the past decade there has been a dramatic increase in the number of infants diagnosed by newborn screening, from less than 10% before 2001 to almost 60% in 2011 [4]. It is expected that the number of those diagnosed conventionally will continue to decrease. Despite this, clinicians need to maintain vigilance in order to identify those with CF missed by newborn screening because of (1) false-negative results, (2) laboratory error, or (3) birth before implementation of newborn screening or in a country without a screening program. Clinical manifestations that should prompt further evaluation for CF include failure to thrive with symptoms of fat malabsorption, chronic productive cough, recurrent pneumonia, nasal polyposis, bronchiectasis, pancreatitis, digital clubbing, dehydration with hyponatremic, hypochloremic metabolic alkalosis, and male infertility (see Box 1). Patients with pancreatic-sufficient CF are at a slightly higher risk of being missed by newborn screening and may present without the nutritional deficiencies seen in pancreatic-insufficient CF.

MANAGEMENT GOALS IN CF

Management goals in CF broadly include optimizing nutritional status and lung health, and preventing and treating comorbidities (Table 1). The care of people with CF requires a multidisciplinary team approach in order to adequately address these issues. Clinical care guidelines are based on evidence from clinical trials, expert consensus, and benchmarking, a tool used by the CFF to identify health care practices associated with the best outcomes and to spread these strategies in order to improve overall care [24]. These guidelines are available for viewing and downloading from the Web site at www.cff.org/treatments/CFCareGuidelines.

Table 1
Management goals in CF

Management goals	Clinical approach	Clinical care guidelines
Nutritional:	High-calorie, high-fat diet	Stallings et al [59], 2008
• Maintain normal growth patterns in children	Nutritional supplements (oral or enteral) for growth deficits	Borowitz et al [22], 2009
○ Goal weight for length ≥50th percentile for infants <2 y old	Behavioral and nutritional intervention as indicated	
○ Goal BMI ≥50th percentile for children ≥2 y old	Pancreatic enzyme replacement therapy for patients with pancreatic insufficiency	
• Maintain normal blood levels of fat-soluble vitamins	CF vitamin containing vitamins A, D, E, and K	
	Salt supplementation: table salt prescribed in infants; older children salt food liberally	
• Prevent hyponatremia and hypochloremia		
Lung health:	Frequent monitoring, particularly in infancy	Borowitz et al [22], 2009
• Minimize lung damage caused by infection, mucus plugging, and inflammation	Avoidance of tobacco smoke	Flume et al [30], 2007
• Maintain lung function (age ≥6 y)	Seasonal influenza vaccination	Flume et al [38], 2009
• Prevent onset of new lung infections	Avoid contact between individuals with CF to reduce transmission of bacteria (unless siblings or close relatives)	
• Detect and treat chronic lung infections	Infection control procedures in CF clinic	
• Prevent and treat pulmonary exacerbations	Daily airway clearance treatments	
	Use of dornase or hypertonic saline	
	Early treatment with antibiotics for any increase in respiratory symptoms	
	Chronic azithromycin when indicated	
	Routine airway cultures at least quarterly	
	Routine spirometry at least twice annually	
Comorbidities:	Obtain regular CF care in a CF Foundation–accredited care center (every 1–2 mo for infants, then every 3 mo after age 1 y)	Debray et al [62], 2011
• Detect and treat complications of CF including:	Annual screening for liver disease, fat-soluble vitamin deficiency, ABPA	Moran et al [63], 2010
○ CF liver disease	Annual oral glucose tolerance testing starting at age 10 y	Stevens et al [64], 2003
○ CF-related diabetes	Referral to ENT, GI, liver, or endocrinology specialists as indicated	Besier et al [65], 2011
○ Nasal polyposis	At least annual assessments by CF-trained social worker or psychologist	
○ Gastrointestinal complications		
○ ABPA		
○ CF-related osteoporosis		
○ Depression		
○ Anxiety		

Abbreviations: ABPA, allergic bronchopulmonary aspergillosis; ENT, ear, nose, and throat; GI, gastrointestinal.

PHARMACOLOGIC AND NONPHARMACOLOGIC STRATEGIES IN CF

Therapies for CF lung disease primarily target the progressive cycle of mucus obstruction; chronic, persistent airway infections; and excessive inflammatory response in an attempt to maintain lung function, reduce pulmonary exacerbations, and slow progression of bronchiectasis and structural lung damage. The use of airway clearance, antibiotics, and nebulized medications to improve mucus clearance has led to significant improvements in survival (see Fig. 1).

Airway clearance

Airway clearance therapies (ACT) are mechanical means of assisting patients in clearing secretions and mucus obstructing the airways. Routine ACT is recommended for all patients with CF to maintain lung health [25]. No single form of ACT has been shown to be superior to others, therefore the modality is chosen based on patient age and preference [25]. The most commonly used forms of airway clearance include chest physiotherapy or percussion and postural drainage, positive expiratory pressure (PEP) or oscillatory PEP, and high-frequency chest compression with a vest device. To optimize mucus clearance, patients perform forced exhalation huff coughs in coordination with ACT to clear sections. Vigorous exercise is also considered to be a form of ACT and is recommended for this reason in addition to its other health-related benefits beyond mucus clearance. ACT is recommended to be performed at least 1 or 2 times daily and is typically increased in frequency during periods of illness.

Airway surface liquid and mucus alteration treatments

The airway surface liquid is dehydrated in CF because of defective chloride transport by the CFTR protein, which impairs mucociliary clearance. Hypertonic saline (HTS) inhalation is a treatment that theoretically helps to hydrate the airways in CF and accelerate mucus clearance and improve lung function [26,27]. HTS is typically pretreated with a bronchodilator to help prevent potential bronchospasm side effects. Inhaled dry-powder mannitol (Bronchitol) similarly is an osmotic agent that is thought to increase surface liquid in the airways [28]. Recombinant human deoxyribonuclease or dornase alpha (Pulmozyme) is a nebulized medication designed to degrade extracellular DNA that accumulates within the CF mucus, thereby reducing mucus viscosity and promoting clearance of secretions [29]. Hypertonic saline and dornase alpha are recommended for chronic use in children 6 years of age and older to improve lung function and reduce exacerbations [30]. At present, dry-powder mannitol is approved for use in Australia and the European Union, but is not yet available in the United States. These inhaled treatments are typically used in conjunction with ACT.

Antimicrobials

As part of CF care, routine surveillance cultures are obtained on a quarterly basis and often during periods of illness. Culture samples are obtained via oropharyngeal swab, collection of spontaneously expectorated or induced sputum, or bronchoscopy with bronchoalveolar lavage. Typical CF pathogens early in life include *Staphylococcus aureus* and *Haemophilus influenzae*. *Pseudomonas aeruginosa* takes over as the primary pathogen in teen and adult years and chronic *P aeruginosa* infection is associated with lower lung function and increased pulmonary exacerbations [31]. *P aeruginosa* has the ability to convert over time to a mucoid phenotype that is more resistant to antibiotics and innate immunity [32]. Eradication of *P aeruginosa* after initial or early detection using inhaled tobramycin is effective in more than 80% of patients, and likely delays the time until chronic infection [33]. Thus, early detection and eradication therapy for *P aeruginosa* is now standard of care. In patients 6 years of age and older who are chronically infected with *P aeruginosa*, the CFF recommends chronic use of inhaled tobramycin [34] or aztreonam (Cayston) [35] every other month because this has been shown to improve pulmonary function, reduce exacerbation, and improve quality of life [30,36]. Other less common CF pathogens that are emerging and are pathogenic at times in the CF population include methicillin-resistant *S aureus*, *Burkholderia cepacia* complex, and nontuberculous mycobacteria, including *Mycobacterium avium* complex and *Mycobacterium abscessus*.

Pulmonary exacerbations
CF is characterized by progressive lung function decline with acute periods of worsened respiratory symptoms known as pulmonary exacerbations. Pulmonary exacerbations are characterized by increased cough, changes in sputum production, shortness of breath, constitutional symptoms, and/or decline in lung function to less than baseline, among other symptoms [37]. Exacerbations are treated with both increased airway clearance and courses of oral or intravenous antibiotics (either at home or in the hospital), typically targeting patients' typical CF pathogens [38]. Key questions yet to be answered include the optimal form of antibiotics to use (ie, oral vs intravenous), duration of treatment, and use of single agents versus combination therapy. Pulmonary exacerbations can lead to residual loss of lung function and decreased quality of life; recurrent exacerbations are associated with more rapid decline in lung function. Thus, detection and early treatment of exacerbations are critical.

Antiinflammatories
Neutrophil-dominated airway inflammation is a hallmark feature of CF lung disease that starts early in life. A major emphasis in CF treatment has therefore been placed on evaluating drugs that target inflammation. Corticosteroids and high-dose ibuprofen are broad spectrum antiinflammatory agents that have been studied in CF and that inhibit proinflammatory signaling. Both have shown clinical benefit [39,40], but side effects and other considerations have limited their use [41,42]. There are currently 2 routinely prescribed CF therapies that alter inflammation, although they are not considered traditional antiinflammatory agents. The first is recombinant human deoxyribonuclease, discussed in further detail earlier. Over a 3-year period, dornase alpha prevented an increase in several markers of lower airway inflammation that

was observed in untreated patients [43]. The second therapeutic agent is azithromycin, a macrolide antibiotic, which has been shown to reduce pulmonary exacerbations and improve lung function in patients with CF without significantly affecting lower airway bacterial density [44,45]. Evidence suggests that azithromycin may act as an antiinflammatory or immunomodulatory agent in patients both with and without chronic *P aeruginosa* infection [45,46]. Targeting inflammation in CF is still an attractive therapeutic approach, but optimizing antiinflammatory effects while minimizing the detrimental impact on host defense remains a key challenge.

CFTR modulators

In an effort to develop drugs that target the underlying defects in the CFTR protein, the CFF established collaborations with biopharmaceutical companies to support early-stage efforts to discover new medicines for CF. This effort has led to the development and clinical trial testing of a novel class of drugs known as CFTR modulators, which target specific CFTR mutations. These drugs have the potential to be disease modifying, extending the lives of individuals with CF by years and possibly even decades.

As noted earlier, a CFTR mutation class system has been developed to help categorize the myriad of CFTR mutations into groupings with similar functional consequences (see Fig. 3) [1]. Mutations in classes I to III typically have minimal protein function, whereas members of classes IV and V retain partial function and are usually associated with lower sweat chloride levels and pancreatic sufficiency. To date, the most successful type of CFTR modulators studied have been potentiators, which open the mutant CFTR channel and augment the activity of the protein at the plasma membrane. A landmark phase II trial of the CFTR potentiator ivacaftor (Kalydeco), which was studied in 40 patients with CF with at least one copy of the G551D mutation, a class III gating mutant, showed impressive improvements in CFTR activity, detected by NPD and sweat chloride testing, resulting in significant changes in lung function [47]. This trial was rapidly followed by 2 pivotal phase III trials in which ivacaftor treatment led to rapid, dramatic, and sustained improvements in forced expiratory volume in 1 second (FEV_1), weight, quality of life, and biomarkers of CFTR function, and reductions in pulmonary exacerbations [48,49]. As a result, in 2012, the US Food and Drug Administration approved ivacaftor for patients with CF aged 6 years and older with the G551D mutation.

Although G551D is present in only about 4% of the US CF population, the dramatic success of ivacaftor has proved that rescue of mutant CFTR is possible, preparing the way for the development and clinical trial testing of additional CFTR modulators that target most patients with CF. Ivacaftor is currently being studied in young patients with CF, aged 2 to 5 years, with the G551D mutation. Based on in vitro data that this drug shows activity in other CFTR mutations, clinical trials were performed in patients with other non-G551D class III gating mutations. In 2014, ivacaftor was approved for use in patients with one of 8 additional class III gating mutations, benefiting an additional 1% of the US CF population.

The next class of CFTR modulators in development and clinical trial testing are correctors of F508del CFTR trafficking defects, which work by increasing F508del CFTR protein at the plasma membrane (see Fig. 3). Vertex Pharmaceuticals has developed 2 F508del correctors that have advanced to clinical trials (VX-809 or lumacaftor, and VX-661). Preclinical testing has shown that combining the CFTR corrector lumacaftor with the potentiator ivacaftor leads to enhanced F508del CFTR activity relative to lumacaftor alone [50]. This finding led to a phase II combination trial of lumacaftor and ivacaftor that showed statistically significant improvements in lung function among adults with CF with 2 copies (homozygous) of the F508del mutation (press release from Vertex Pharmaceuticals, unpublished data, June 28, 2012). These findings provided the basis for 2 large phase III trials that are currently investigating the safety and efficacy of combination therapy in patients with CF homozygous for F508del. Results from these phase III trials are expected by the end of 2014. Combination therapy with a CFTR corrector and potentiator, if successful, has the potential to benefit approximately 75% of the US CF population.

The CFTR modulator program also includes treatment strategies directed toward suppression of premature termination codons (class I mutations) (see Fig. 3), present in approximately 10% of US patients with CF. The discovery that aminoglycoside antibiotics can allow the ribosome to read through premature termination codons resulting in full-length functional protein [51] has led to investigations of the small molecule ataluren (PTC124) by PTC Therapeutics. Following a series of phase II trials that showed modest improvements in primary outcomes [52,53], a large phase III trial failed to show a significant improvement in FEV_1, the primary end point, but did show a small effect on lung function in a predefined subset of individuals who were not treated with inhaled antibiotics, which are purported to alter the efficacy of ataluren [54]. Although the clinical status of ataluren remains uncertain at present, studies involving other compounds with translational read-through properties are proceeding [55].

Lung transplant

Although a rare occurrence in pediatrics, bilateral lung transplant is an option to consider for patients with CF who develop severe bronchiectasis and end-stage lung disease. Referral for transplant should be considered for patients with an FEV_1 consistently less than 30% of predicted or a rapid decline in FEV_1, increased frequency or severity of pulmonary exacerbations, recurrent episodes of massive hemoptysis, and/or recurrent or refractory pneumothorax [56]. Other factors included in the pretransplant assessment include oxygen dependency, hypercapnia, and pulmonary hypertension, as well as the patients' infectious history and CF comorbidities [56]. In 2011, there were about 75 pediatric lung transplants worldwide for an indication of CF reported to the Registry for the International Society for Heart and Lung Transplantation [57]. Survival following CF pediatric lung transplant from 1990 to 2011 is estimated to be 80% at 1 year, 50% at 5 years, and 33% at 10 years after transplantation. Median survival for pediatric CF transplant is 4.7 years [57]. Lung transplant for CF-related bronchiectasis and lung disease is more common in adults, with more than 600 transplants performed worldwide in 2011 [58]. Survival is slightly better at about 85% at 1 year, 60% at 5 years, and 45% at 10 years after transplantation. Median survival for adult CF transplant is 7.8 years [58].

Nutrition
The goal of nutritional therapy in CF is to maintain normal growth velocity throughout childhood and normal weight in adulthood [59]. Population-based studies show improved lung function and survival in those with higher weight for height and body mass index (BMI). Based on studies showing that optimal growth is associated with improved lung function, the stated goal for infants is to maintain weight for height greater than the 50th percentile and children aged 2 years and older to maintain BMI greater than the 50th percentile. In order to achieve optimal growth, children with CF require a high-calorie (typically 110%–200% of normal recommended caloric intake) and high-fat (40% of calories from fat is recommended) diet. Oral or gastrostomy tube supplements are often required in order to meet caloric goals. For patients with CF who are pancreatic insufficient (85%–90% of the CF population), pancreatic enzyme replacement therapy (PERT) is required in order to adequately absorb complex carbohydrates, fat, and protein. Enzymes are taken before all meals, snacks, supplements, and enteral feedings.

Patients with CF are at risk for fat-soluble vitamin and zinc deficiency caused by malabsorption. A CF-specific multivitamin is recommended for all people with CF. Zinc supplementation should be considered in children who are not growing adequately. Fat-soluble vitamin levels for vitamins A, D, and E are measured annually, and additional vitamin supplements are prescribed as needed. The CFF recommends a minimal 25-hydroxyvitamin D concentration of 30 ng/mL (75 nmol/L) for vitamin D sufficiency in CF [60]. Vitamin K status is more difficult to assess, but serum prothrombin time increase in a patient with CF strongly suggests vitamin K deficiency and is generally treated with additional supplementation. Daily supplementation with salt is also critical for people with CF, to prevent against hyponatremic, hypochloremic dehydration, and other electrolyte abnormalities. Chronic salt depletion can also contribute to failure to thrive, and should be considered in children with CF who are not growing adequately. A child presenting with unexplained hypochloremic metabolic alkalosis should be evaluated for CF, because this condition strongly suggests CF.

ACCREDITED CF CLINICAL CARE CENTERS AND SURVEILLANCE
The CFF is responsible for accrediting and funding the more than 110 pediatric and adult CF care centers across the United States. In addition, the CFF oversees the publication and dissemination of consensus CF care guidelines and

supporting many CF-related research efforts. Following diagnosis through newborn screen, the CFF recommends that infants be evaluated at an accredited CF care center, with the goal of an initial visit within 24 to 72 hours of diagnosis [61]. At that visit families receive comprehensive education regarding the CF diagnosis and CF-specific cares. In addition, treatments including salt supplementation, CF vitamins, and PERT are initiated. In the first year of life, there is much collaboration between the primary care provider and the CF care center, and visits are meant to complement one another. In addition to the standard pediatric visits, it is recommended that infants are followed monthly at the CF care center for the first 6 months of life, then every 1 to 2 months until 1 year. After 1 year of age, the CFF recommends that all patients with CF be followed at an accredited CF care center on a quarterly basis. Surveillance cultures are performed quarterly and, when capable, patients undergo routine spirometry for monitoring purposes at least twice annually. Care is provided with a multidisciplinary team approach, including pulmonologists trained in CF care, advance practice providers, nurses, respiratory therapists, dieticians, and social workers. Other consultants that patients may see regularly include otolaryngologists, endocrinologists, gastroenterologists, and liver specialists to assist in managing the comorbidities in CF. Mental health issues (eg, depression and anxiety) are increasingly recognized as important contributors to impaired quality of life and decreased adherence to medical therapy. Thus, the importance of mental health screening and psychiatry/psychology availability in CF care centers is becoming clear. Patients with CF should also maintain a relationship with a primary care provider for routine cares and immunizations provided on a standard schedule.

SUMMARY

CF is a genetic, life-shortening, multisystem disease that is most commonly diagnosed through newborn screen performed in all 50 states in the United States. In the past, therapies for CF lung disease have primarily targeted the downstream effects of a dysfunctional CFTR protein. Newer CFTR modulator therapies, targeting the basic defect in CF, are available for a limited group of people with CF, and offer the hope of improved treatment options for many more people with CF in the near future. Best practice is directed by consensus clinical care guidelines from the CFF and is provided with a multidisciplinary approach by the team at the CF care center and the primary care office.

References

[1] Welsh MJ, Ramsey BW, Accurso FJ, et al. Cystic fibrosis. In: Scriver CR, Beadudet AL, Valle D, et al, editors. The metabolic and molecular bases of inherited disease. New York: McGraw-Hill; 2001. p. 521–88.

[2] Anselmo MA, Lands LC. Cystic fibrosis: overview. In: Taussig LM, Landau LI, editors. Pediatric respiratory medicine. 2nd edition. Philadelphia: Mosby; 2008. p. 845–57.

[3] Andersen DH. Cystic fibrosis of the pancreas and its relation to celiac disease. Am J Dis Child 1938;56:344–99.

[4] Cystic Fibrosis Foundation patient registry: 2012 annual data report to the center directors. Bethesda, MD: Cystic Fibrosis Foundation; 2013.

[5] Cohen-Cymberknoh M, Shoseyov D, Kerem E. Managing cystic fibrosis: strategies that increase life expectancy and improve quality of life. Am J Respir Crit Care Med 2011;183: 1463–71.

[6] Clancy JP, Jain M. Personalized medicine in cystic fibrosis: dawning of a new era. Am J Respir Crit Care Med 2012;186:593–7.

[7] Grosse SD, Boyle CA, Botkin JR, et al. Newborn screening for cystic fibrosis: evaluation of benefits and risks and recommendations for state newborn screening programs. MMWR Recomm Rep 2004;53:1–36.

[8] Comeau AM, Accurso FJ, White TB, et al. Guidelines for implementation of cystic fibrosis newborn screening programs: Cystic Fibrosis Foundation workshop report. Pediatrics 2007;119:e495–518.

[9] Rosenstein BJ, Cutting GR. The diagnosis of cystic fibrosis: a consensus statement. Cystic Fibrosis Foundation Consensus Panel. J Pediatr 1998;132:589–95.

[10] Farrell PM, Rosenstein BJ, White TB, et al. Guidelines for diagnosis of cystic fibrosis in newborns through older adults: Cystic Fibrosis Foundation consensus report. J Pediatr 2008;153:S4–14.

[11] Hammond KB, Abman SH, Sokol RJ, et al. Efficacy of statewide neonatal screening for cystic fibrosis by assay of trypsinogen concentrations. N Engl J Med 1991;325: 769–74.

[12] LeGrys VA, Applequist R, Briscoe DR, et al. Sweat testing: sample collection and quantitative chloride analysis; approved guideline—third edition. CLSI document C34-A3. Wayne, PA: Clinical and Laboratory Standards Institute; 2009.

[13] Highsmith WE, Burch LH, Zhou Z, et al. A novel mutation in the cystic fibrosis gene in patients with pulmonary disease but normal sweat chloride concentrations. N Engl J Med 1994;331:974–80.

[14] Moskowitz SM, Chmiel JF, Sternen DL, et al. Clinical practice and genetic counseling for cystic fibrosis and CFTR-related disorders. Genet Med 2008;10:851–68.

[15] Rogan MP, Stoltz DA, Hornick DB. Cystic fibrosis transmembrane conductance regulator intracellular processing, trafficking, and opportunities for mutation-specific treatment. Chest 2011;139:1480–90.

[16] Paranjape SM, Zeitlin PL. Atypical cystic fibrosis and CFTR-related diseases. Clin Rev Allergy Immunol 2008;35:116–23.

[17] Thauvin-Robinet C, Munck A, Huet F, et al. The very low penetrance of cystic fibrosis for the R117H mutation: a reappraisal for genetic counselling and newborn screening. J Med Genet 2009;46:752–8.

[18] Cutting GR. Modifier genes in Mendelian disorders: the example of cystic fibrosis. Ann N Y Acad Sci 2010;1214:57–69.

[19] Borowitz D, Durie PR, Clarke LL, et al. Gastrointestinal outcomes and confounders in cystic fibrosis. J Pediatr Gastroenterol Nutr 2005;41:273–85.

[20] Zielenski J. Genotype and phenotype in cystic fibrosis. Respiration 2000;67:117–33.

[21] Castellani C. CFTR2: how will it help care? Paediatr Respir Rev 2013;14(Suppl 1):2–5.

[22] Borowitz D, Parad RB, Sharp JK, et al. Cystic Fibrosis Foundation practice guidelines for the management of infants with cystic fibrosis transmembrane conductance regulator-related metabolic syndrome during the first two years of life and beyond. J Pediatr 2009;155: S106–16.

[23] De Boeck K, Kent L, Davies J, et al. CFTR biomarkers: time for promotion to surrogate endpoint. Eur Respir J 2013;41:203–16.

[24] Schechter MS. Benchmarking to improve the quality of cystic fibrosis care. Curr Opin Pulm Med 2012;18:596–601.

[25] Flume PA, Robinson KA, O'Sullivan BP, et al. Cystic fibrosis pulmonary guidelines: airway clearance therapies. Respir Care 2009;54:522–37.

[26] Donaldson SH, Bennett WD, Zeman KL, et al. Mucus clearance and lung function in cystic fibrosis with hypertonic saline. N Engl J Med 2006;354:241–50.

[27] Elkins MR, Robinson M, Rose BR, et al. A controlled trial of long-term inhaled hypertonic saline in patients with cystic fibrosis. N Engl J Med 2006;354:229–40.

[28] Aitken ML, Bellon G, De Boeck K, et al. Long-term inhaled dry powder mannitol in cystic fibrosis: an international randomized study. Am J Respir Crit Care Med 2012;185: 645–52.

[29] Fuchs HJ, Borowitz DS, Christiansen DH, et al. Effect of aerosolized recombinant human DNase on exacerbations of respiratory symptoms and on pulmonary function in patients with cystic fibrosis. The Pulmozyme Study Group. N Engl J Med 1994;331:637–42.

[30] Flume PA, O'Sullivan BP, Robinson KA, et al. Cystic fibrosis pulmonary guidelines: chronic medications for maintenance of lung health. Am J Respir Crit Care Med 2007;176: 957–69.

[31] Emerson J, Rosenfeld M, McNamara S, et al. Pseudomonas aeruginosa and other predictors of mortality and morbidity in young children with cystic fibrosis. Pediatr Pulmonol 2002;34:91–100.

[32] Li Z, Kosorok MR, Farrell PM, et al. Longitudinal development of mucoid Pseudomonas aeruginosa infection and lung disease progression in children with cystic fibrosis. JAMA 2005;293:581–8.

[33] Treggiari MM, Retsch-Bogart G, Mayer-Hamblett N, et al. Comparative efficacy and safety of 4 randomized regimens to treat early Pseudomonas aeruginosa infection in children with cystic fibrosis. Arch Pediatr Adolesc Med 2011;165:847–56.

[34] Ramsey BW, Pepe MS, Quan JM, et al. Intermittent administration of inhaled tobramycin in patients with cystic fibrosis. Cystic Fibrosis Inhaled Tobramycin Study Group. N Engl J Med 1999;340:23–30.

[35] McCoy KS, Quittner AL, Oermann CM, et al. Inhaled aztreonam lysine for chronic airway Pseudomonas aeruginosa in cystic fibrosis. Am J Respir Crit Care Med 2008;178:921–8.

[36] Mogayzel PJ Jr, Naureckas ET, Robinson KA, et al. Cystic fibrosis pulmonary guidelines. Chronic medications for maintenance of lung health. Am J Respir Crit Care Med 2013;187:680–9.

[37] Goss CH, Burns JL. Exacerbations in cystic fibrosis. 1: Epidemiology and pathogenesis. Thorax 2007;62:360–7.

[38] Flume PA, Mogayzel PJ Jr, Robinson KA, et al. Cystic fibrosis pulmonary guidelines: treatment of pulmonary exacerbations. Am J Respir Crit Care Med 2009;180:802–8.

[39] Eigen H, Rosenstein BJ, FitzSimmons S, et al. A multicenter study of alternate-day prednisone therapy in patients with cystic fibrosis. Cystic Fibrosis Foundation Prednisone Trial Group. J Pediatr 1995;126:515–23.

[40] Konstan MW, Byard PJ, Hoppel CL, et al. Effect of high-dose ibuprofen in patients with cystic fibrosis. N Engl J Med 1995;332:848–54.

[41] Lai HC, FitzSimmons SC, Allen DB, et al. Risk of persistent growth impairment after alternate-day prednisone treatment in children with cystic fibrosis. N Engl J Med 2000;342:851–9.

[42] Lands LC, Milner R, Cantin AM, et al. High-dose ibuprofen in cystic fibrosis: Canadian safety and effectiveness trial. J Pediatr 2007;151:249–54.

[43] Paul K, Rietschel E, Ballmann M, et al. Effect of treatment with dornase alpha on airway inflammation in patients with cystic fibrosis. Am J Respir Crit Care Med 2004;169: 719–25.

[44] Saiman L, Marshall BC, Mayer-Hamblett N, et al. Azithromycin in patients with cystic fibrosis chronically infected with Pseudomonas aeruginosa: a randomized controlled trial. JAMA 2003;290:1749–56.

[45] Saiman L, Anstead M, Mayer-Hamblett N, et al. Effect of azithromycin on pulmonary function in patients with cystic fibrosis uninfected with Pseudomonas aeruginosa: a randomized controlled trial. JAMA 2010;303:1707–15.

[46] Ratjen F, Saiman L, Mayer-Hamblett N, et al. Effect of azithromycin on systemic markers of inflammation in cystic fibrosis patients uninfected with *Pseudomonas aeruginosa*. Chest 2012;142(5):1259–66.

[47] Accurso FJ, Rowe SM, Clancy JP, et al. Effect of VX-770 in persons with cystic fibrosis and the G551D-CFTR mutation. N Engl J Med 2010;363:1991–2003.

[48] Ramsey BW, Davies J, McElvaney NG, et al. A CFTR potentiator in patients with cystic fibrosis and the G551D mutation. N Engl J Med 2011;365:1663–72.

[49] Davies JC, Wainwright CE, Canny GJ, et al. Efficacy and safety of ivacaftor in patients aged 6 to 11 years with cystic fibrosis with a G551D mutation. Am J Respir Crit Care Med 2013;187:1219–25.

[50] Van Goor F, Hadida S, Grootenhuis PD, et al. Correction of the F508del-CFTR protein processing defect in vitro by the investigational drug VX-809. Proc Natl Acad Sci U S A 2011;108:18843–8.

[51] Bedwell DM, Kaenjak A, Benos DJ, et al. Suppression of a CFTR premature stop mutation in a bronchial epithelial cell line. Nat Med 1997;3:1280–4.

[52] Kerem E, Hirawat S, Armoni S, et al. Effectiveness of PTC124 treatment of cystic fibrosis caused by nonsense mutations: a prospective phase II trial. Lancet 2008;372:719–27.

[53] Sermet-Gaudelus I, Boeck KD, Casimir GJ, et al. Ataluren (PTC124) induces cystic fibrosis transmembrane conductance regulator protein expression and activity in children with nonsense mutation cystic fibrosis. Am J Respir Crit Care Med 2010;182:1262–72.

[54] Rowe S, Sermet-Gaudelus I, Konstan M, et al. Results of the phase 3 study of ataluren in nonsense mutation cystic fibrosis (NMCF). Pediatr Pulmonol Suppl 2012;35:A193.

[55] Xue X, Mutyam V, Tang L, et al. Synthetic aminoglycosides efficiently suppress cystic fibrosis transmembrane conductance regulator nonsense mutations and are enhanced by ivacaftor. Am J Respir Cell Mol Biol 2014;50(4):805–16.

[56] Braun AT, Merlo CA. Cystic fibrosis lung transplantation. Curr Opin Pulm Med 2011;17: 467–72.

[57] Benden C, Edwards LB, Kucheryavaya AY, et al. The Registry of the International Society for Heart and Lung Transplantation: sixteenth official pediatric lung and heart-lung transplantation report–2013; focus theme: age. J Heart Lung Transplant 2013;32:989–97.

[58] Yusen RD, Christie JD, Edwards LB, et al. The Registry of the International Society for Heart and Lung Transplantation: thirtieth adult lung and heart-lung transplant report–2013; focus theme: age. J Heart Lung Transplant 2013;32:965–78.

[59] Stallings VA, Stark LJ, Robinson KA, et al. Evidence-based practice recommendations for nutrition-related management of children and adults with cystic fibrosis and pancreatic insufficiency: results of a systematic review. J Am Diet Assoc 2008;108:832–9.

[60] Tangpricha V, Kelly A, Stephenson A, et al. An update on the screening, diagnosis, management, and treatment of vitamin D deficiency in individuals with cystic fibrosis: evidence-based recommendations from the Cystic Fibrosis Foundation. J Clin Endocrinol Metab 2012;97:1082–93.

[61] Borowitz D, Robinson KA, Rosenfeld M, et al. Cystic Fibrosis Foundation evidence-based guidelines for management of infants with cystic fibrosis. J Pediatr 2009;155:S73–93.

[62] Debray D, Kelly D, Houwen R, et al. Best practice guidance for the diagnosis and management of cystic fibrosis-associated liver disease. J Cyst Fibros 2011;10(Suppl 2):S29–36.

[63] Moran A, Brunzell C, Cohen RC, et al. Clinical care guidelines for cystic fibrosis-related diabetes: a position statement of the American Diabetes Association and a clinical practice guideline of the Cystic Fibrosis Foundation, endorsed by the Pediatric Endocrine Society. Diabetes Care 2010;33:2697–708.

[64] Stevens DA, Moss RB, Kurup VP, et al. Allergic bronchopulmonary aspergillosis in cystic fibrosis–state of the art: Cystic Fibrosis Foundation Consensus Conference. Clin Infect Dis 2003;37(Suppl 3):S225–64.

[65] Besier T, Born A, Henrich G, et al. Anxiety, depression, and life satisfaction in parents caring for children with cystic fibrosis. Pediatr Pulmonol 2011;46:672–82.

Advances in Pediatrics 61 (2014) 245–260

ADVANCES IN PEDIATRICS

Pediatrics in Disasters
Evaluation of a Global Training Program

Lindsey Cooper, MD[a], Hongyan Guan, MD, PhD[b],
Ana A. Ortiz-Hernández, MD[c], Beatriz Llamosas Gallardo, MD[c],
Genesis Rivera, MD[d], Joseph Wathen, MD[a],
Benjamin Shulman, BA[e], Stephen Berman, MD[a],*

[a]University of Colorado Denver, Center for Global Health-Colorado School of Public Health, 13199 East
Montview Boulevard, Aurora, CO 80045, USA; [b]Department of Early Childhood Development, Capital
Institute of Pediatrics, Chaoyang District, Beijing 100020, China; [c]Emergency Department, Instituto
Nacional de Pediatria Insurgentes Sur 3700 C, D. F04530, México; [d]St. Luke's College of Medicine,
Quezon City, Phillippines; [e]Department of Biostatistics and Informatics, Colorado School of Public
Health, 13199 East Montview Boulevard, Aurora, CO 80045, USA

Keywords

- PEDS in disaster • Pediatric disaster education • Evaluation • Efficacy • Outcomes
- Disaster training program • American Academy of Pediatrics

Contributors' statements

Dr Lindsey Cooper designed the 6 month evaluation instruments for the PEDS in
Disaster course. She conducted much of the data evaluation in partnership
with international sites. She drafted the initial manuscript, incorporated the revisions of all authors, and approved the manuscript as submitted.

Dr Hongyan Guan administered the evaluation tools after teaching and organizing the PEDS courses in China. She then carried out a data analysis with
Dr Cooper. She critically evaluated and approved the final manuscript as
submitted.

(continued on next page)

Funding Source: No external funding source was secured for this study.
Financial Disclosure: The authors have no financial relationships relevant to this article to disclose.
Conflict of Interest: The authors have no conflicts of interest to disclose.

*Corresponding author. *E-mail address:* stephen.berman@childrenscolorado.org

0065-3101/14/$ – see front matter
http://dx.doi.org/10.1016/j.yapd.2014.03.003 © 2014 Elsevier Inc. All rights reserved.

(continued)

Dr Ana A. Ortiz Hernandez was involved in designing educational tools used in Mexico, as well as teaching and organizing the PEDS course. She was involved in data collection and evaluation with Dr Cooper. She critically evaluated and approved the final manuscript as submitted.

Dr Beatriz Llamosas Gallardo was involved in teaching and organizing the PEDS course in Mexico. She was also involved in data collection and review of the results. She critically evaluated and approved the final manuscript as submitted.

Dr Genesis Rivera was involved in teaching and organizing the first PEDS course in the Philippines. He was involved in adapting the curriculum to a new context. He was also involved in data collection and review of the results. He critically evaluated and approved the final manuscript as submitted.

Dr Joseph Wathen was involved in teaching, curriculum design, and organizing the PEDS courses. He was involved in data evaluation and design of the figures. He critically evaluated and approved the final manuscript as submitted.

Benjamin Shulman was involved in statistical design and evaluation of both qualitative and quantitative data. He assisted Dr Cooper in the design of the figures. He critically evaluated and approved the final manuscript as submitted.

Dr Stephen Berman designed the PEDS course evaluative instruments with Dr Cooper. He was involved in course design, organization, and teaching of the PEDS course. He was involved in data collection and critical appraisal with Dr Cooper. He was instrumental in the writing of the initial manuscript with Dr Cooper and approved the final manuscript as submitted.

Key points

- This report describes the experience and evaluations available in the 20 Pediatrics in Disasters (PEDS) training courses held between 2008 and 2013 in 13 low income countries.

- Pre and post-testing documented cognitive gains, satisfaction with the course was high, the material was considered very useful and participation motivated involvement in disaster-related activities.

- Obtaining stronger support from ministries of health and other governmental agencies will be necessary to disseminate this course in LMICs.

Abbreviations

AAP	American Academy of Pediatrics
ACINDES	Association for Health Research and Development
ALAPE	Latin American Pediatric Society
ATLS	Advanced Trauma Life Support
LMIC	Low- and middle-income countries
MOH	Ministry of Health
PAHO	Pan American Health Organization
PBL	Problem-based learning
PEDS	Pediatrics in Disasters

What is known on this subject: There are few evaluations of pediatric disaster training programs. Most evaluations are of small programs with limited curricula and audience.

What this study adds: We assess the cognitive gains in disaster-related knowledge associated with participation in the course and the usefulness of the training. The follow-up assessment in a subset of the courses documents post-course participation in disaster planning, training, and response.

INTRODUCTION

From the earthquakes in Haiti, Chile, and China to floods in Pakistan and the deadly Asian tsunami, natural disasters have increasingly caused unimaginable levels of destruction and death. In 2009, there was nearly one natural disaster daily somewhere in the world, killing an estimated 10,655 persons and affecting 119 million others through loss of homes or livelihoods [1]. Complex humanitarian emergencies resulting from an international or civil war continue to increase in frequency.

Although a quarter of the world's population is younger than 5 years, 50% of the victims of man-made and natural disasters are children [2]. Children are disproportionately victims of both man-made and natural disasters, as their vulnerability has physiologic, psychological, and developmental determinants. Despite their increased risk, children are more likely to be unaware of danger and often fail to recognize the meaning of their own distress. Therefore, they often fail to quickly seek help.

Disaster plans often fail to adequately consider the emotional vulnerability of children and adolescents. The severity of emotional reactions is influenced by the psychosocial developmental stage, individual characteristics, degree of emotional and affective dependency on adults, and previous experiences. Reunification of children and adolescents with their families as soon as possible is critical following a disaster. Failure to achieve reunification also increases concerns about child and youth safety and security.

Pediatricians must ensure that local, regional, and national disaster preparedness planning meets the specific needs of children and adolescents. In addition, pediatricians need to be an important source of information, support, and help for the community, school, families, and children. To do this effectively, pediatricians must be trained and motivated to take on these tasks. Hurricane Katrina demonstrated that even high-income countries like the United States have gaps in pediatric disaster preparedness and problems in response [3]. We have learned that there is a need to improve pediatric disaster preparedness at all levels of medical training [4–6], as well as for a wide range of disaster relief workers worldwide [7].

The American Academy of Pediatrics (AAP) in partnership with the Johnson and Johnson Leadership Institute created a task force in 2004 to develop the Pediatrics in Disasters program to address this training need in LMICs. The training course was designed with input from the World Health Organization

(WHO), the Pan American Health Organization (PAHO), the United States Military, and the Association for Health Research and Development.

The course, delivered during 3 or 4 days, includes lectures with standardized PowerPoint presentations and notes, as well as small group problem-based learning (PBL) exercises. The small group PBL exercises reinforce the lecture presentations through role playing, case discussions, and clinical skills practice workshops. The course finishes with a mass casualty simulation that allows participants to apply the skills of organization, communication, triage, and the care of trauma victims. The course design emphasizes active learning through repetitive exposure, demonstration of technical skills, and participation in problem-based exercises. The 10 modules covered in the international course are displayed in Box 1. The manual can be found at: http://www.aap.org/en-us/advocacy-and-policy/aap-health-initiatives/Children-and-Disasters/Pages/Pediatric-Education-in-Disasters-Manual.aspx [2].

The PEDS program has 3 main aims. First, motivate pediatric health professionals in LMICs to participate in pediatric disaster planning and response activities for their communities by providing training that they consider useful and valuable. Second, establish national PEDS training centers in LMICs to disseminate the training throughout the country, especially in areas prone to natural events. Third, facilitate collaborative training among professional societies, hospitals, medical schools, and governmental agencies, as well as disaster preparedness planning. This report describes the available findings of a structured evaluation of the PEDS course to assess how well the 3 aims have been met.

METHODS

PEDS course evaluation components

Table 1 describes the PEDS courses. Nineteen of these courses had 730 participants. All courses were 4 days except for Vietnam (2010), Haiti, Cambodia, and Indonesia (3 days) and Vietnam 2011 (2 days). The evaluation components included (1) precourse and postcourse testing of cognitive knowledge,

---

Box 1: Course modules in the Pediatrics in Disasters course

1. Disasters and their effects on the population: key concepts
2. Preventive medicine in humanitarian emergencies
3. Planning and triage in the disaster scenario
4. Pediatric trauma
5. Management of prevalent infections in children after a disaster
6. Diarrhea and dehydration
7. Delivery and immediate neonatal care
8. Nutrition and malnutrition
9. The emotional impact of disasters in children and their families
10. Toxic exposures

Table 1

Course summary and available evaluative elements from 19 courses held from 2008 to 2013 with 730 participants

Course location	Course date	Participants	Course sponsorship	Pretest data	Postcourse test data	Immediate course evaluation	Long-term survey data
Panama: Panama City	2008	33	Children's Hospital of Panama, ALAPE		X	X	X
Mexico: Mexico City	2008	31	Instituto Nacional de Pediatria				
China: Beijing	2008	75	Provincial Health Bureau, MOH	X	X	X	X (54 of 75 responses)
Ecuador: Quito	2009	29	Children's Hospital Baca Ortiz, MOH		X		X
Peru: Lima	2009	35	Pediatric Society		X		X
Vietnam: Ho Chi Minh City	2009	46	Project Vietnam, Medical School				X
China: Sichuan	2010	25	UNICEF/WHO, MOH	X	X	X	X (14 of 25 responses)
Panama: David	2010	24	Panamanian Social Security Hospital System, Pediatric Society		X	X	
Vietnam: Da Nang	2010	39	Project Vietnam, Local Hospital, MOH				X
Mexico: Mexico City	2010	25	Pediatric Society, Instituto Nacional Pediatria	a	X	X	X (15 of 25 responses)
China: Beijing	2011	35	Provincial Health Bureau, MOH	X	X		X
Colombia: Cali	2011	31	Pediatric Society, Universidad de Valle		X		X
Philippines: Manila	2011	30	Pediatric Societies	X	X	X	X (15 of 30 responses)
Vietnam: Hanoi	2011	43	Project Vietnam, MOH				X
Nicaragua: Managua	2011	26	MOH, PAHO	X	X	X	X
Mexico: Mexico City	2012	35	Pediatric Society, Instituto Nacional Pediatria	a	X	X	X (14 of 35 responses)
Haiti: Port au Prince	2012	72	Pediatric Society, PAHO, MOH	X	X	X	
Indonesia: Bandung	2013	59	Pediatric Society, Universitas Padjadjaran, Critical Care Working Group	X	X	X	
Cambodia: Phnom Penh	2013	37	University of Health Sciences, Phnom Penh, Cambodia, National Pediatric Hospital	a			
Haiti: Laborde	2013		MOH, UNICEF				

Abbreviations: ALAPE, Latin American Pediatric Society; UNICEF, United Nations Children's Fund.

a Pretest data excluded because of having answers or using the manual.

(2) assessments of satisfaction and usefulness of the overall course and its specific components (lectures and PBL exercises for each module) immediately after completion of the course and at least 6 months later, (3) identification and survey of participants who subsequently engaged in disaster response or planning activities, and (4) surveys of local course directors to determine factors promoting or undermining dissemination of the training. All courses had an agenda that included a precourse test and an immediate postcourse test, as well as formal evaluations of lectures, PBL exercises, and the final simulation. However, because of language barriers or lack of administrative support at certain sites and/or disorganization, these evaluative components were not obtained in all courses. Table 1 describes the evaluation components that were available from each of the courses.

Precourse and postcourse cognitive testing

Precourse testing data were available for 7 courses, whereas postcourse testing data were available for 14 courses (see Table 1). Precourse disaster knowledge was assessed with a pretest consisting of 2 multiple choice questions from each of the 10 modules for a total of 20 questions. Postcourse disaster knowledge was assessed on the final course day with a 60 multiple choice question test covering material from all course modules. All questions from the pretest were incorporated into the posttest. Pretest results were excluded in 2 courses (Mexico 2012, Cambodia): one in which participants had access to the manual and the other in which participants had access to the answer key on the Internet. Some course directors preferred that the results of cognitive testing be presented without course identifiers. Therefore, the results of cognitive testing are presented as course numbers by region.

Immediate postcourse satisfaction and usefulness assessments

The immediate postcourse assessment used a 5-point Likert scale ranging from 1 to 5 (poor, fair, good, very good, and excellent). The overall course evaluation addressed the following questions: (1) How well were the course objectives accomplished? (2) How well did you achieve your objectives in taking the course? (3) Did you receive new information? (4) How relevant and applicable was the course content? (5) How useful was the material? These data were available for 8 courses. Participants also used the 5-point Likert scale to assess the usefulness of the lectures and PBL exercises. These data were available for 10 courses.

Long-term follow-up assessment

The long-term assessment was administered at least 6 months after completion of the course through the Research Electronic Data Capture secure online survey system [8] The survey was sent to Beijing and Sichuan participants 2 years and 1 year after course completion, respectively; other sites completed the survey 6 months after the course. Collected information included course location and dates, age, sex, professional discipline, and usual practice setting. It also assessed respondents' involvement in disaster planning and response before and after the course. The survey assessed whether respondents had used the course manual in their daily medical work and which modules were most useful. Respondents indicated their level of interest in a range of disaster topics by assigning individual integer percentage values (eg, 1%, 2%…99%, 100%). Finally, the follow-up survey included free-text fields in which respondents were asked to suggest potential new content areas and course changes. These free text responses were categorized by theme by 2 researchers independently and decided by collaboration. Although the participants of all courses held before 2012 were surveyed, the response rate was only more than 20% from 5 courses, China 2008, China 2010, Mexico 2010, Mexico 2011, and the Philippines 2011. Responses from other courses were not included in the analysis because of poor response rates.

Surveys of LMIC PEDS course directors

Course directors were surveyed on factors influencing the dissemination of the training such as governmental and or institutional support, faculty support, and funding. Survey questions were developed through a panel of educational experts. Responses were categorized by theme by 2 researchers independently and decided by collaboration.

Statistical sampling, sample size, and analytical plan

Descriptive statistics (means with confidence intervals) were calculated to summarize participants' performance on precourse and postcourse cognitive skills testing using Excel statistical package (Redmond, WA, USA). Descriptive statistics (means) were also calculated to summarize response frequencies for the 5-point Likert scale questions, by country. Paired t-tests were performed on Likert score averages for each module (lecture vs PBL) for each country to help determine whether there was a preferred mode of learning. Free-text responses from the long-term follow-up survey were qualitatively coded by 2 independent investigators, classified into thematic groups, and tallied by thematic group.

The analysis of variance (ANOVA) test was used to test for group differences between LMIC sites in level of interest in learning about particular disaster types on a scale from 0% to 100%. A separate ANOVA was carried out for each category of disaster (epidemic, geophysical, hydrologic, meteorologic, and climatological). A linear model was then used to estimate differences in scores for type of disaster within each site. All components of this structured evaluation were submitted to and approved (or considered exempt) for use by the University of Colorado Combined Institutional Review Board Committee.

RESULTS

Aim 1: Motivate pediatric health professionals in LMICs to participate in pediatric disaster planning and response activities for their communities by providing training that they consider useful and valuable.

Participants gained knowledge from the course based on the performance scores on precourse and postcourse examinations (Table 2). In Asia, the

Table 2
Results of pretesting and posttesting by region

Location	Average pretest score (%)	Average posttest score (%)
Asia		
Course 1	56	70
Course 2	57	72
Course 3	49	65
Course 4	56	73
Course 5	46	71
Latin America & Caribbean		
Course 6	N/A	69
Course 7	N/A	69
Course 8	N/A	78
Course 9	N/A	73
Course 10	N/A	75
Course 11	26	63
Course 12	38	55
Course 13	42	63

precourse examination scores ranged from 46% to 57%, whereas the scores in Latin America/Caribbean were 26%, 38% and 42% (data available for 3 of 8 courses). Posttest scores were available on 509 of the 730 (70%) participants. The posttest examination scores in Asia ranged from 65% to 73%, whereas the scores in Latin America/Caribbean ranged from 55% to 78%. The average posttest score was 70% or higher in 8 of the 13 courses, and 2 courses had an average score of 69%. The average percent increase in scores from pretest to posttest for courses with data was 20%.

For the course to be replicated, course participants (also potential trainers for future courses) would need to value the course material and design. Therefore, having positive course evaluation data would be critical for promoting replication of the course throughout the country. For the 9 courses (China [2], Panama [2], Mexico [2], Philippines [1], Nicaragua [1], and Haiti [1]) with overall course evaluation data, the 5-point Likert scores for course objectives accomplished ranged from 4.1 to 4.9, for personal objectives achieved 4.0 to 4.8, for expectations exceeded 4.1 to 4.9, for amount of new information 4.0 to 4.9, for relevance and applicability 4.0 to 4.8, and for overall usefulness 4.1 to 5.0 (Table 3). The lectures with standardized slides and notes, as well as the problem-based exercises were consistently rated highly. Average Likert scores for lectures and PBL sessions are shown in Table 4 for 9 courses (China [2], Panama, Mexico [2], Philippines, Nicaragua, Indonesia, and Haiti). PBL sessions were rated slightly higher than lectures in China, the Philippines, and Nicaragua, whereas lectures were rated slightly higher in Panama, Haiti, and Indonesia. Both PBL sessions and lecture presentations were rated more than 4 on the Likert scale in all courses except Indonesia. In Sichuan, China, there was significant preference (all P values <.0005) for PBL sessions for 3 modules, nutrition/malnutrition, toxic exposures, and delivery/neonatal care

Table 3
Overall course evaluations for 315 of 730 (43%) of course participants

General course information			Averages from course evaluations					
Course location	Course date	Number of participants	Course objectives accomplished	Personal objectives achieved	Expectations exceeded	Amount of new information	Relevance and applicability	Usefulness overall
Panama	2008	33	4.8	4.8	4.8	4.9	4.9	4.8
China: Beijing	2008	75	4.5	4.5	4.0	4.0	4.1	4.6
China: Sichuan	2010	30	4.2	4.3	4.1	4.6	4.0	4.3
Panama	2010	24	4.8	4.8	4.9	5.0	4.8	5.0
Mexico	2010	25	4.9	4.7	4.6	4.9	4.8	4.5
Philippines	2011	30	4.6	4.5	4.4	4.8	4.8	4.7
Nicaragua	2011	26	4.8	4.7	4.7	4.8	4.7	4.9
Mexico	2012	35	4.9	4.8	4.7	4.8	4.9	4.9
Haiti	2013	72	4.1	4.0	4.1	4.4	4.1	4.1

Ratings based on 5-point Likert scale (1 = poor, 5 = excellent).

Table 4
Usefulness of lectures and problem-based learning exercises by module

Lectures and PBLs	Beijing 2008	Sichuan 2010	Panama 2010	Mexico 2010	Philippines 2011	Nicaragua 2011	Mexico 2012	Haiti 2013	Indonesia 2013
Module 1: Key Concepts	4.3	4.4	4.5	4.5	4.6	4.9	4.8	4.4	3.9
Module 2: Preventive Medicine	4.4	4.5	4.6	4.6	4.7	4.8	4.7	4.1	4.0
Module 2: PBL	4.4	4.3	4.4	4.4	4.5	4.7	4.7	4.4	3.6
Module 3: Planning and Triage	4.5	4.4	4.6	4.5	4.7	4.8	4.8	4.5	3.9
Module 3: PBL	4.5	4.5	4.0	5.0	4.7	4.9	4.8	4.0	3.4
Module 4: Pediatric Trauma	4.2	4.1	4.8	4.8	4.5	4.6	4.9	4.5	3.9
Module 4: PBL	3.9	4.2	4.7	4.7	4.6	4.8	4.8	4.3	3.5
Module 5: Prevalent Infections	4.3	4.3	4.7	4.7	4.7	4.7	4.6	4.4	3.75
Module 5: PBL	4.4	4.4	4.5	4.5	4.7	4.9	4.7	4.3	No data
Module 6: Diarrhea & Dehydration	4.4	4.4	4.7	4.7	4.7	4.8	No data	4.6	3.8
Module 6: PBL	4.5	4.7	4.7	4.7	4.7	4.8	4.8	5.0	No data
Module 7: Neonatal Care	4.2	*4.2	4.6	4.6	4.6	4.5	4.8	5.0	No data
Module 7: PBL	4.4	*4.6	4.6	4.6	4.7	4.9	4.7	No data	No data
Module 8: Malnutrition	4.3	*4.3	4.4	4.4	4.6	4.3	4.7	4.5	4.1
Module 8: PBL	4.5	*4.95	4.5	4.5	4.6	4.9	4.7	No data	4.0
Module 9: Emotional Impact	4.3	4.4	4.8	4.8	4.4	4.7	4.6	No data	4.1
Module 9: PBL	4.5	4.6	4.5	4.5	4.6	4.8	4.6	No data	4.2
Module 10: Toxic Exposures	4.2	*4.1	4.5	4.5	4.5	4.5	4.7	No data	No data
Module 10: PBL	4.6	*4.7	4.6	4.6	4.5	4.7	4.9	No data	No data

Average score based on Likert scale of 1–5, 1 = poor and 5 = excellent.
* P<.0005 for preference for PBL over lecture in Sichuan, China, for 3 modules: Neonatal Care, Malnutrition, and Toxic Exposures.

and a trend toward a preference of PBL for the diarrhea/dehydration module ($P = .07$). None of the other courses had significant preferences for PBL versus lecture for any of the modules.

Follow-up survey assessments with response rates higher than 20% were available from 5 courses: Mexico (2), China (2), and the Philippines (1). These courses with follow-up survey assessments included 184 of 730 (25%) total participants. Response rates to the long-term follow-up survey varied between 43% in Mexico City, Mexico, and 76% in Beijing, China. General and emergency department pediatricians accounted for most of the respondents in the courses held in Mexico and the Philippines. In China, the preventive medicine/public health physician participants made up the largest group. There were lesser numbers of surgeons, psychologists, and nurse respondents. Respondents worked in a wide range of hospital and outpatient facilities in both the private and public sectors. The free-text responses were coded and grouped by theme. The acquisition of clinical skills (14 of 29 responses) and disaster preparedness planning (9 of 29 responses) were most often cited as the most useful elements of the course. Most respondents indicated that the modules were useful in their everyday work (23 of 52 responses), and 22% of these respondents (5 of 23 responses) noted usefulness of the material in designing educational lectures. Respondents indicated interest in enhancing their clinical skills (27 of 70 responses), disaster preparedness planning (17 of 70 responses), and understanding psychological health (14 of 70 responses). A large percentage of respondents in China (63%), Mexico (79%), and the Philippines (93%) indicated that they referred to the PEDS course manual on a regular basis. The respondents across all sites ranked the most useful modules as Planning/Triage and Emotional Impact (43 respondents with these in their top 3 selections) followed by Preventative Medicine (not preventative) and Dehydration/Diarrhea (25 top 3 selections) (Fig. 1). Participants from Mexico rated the Neonatal Care highly, whereas the Chinese rated the Nutrition module highly. Respondents also indicated their level of interest in epidemics (viral and bacterial), geophysical (earthquake, volcano, and earth movements), hydrological (flood), meteorologic (cyclones and hurricanes), and climatological disasters (drought and wildfire). Participants in Sichuan indicated a slightly higher interest in epidemics, geophysical events, and hydrological events than meteorologic or climatological events. Participants in Mexico had more interest in geophysical events than in other disaster types. However, these differences were not statistically significant. For each country, a linear regression model was used to estimate differences in scores for type of disaster within each site. After multivariate analysis, there was not a significant difference in educational interests of various disaster types within a country.

There were 20 individuals who indicated postcourse involvement in either disaster planning or response activities on the long-term survey from 5 courses (China, Mexico, and Philippines). China had 12 individuals involved in such activities (5 were involved before and after course, 7 only after course); Mexico

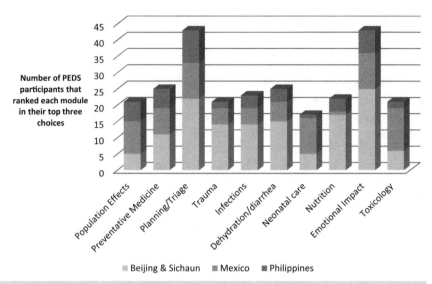

Fig. 1. Ranking of course modules by PEDS participants.

had 4 (2 were involved before and after course, 2 after course); and the Philippines had 4 (1 was involved before and after course, 3 after course). After courses in China, Mexico, and the Philippines, 55% of the participants who were involved in disaster-related activities were involved for the first time. Postcourse involvement in disaster preparation and/or response included disaster preparedness at the community or hospital level, involvement in disaster response activities, disaster-related research activities, and becoming an instructor in a disaster training course. Many of the Chinese participants (7 of 12) became course instructors.

Aim 2: Establish national PEDS training centers in LMICs to disseminate the training throughout the country, especially in areas prone to natural events.

National PEDS training centers were established in 12 LMICs between 2008 and 2013. These centers agreed to hold at least 1 train the trainer course a year and enlist additional hospitals and organizations to carry out their own courses. Six of the national PEDS training centers organized subsequent PEDS courses as agreed (China, Haiti, Mexico, Panama, Philippines, and Vietnam). Indonesia is planning a follow-up course in February 2014. Of these 6 national centers, 5 had support of a governmental agency; 4 of the MOH, 1 of the social security agency, and 1 of the national institute of health. Only the Philippines replicated the course through the Philippine Pediatric Society without government support.

National center course directors were responsible for obtaining faculty, selecting participants, arranging the venue, and implementing the initial course with the assistance of a visiting faculty member from the University of Colorado Center for Global Health. Subsequent courses did not require the attendance of a visiting faculty member, but when requested, the authors tried to send an observer to provide support. Most national course directors (5 of 8 respondents) were initially contacted and recruited by the AAP. Two of these were also contacted by a local pediatric society. Most course directors (6 of 8) were selected because of their experience with educational programs. The ability to disseminate the course throughout the country was limited by a lack of funding according to all the respondents. Additional dissemination limiting factors included the lack of commitment from the local sponsoring organization, constraints on the director's time that would be needed to organize additional courses, and difficulty obtaining faculty. Four course directors thought that local ministries of health should provide financial assistance for future courses. Others suggested that additional support from PAHO or the AAP would be helpful. When asked how the AAP could assist with future courses, everyone noted the need for providing instructors who would help organize and deliver the course. Two countries that failed to replicate the course indicated interest in continuing the program but lacked administrative support/funding and support from local pediatric societies.

Aim 3: Facilitate collaboration for the training among professional societies, hospitals, medical schools, and governmental agencies to improve coordination related to pediatric disaster preparedness planning and response.

Among the 20 LMIC courses, 9 had the ministry of health cosponsor, 7 had a children's hospital cosponsor, 8 had a local pediatric society cosponsor, 4 had a school of medicine cosponsor, 4 had a WHO/United Nations Children's Fund cosponsor, 6 had a general hospital sponsor, and 3 had a nongovernmental organization cosponsor.

DISCUSSION

Although there is an extensive literature describing disaster preparedness training, few formal evaluations of existing programs have been published [4]. Most existing pediatric courses have a narrow focus on resuscitation and initial stabilization of pediatric patients. These include Pediatric Advanced Life Support [9], Pediatric Disaster Life Support [10], and Advanced Pediatric Life Support [11]. The Neonatal Resuscitation Program has become a standard in neonatal care in the United States [12,13]. A more basic neonatal resuscitation program designed for LMICs, called Helping Babies Breathe has been widely disseminated and has undergone extensive evaluation in the developing world to determine posttraining neonatal resuscitation skills [14]. PEDS differs from these programs in that it targets LMICs and includes a more comprehensive curriculum incorporating clinical, public health, and mental health components. PEDS most closely resembles an adult curriculum offered in the United States (as well as in international sites) through the National Disaster Life Support Foundation, Inc, which has courses ranging from core public health concepts to basic and advanced life support [15]. An initial in-depth look at the implementation of the PEDS course in China revealed a variety of postcourse activities including teaching, research, and direct disaster response in the community suggesting that PEDS is meeting its aims [16]. This article explores the effect of the PEDS course at the other sites and in China.

Relative to the first aim, pretesting and posttesting documented cognitive gains, satisfaction with the course was high, and the material was considered useful. Participation motivated involvement in disaster-related activities. After courses in China, Mexico, and the Philippines, 55% of the participants who were involved in disaster-related activities were involved for the first time. The number of participants involved may be a reflection of the occurrence of events in their region and/or government policies that provided opportunities to become involved in planning and response.

One of the added benefits of the courses was the training of local faculty as facilitators in PBL experiences. After the course, several facilitators planned to incorporate the PBL approach into medical school curriculum. The responses also indicated that participants from all countries liked a general approach to course material and had no preference for learning according to specific disaster type (epidemics, geophysical, hydrological, meteorologic, and climatological disasters). However, participants would have liked the PBL scenarios to be more relevant to local conditions.

Related to the second aim, more than half of the national training centers held additional courses or are planning additional courses. Survey of course directors indicated the need for governmental funding for the subsequent courses, as well as support for the course director's time. Because the course is comprehensive and requires a diverse faculty, it is also important to have a close collaboration with a children's hospital, medical school, and/or professional society to obtain the necessary faculty. A high level of satisfaction with the training and belief that the material is useful and valuable is not sufficient to promote dissemination of the training throughout the country. One of the most effective ways to overcome the constraints of funding and leadership is to have the training program integrated into the MOH division responsible for disaster planning and response. The administrative support of regional WHO offices can also assist in accomplishing these goals. It seems that in most cases, countries that have disseminated the training have had support and collaboration of the MOH or another governmental agency.

Relative to the third aim, organizing the courses seemed to facilitate collaboration among professional societies, hospitals, medical schools, and governmental agencies in the hope to improve pediatric disaster preparedness and response. In organizing the courses, each local course director was encouraged to reach out to these potential collaborators to cosponsor the training and serve as faculty in the course. Several of the course directors commented to an author (S.B.) that the course provided the first opportunity for collaboration with cosponsors. The authors did not determine to what extent these collaborations continued and if the coordination around sponsoring the course led to improvements in disaster planning and response.

STUDY LIMITATIONS

The impact of the training program on actual disaster planning and response was not directly measured. Changes in regional or national pediatric-related disaster planning documents or other changes in government disaster-related policies were not analyzed. The analysis of pretest and posttest scores indicates that participants acquired new disaster-related knowledge in the short term, but the long-term retention of this knowledge was not assessed.

Complete data elements from all courses could not be obtained because of communication difficulties and lack of local resources to collect and collate data. The response rates to the long-term survey were varied, and only 5 of the 13 courses surveyed could be included. Therefore, it is difficult to know if the results may be generalized to all course participants and all courses. Low response rates may be due to a variety of reasons, including the lack of Internet access and busy schedules. Course demographic information is incomplete because of inconsistent survey response rates and because not all participants were surveyed. The true incidence of postcourse disaster participation is not known, as this relies on survey completion. In addition, the China follow-up surveys were carried out much later than the other courses. Survey work is subject to recall bias, because of the time interval between the intervention and the evaluation.

SUMMARY

The findings of this evaluation document partial success for the PEDS training program to achieve its 3 aims. It will take several years for the dissemination of this program to reach a critical mass of pediatricians and other physicians in many LMICs. Obtaining stronger support from MOHs and other governmental agencies is necessary to achieve this goal. Another additional approach would be to integrate the training into medical school and residency programs.

References

[1] The International Disaster Database. Centre for Research on the Epidemiology of Disasters (CRED). Available at: http://www.cred.be. Accessed November 16, 2012.

[2] Pediatric education in disasters manual. 2008. Available at: http://www.aap.org/en-us/advocacy-and-policy/aap-health-initiatives/Children-and-Disasters/Pages/Pediatric-Education-in-Disasters-Manual.aspx. Accessed June 3, 2013.

[3] Dolan M, Krug SE. Pediatric disaster preparedness in the wake of Katrina: lessons to be learned. Pediatr Emerg Care 2006;7:59–66.

[4] Ablah E, Tinius AM, Konda K. Pediatric emergency preparedness training: are we on a path toward national dissemination? J Trauma 2009;67(Suppl 2):S152–8.

[5] Cicero M, Baum CR. Pediatric disaster preparedness: best planning for the worst-case scenario. Pediatr Emerg Care 2008;24(7):478–84.

[6] Cicero MX, Blake E, Gallant N, et al. Impact of an educational intervention on residents' knowledge of pediatric disaster medicine. Pediatr Emerg Care 2009;25(7):447–51.

[7] Walker P, Hein K, Russ C, et al. A blueprint for professionalizing humanitarian assistance. Health Aff (Millwood) 2010;29(12):2223–30.

[8] Harris PA, Taylor R, Thielke R, et al. Research electronic data capture (REDCap) - a metadata-driven methodology and workflow process for providing translational research informatics support. J Biomed Inform 2009;42(42):377–81.

[9] Pediatric Advanced Life Support (PALS) American Heart Association. Available at: http://www.heart.org/HEARTORG/CPRAndECC/HealthcareTraining/Pediatrics/Pediatric-Advanced-Life-Support-PALS_UCM_303705_Article.jsp. Accessed August 10, 2012.

[10] E Aghababian. Pediatric Disaster Life Support (PDLS). Available at: http://www.umassmed.edu/cme/courses/pdls/index.aspx?linkidentifier=id&itemid=75640. Accessed August 10, 2012.

[11] Advanced Pediatric Life Support (APLS). American College of Emergency Physicians. Available at: http://www.aplsonline.com/default.aspx. Accessed August 10, 2012.

[12] Neonatal Resuscitation Program (NRP). 2011. Available at: http://www2.aap.org/nrp/. Accessed November 16, 2012.

[13] Wu TJ, Carlo WA. Neonatal resuscitation guidelines 2000: framework for practice. J Matern Fetal Neonatal Med 2002;11(1):4–10.

[14] Goudar S, Somannavar M, Clark R, et al. Stillbirth and newborn mortality in India after Helping Babies Breathe training. Pediatrics 2013;131(2):e344–52. Available at: http://pediatrics.aappublications.org/content/early/2013/o1/15/peds.2012-2112. Accessed October 1, 2013.

[15] National Disaster Life Support. National Disaster Life Support Foundation, Inc. 2012. Available at: http://www.ndlsf.org/. Accessed August 10, 2012.

[16] Cooper L, Guan H, Ventre K, et al. Evaluating the efficacy of the AAP "Pediatrics in Disaster" course: the Chinese experience. Am J Disaster Med 2012;7(3):231.

Advances in Pediatrics 61 (2014) 261–269

ADVANCES IN PEDIATRICS

ELSEVIER
MOSBY

Prevention and Management of Pediatric Obesity
A Multipronged, Community-Based Agenda

Alan Shapiro, MD[a], Sandra Arevalo, MPH, RD, CDE[b],
Altagracia Tolentino, MD[b], Hildred Machuca, DO[b],
Jo Applebaum, MPH[a],*

[a]Children's Health Fund and Community Pediatric Programs, Montefiore Medical Center, 853 Longwood Avenue, Bronx, NY 10459, USA; [b]Center for Child Health and Resiliency, Montefiore Medical Center, 890 Prospect Avenue, Bronx, NY 10459, USA

Keywords
- Pediatric obesity - Prevention - Intervention - Primary care - Nutrition education

Key points
- Although childhood obesity rates have stabilized in the last decade, 17% of US children are obese, and poor minority children remain disproportionately affected.
- Community health centers, with their family-centered approach, are ideally situated to play a leading role in prevention and intervention of childhood obesity in the poor communities they serve. Public–private partnerships enhance resources for community health centers, enabling more intensive focus on interventions that address the most prevalent health conditions in these communities.
- Starting Right, an example of such a partnership, is a guideline-based, multidisciplinary, multicomponent initiative for screening, prevention, and treatment of pediatric obesity at an inner city community health center. The initiative aims to build capacity at the individual, family, health center, and community level. Universal screening, messaging throughout the life cycle, and innovative interventions appear to be making an impact.

INTRODUCTION

National surveillance data show that obesity prevalence among US children has stabilized over the past decade at nearly 17% [1]. Although encouraging, these

*Corresponding author. Community Pediatric Programs, Montefiore Medical Center, 853 Longwood Avenue, 2nd Floor, Bronx, NY 10459. *E-mail address:* jappleba@montefiore.org

0065-3101/14/$ – see front matter
http://dx.doi.org/10.1016/j.yapd.2014.03.008 © 2014 Elsevier Inc. All rights reserved.

rates place millions of children at risk for associated chronic health conditions, and poor minority children are disproportionately affected. According to 2009 to 2010 national data, 24% of non-Hispanic black and 21% of Hispanic children were obese compared with 14% of non-Hispanic white children. These disparities persist across all age groups, and present as early as 2 to 5 years of age. Recent reports suggest childhood obesity rates are decreasing in New York City, but predominantly among white children [2]. From 2010 to 2011, the highest obesity rates were seen in Hispanic (27%) and black (21%) children living in high-poverty neighborhoods (ie, ≥30% of residents living below federal poverty level).

Developed by the Children's Health Fund (CHF) in partnership with the Children's Hospital at Montefiore, the Center for Child Health and Resiliency (CCHR) and the South Bronx Health Center (SBHC) are federally qualified health centers serving the nation's poorest congressional district. In this community, a staggering 47% of families with children live below the federal poverty level; 71% of residents are Hispanic, and 26% are black. Thirty-one percent are children under age 18 years (vs 22% in NYC overall) [3]. The South Bronx has among the lowest concentration of grocery stores, and smallest proportion of land used for parks and recreation, of any New York City neighborhood [4,5]. Furthermore, children in this community engage in less physical activity than recommended [6], spending more time at home while parents work long hours and/or multiple jobs–a 21st century version of the latchkey kids. Not surprisingly given this context, the South Bronx has a disproportionately high prevalence of obesity and type 2 diabetes, and low rates of health-promoting behaviors [7]. Of 42 New York City neighborhoods, the communities served by CCHR rank last in most key health indicators [8,9].

To advance the community health center's mission of closing the gap in health disparities, CCHR develops and evaluates interventions that address these conditions in the community it serves [10]. In response to the surge in childhood obesity, Starting Right was launched in 2001 as a guideline-based, multidisciplinary, multicomponent initiative designed as front-line screening, prevention, and treatment of pediatric obesity in a busy primary care setting [11–13]. The initiative consists of interventions that build capacity at the individual, family, health center, and community level. This report describes the elements of Starting Right adopted by an inner city community health center and the population served, consisting of children and families living primarily in public housing in the South Bronx. It also discusses preliminary outcome findings.

SETTING

The South Bronx Health Center (SBHC) was established in 1993 by CHF/Montefiore to serve children and their families in one of New York City's most densely concentrated public housing neighborhoods and a federally designated Health Provider Shortage Area. In 2011, CHF and Montefiore opened the Center for Child Health and Resiliency, providing family-focused, comprehensive primary care to approximately 3500 pediatric patients (0–19 years) annually. In 2010, 42% of children aged 10 to 19 years seen at this clinic were overweight (18%) or obese (24%), and 70% of them had multiple risk factors for type 2 diabetes. In addition to primary care, CCHR provides colocated nutrition, mental health, health education, and case management services.

STARTING RIGHT

Starting Right's goals are to intervene as early as possible to prevent childhood obesity. Primary care providers are well-positioned for front-line identification of children at risk, yet clinician adoption of screening guidelines remains suboptimal in primary care practice [14,15]. Studies show that providers believe obesity prevention and treatment are important and that they have a role to play in intervention [16,17]. However, pediatric primary care providers are reluctant to address obesity due to lack of time and resources, unfamiliarity with guidelines, and the perception that interventions are either unavailable or ineffective [17].

The Starting Right initiative addresses these barriers with its 4 key components: tools and training for improved screening and treatment, culturally appropriate nutrition education materials and counseling, targeted group interventions, and community partnerships. The multidisciplinary team includes primary care providers, nurses, registered dietitians, a health educator, and public health professionals to support intervention design and evaluation. CCHR has a dedicated evaluation team to conduct continuous quality improvement and assess intervention effectiveness, with an emphasis on using health information technology.

INITIATIVE COMPONENTS

Pediatric primary care screening and treatment

At the core of Starting Right is putting into practice complex, nationally accepted guidelines in a primary care setting in which patients have multiple medical and psychosocial issues. Starting Right's clinical leadership, a pediatrician and a registered dietitian, conduct trainings on the latest guidelines and develop tools to facilitate screening, assessment, and referral in the primary care visit. Protocols have been implemented to: (1) universally screen for overweight/obesity by determining body mass index (BMI) percentile; (2) counsel families about nutrition and physical activity regardless of children's weight status; (3) assess risk factors for obesity-related comorbid conditions, such as cardiovascular disease, type 2 diabetes, and nonalcoholic fatty liver disease; and (4) refer to subspecialty care as appropriate [12,13,18].

In 2003, based on then-current American Diabetes Association and Expert Committee recommendations for screening and treatment of pediatric obesity [11,19], the Starting Right team developed a template that was incorporated into the paper medical record to guide providers through the screening process. The template was then revised according to 2007 Expert Committee recommendations [12]. In response to guidelines issued by the National Heart, Lung, and Blood Institute in 2011 for screening and management of cardiovascular risk in children, the authors developed a new algorithm to translate the latest evidence into routine primary care (Fig. 1) [13,20,21]. To the authors'

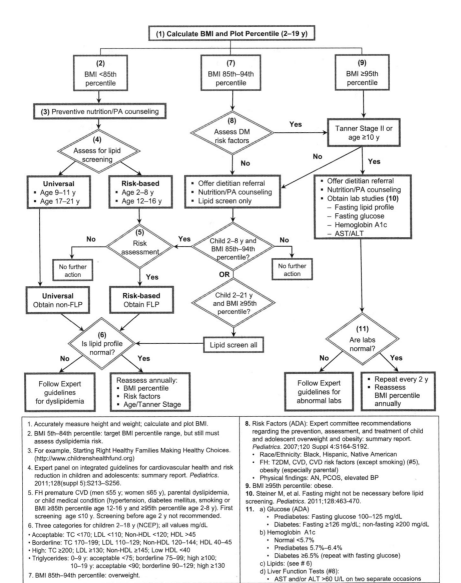

1. Accurately measure height and weight; calculate and plot BMI.
2. BMI 5th–84th percentile: target BMI percentile range, but still must assess dyslipidemia risk.
3. For example, Starting Right Healthy Families Making Healthy Choices. (http://www.childrenshealthfund.org)
4. Expert panel on integrated guidelines for cardiovascular health and risk reduction in children and adolescents: summary report. *Pediatrics.* 2011;128(suppl 5):S213–S256.
5. FH premature CVD (men ≤55 y; women ≤65 y), parental dyslipidemia, or child medical condition (hypertension, diabetes mellitus, smoking or BMI ≥85th percentile age 12-16 and ≥95th percentile age 2-8 y). First screening age ≤10 y. Screening before age 2 y not recommended.
6. Three categories for children 2–18 y (NCEP); all values mg/dL
- Acceptable: TC <170; LDL <110; Non-HDL <120; HDL >45
- Borderline: TC 170–199; LDL 110–129; Non-HDL 120–144; HDL 40–45
- High: TC ≥200; LDL ≥130; Non-HDL ≥145; Low HDL <40
- Triglycerides: 0–9 y: acceptable <75; borderline 75–99; high ≥100;
              10–19 y: acceptable <90; borderline 90–129; high ≥130
7. BMI 85th–94th percentile: overweight.

8. Risk Factors (ADA): Expert committee recommendations regarding the prevention, assessment, and treatment of child and adolescent overweight and obesity: summary report. *Pediatrics.* 2007;120 Suppl 4:S164-S192.
   - Race/Ethnicity: Black, Hispanic, Native American
   - FH: T2DM, CVD, CVD risk factors (except smoking) (#5), obesity (especially parental)
   - Physical findings: AN, PCOS, elevated BP
9. BMI ≥95th percentile: obese.
10. Steiner M, et al. Fasting might not be necessary before lipid screening. *Pediatrics.* 2011;128:463-470.
11. a) Glucose (ADA)
     - Prediabetes: Fasting glucose 100–125 mg/dL
     - Diabetes: Fasting ≥126 mg/dL; non-fasting ≥200 mg/dL
    b) Hemoglobin A1c
     - Normal <5.7%
     - Prediabetes 5.7%–6.4%
     - Diabetes ≥6.5% (repeat with fasting glucose)
    c) Lipids: (see # 6)
    d) Liver Function Tests (#8):
     - AST and/or ALT >60 U/L on two separate occasions

Fig. 1. Screening algorithm for childhood overweight, obesity, and comorbidities based on 2011 Guidelines for Cardiovascular Health and Risk Reduction in Children and Adolescents National Heart, Lung, and Blood Institute. *Abbreviations:* ALT, alanine aminotransferase; AN, acanthosis nigricans; AST, aspartate aminotransferase; BMI, body mass index; BP, blood pressure; CVD, cardiovascular disease; DM, diabetes mellitus; FH, family history; FLP, fasting lipid profile; HDL, high-density lipoprotein; LDL, low-density lipoprotein; PA, physical activity; PCOS, polycystic ovary syndrome; TC, total cholesterol. (*Courtesy of* The National Heart, Lung, and Blood Institute, Bethesda, MD.)

knowledge, an algorithm reflecting these guidelines has not been published previously. These guidelines have been incorporated into templates for the electronic medical record adopted by CCHR and its hospital affiliate.

As part of performance improvement, chart reviews were conducted before and after provider training and implementation of each version of the screening protocol. Providers received feedback and retraining as needed to improve screening and documentation, which are essential components of performance improvement. Results show a marked increase in documentation of BMI percentile after implementation of the Starting Right template from 2004 to 2005 (Fig. 2); by 2008, 99% of children aged 2 to 19 years had BMI percentile documented at their well child care visit. As of 2012, HRSA requires federally qualified health centers to report annually on the percentage of children aged 3 to 17 years seen for any type of primary care visit, with BMI percentile documented [14]. Using standardized measures enables comparison with national averages. For children seen at CCHR in 2012, 93% had their BMI percentile documented, compared with 46% of Medicaid and 45% of commercially insured patients (2011 data) [14].

Nutrition education and counseling

CCHR primary care providers counsel families about nutrition and physical activity across the lifecycle, from pregnancy through adolescence and adulthood, using Starting Right's low-literacy, culturally appropriate health education materials published in English and Spanish (available at childrenshealthfund.org) [22]. These materials target pregnant women, families with young children, and adolescents.

Children and their families also are referred internally to a registered dietitian for nutrition and lifestyle counseling. Using motivational interviewing techniques [12,23], the dietitian assesses family members' readiness to make

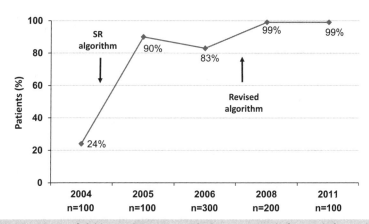

Fig. 2. Percentage of children with BMI percentile documentation before and after implementing the Starting Right (SR) screening protocol and template. Analyses of random samples of children, aged 2 to 19 years, seen for a well child care visit in the measurement year.

changes and helps them set relevant, attainable, and measurable goals. Counseling is informed by years of experience providing care for a diverse community and results of qualitative research conducted among overweight youth and their parents at CCHR. Focus groups emphasized numerous barriers to healthy eating and physical activity: conflicting family needs/preferences; lack of knowledge/skills; financial constraints; limited access to healthy foods and safe outdoor spaces; long work hours; and emotional distress as both a contributor and consequence of overeating and overweight [24]. Moreover, in the local community, cultural norms favor larger body types and discourage weight loss, which could signify poverty, weakness, illness, or drug use.

To enhance acceptance of nutrition referral, the dietitian is called into the examination room by the primary care provider to meet the child and his or her family (meet and greet model) and, when feasible, the dietician conducts a nutrition counseling session immediately following the primary care visit. Tandem visits jump start individual nutrition education and enhance adherence to nutrition-related recommendations. Results of preliminary analysis among 96 overweight/obese children with at least 2 nutrition counseling sessions suggest that over an average of 9.7 months, BMI percentile decreased in 60.4% of patients (mean change of −1.7 percentile).

Group interventions

Health & Fitness Group

Concomitant with universal BMI screening, Starting Right launched a community-based intervention in 2005 to address nutrition education and physical activity among overweight or obese children aged 10 to 14 years. To destigmatize the program, and broaden its reach as obesity prevention and treatment, Health & Fitness was expanded in 2010 to include children aged 6 to 14 years regardless of weight status and integrated into an after-school program at a local public housing community center. The program is open to health center patients and nonpatient public housing residents. This community partnership connects CCHR patients with a free recreational facility and provides essential nutrition education to children and families living in public housing.

Over the 12 weekly sessions, the program's health educator delivers 45-minute age-appropriate, interactive, culturally sensitive nutrition lessons that address food groups, balanced meals, portions, drinks, nutrition facts labels, and healthy fast food options. Children also participate in preparing healthy snacks and taste tests of fruits, vegetables, and low-fat milk. Health & Fitness then devotes 45 minutes each session to physical activity facilitated by a certified fitness instructor. Children are encouraged to perform at least 60 minutes of exercise daily, utilize the community recreational center throughout the week, and limit sedentary activity [12].

To evaluate effectiveness, all children complete an age-appropriate, pre-/postintervention questionnaire tailored to the curriculum to assess changes in knowledge and behavior. Based on preliminary results among 92 children, 82% showed improvement in knowledge, and among a subset of older children,

59% increased physical activity behaviors. Change in pre-/postintervention BMI percentile is also assessed. Because children seen at CCHR may be referred by the dietitian or their primary care provider, 59% of participants thus far were overweight (12%) or obese (47%). Among overweight/obese children who completed the program (n = 42), 60% had a decrease in BMI percentile (mean change of –2.6 percentile). Among healthy weight children, 92% maintained BMI below the 85th percentile. This evaluation is ongoing; the authors also plan to assess the effect on BMI status of individual nutrition counseling and group intervention compared with primary care visits alone.

Group prenatal and well baby care
A paradigm shift from traditional one-on-one care to a group primary care model for pregnant women and in early childhood affords a key prevention strategy to address healthy lifestyle for both mother and baby. Group care provides pregnant women and new mothers with intensive health education, social support, and more time with health professionals than traditional visits. CCHR offers group prenatal care and group well baby care as an alternative to one-on-one prenatal and pediatric visits for the first 18 months. The group care model is based on Centering Pregnancy [25], adapted for the needs and priorities of the CCHR population. During 90- to 120-minute sessions, groups of 8 to 10 women receive prenatal care from women's health providers, and 8 to 10 mother/baby dyads receive well child care from pediatricians, following the routine schedule for prenatal and well child care visits. Fathers or coparents, other family members, and friends are encouraged to attend. Multidisciplinary specialists, including mental health professionals, cofacilitate the group at predetermined sessions to foster stress management, coping, and conflict resolution skills. The registered dietitian has a critical role in providing nutrition messaging, including breastfeeding, introduction of solid foods, and healthy eating for the entire family, and conducting interactive cooking demonstrations at every session.

To date, approximately 400 pregnant women and 90 mother/baby dyads have participated in group care. Outcomes being tracked include breastfeeding initiation and duration, appropriate introduction of solid foods, prenatal weight gain, postpartum weight retention, and children's BMI percentile. Preliminary analyses suggest more favorable results for group compared with traditional care at SBHC/CCHR and with national averages. Of note, among children who participated in group well baby care (n = 36), 2.8% were overweight or obese (≥85th percentile) at age 2 years compared with 15.7%% of 2-year-olds seen at CCHR (n = 356) over the same time period. Ongoing evaluation will further elucidate the effect of group compared with traditional care on primary obesity prevention and other key outcomes.

Partnerships
Partnerships with community-based organizations, private foundations, and local and federal government agencies are essential to developing and sustaining childhood obesity programs. Starting Right's Health & Fitness Group

has been conducted at a police athletic league, a local middle school, and since 2010 in a public housing recreation center. Each partnership permitted children from the host site (nonpatients) to participate, increasing community access to nutrition education and physical activity. Such partnerships build community capacity, promoting healthier communities at the population level [26]. Partnerships with private foundations and government agencies also help to generate resources for the program. Recently, CCHR was chosen to participate in a collaboration of hospital-affiliated community health centers, the New York City Department of Health and Mental Hygiene, and other key stakeholders to improve the health of local communities by increasing access to healthy foods and safe environments for physical activity.

IMPLICATIONS

In addressing health disparities, community health centers, the original medical home, have the unique vantage point as agents of change at the individual, family, and community level. Functioning as beacons in underserved neighborhoods, community health centers garner trust that can be leveraged to tackle etiologically complex conditions such as obesity. Creating culturally sensitive, interactive educational materials helps to narrow the information gap between primary care providers and the population served and encourages behavior change. Moreover, public-private partnerships enhance resources for often financially strapped health centers, enabling more intensive focus on prevalent health conditions that disproportionately affect poor communities.

Starting Right is an example of such a partnership. This multicomponent initiative that provides universal screening, messaging throughout the life cycle, and innovative interventions appears to be making an impact. Governmental, medical, public health, and other nongovernmental bodies have put into action policies and recommendations to reverse the obesity epidemic and mitigate the rise of comorbid conditions. Community health centers, with their family-centered approach, should play a leading role in the prevention and intervention of childhood obesity in the poor communities they serve. Failure to do so will widen the gap in health disparities and result in adverse health outcomes for generations to come.

References

[1] Ogden CL, Carroll MD, Kit BK, et al. Prevalence of obesity and trends in body mass index among US children and adolescents, 1999-2010. JAMA 2012;307(5):483–90.

[2] Centers for Disease Control and Prevention (CDC). Obesity in K-8 students - New York City, 2006-07 to 2010-11 school years. MMWR Morb Mortal Wkly Rep 2011;60(49):1673–8.

[3] U.S. Census Bureau, 2008-2010 American Community Survey. Available at: http://www.nyc.gov/html/dcp/html/neigh_info/bx02_info.shtml. Accessed January 8, 2013.

[4] New York City, Department of City Planning. Going to market: New York City's neighborhood grocery store and supermarket shortage. Available at: http://www.nyc.gov/html/dcp/html/supermarket/index.shtml. Accessed January 8, 2013.

[5] New York City, Department of City Planning. Community district needs for fiscal year 2010: the Bronx. DCP #08–05, December 2008. Available at: http://home2.nyc.gov/html/dcp/pdf/pub/bxneeds_2010.pdf. Accessed January 8, 2013.

[6] Matte T, Ellis JA, Bedell J, et al. Obesity in the South Bronx: a look across generations. New York: New York City Department of Health and Mental Hygiene; 2007.

[7] Goranson C, Jasek J, Olson C, et al. New York city community health survey atlas, 2009. New York: New York City Department of Health and Mental Hygiene; 2010.

[8] Olson EC, Van Wye G, Kerker B, et al. Take care Hunts Point and Mott Haven. NYC community health profiles. 2nd edition. 2006;7(42):1–16. Available at: http://www.nyc.gov/html/doh/downloads/pdf/data/2006chp-107.pdf. Accessed April 16, 2014.

[9] Olson EC, Van Wye G, Kerker B, et al. Take care Highbridge and Morrisania. NYC community health profiles. 2nd edition. 2006;6(42):1–16. Available at: http://www.nyc.gov/html/doh/downloads/pdf/data/2006chp-107.pdf. Accessed April 16, 2014.

[10] Shapiro A, Gracy D, Quinones W, et al. Putting guidelines into practice: improving documentation of pediatric asthma management using a decision-making tool. Arch Pediatr Adolesc Med 2011;165(5):1–7.

[11] Barlow SE, Dietz WH. Obesity evaluation and treatment: expert committee recommendations. The Maternal and Child Health Bureau, Health Resources and Services Administration and the Department of Health and Human Services. Pediatrics 1998;102(3):E29.

[12] Barlow SE, Expert Committee. Expert committee recommendations regarding the prevention, assessment, and treatment of child and adolescent overweight and obesity: summary report. Pediatrics 2007;120(Suppl 4):S164–92.

[13] Expert Panel on Integrated Guidelines for Cardiovascular Health and Risk Reduction in Children and Adolescents, National Heart, Lung, and Blood Institute. Expert panel on integrated guidelines for cardiovascular health and risk reduction in children and adolescents: summary report. Pediatrics 2011;128(Suppl 5):S213–56.

[14] National Committee for Quality Assurance. The state of healthcare quality. 2012. Available at: http://www.ncqa.org/Portals/0/State%20of%20Health%20Care/2012/SOHC_Report_Web.pdf. Accessed April 16, 2014.

[15] Liang L, Meyerhoefer C, Wang J. Obesity counseling by pediatric health professionals: an assessment using nationally representative data. Pediatrics 2012;130(1):67–77.

[16] Leverence RR, Williams RL, Sussman A, et al. Obesity counseling and guidelines in primary care: a qualitative study. Am J Prev Med 2007;32(4):334–9.

[17] Klein JD, Sesselberg TS, Johnson MS, et al. Adoption of body mass index guidelines for screening and counseling in pediatric practice. Pediatrics 2010;125(2):265–72.

[18] American Diabetes Association. Standards of medical care in diabetes—2012. Diabetes Care 2012;35(Suppl 1):S11–63.

[19] American Diabetes Association. Type 2 diabetes in children and adolescents. Pediatrics 2000;105(3):671–80.

[20] Daniels SR, Greer FR, Committee on Nutrition. Lipid screening and cardiovascular health in childhood. Pediatrics 2008;122(1):198–208.

[21] Steiner MJ, Skinner AC, Perrin EM. Fasting might not be necessary before lipid screening: a nationally representative cross-sectional study. Pediatrics 2011;128(3):463–70.

[22] Children's Health Fund. Starting Right health education materials. Available at: http://www.childrenshealthfund.org/healthcare-for-kids/health-education-materials/starting-right. Accessed March 18, 2014.

[23] Schwartz RP, Hamre R, Dietz WH, et al. Office-based motivational interviewing to prevent childhood obesity: a feasibility study. Arch Pediatr Adolesc Med 2007;161(5):495–501.

[24] Larkin M, Applebaum J, Goldsmith S, et al. Double drama: emotional aspects of obesity and behavior change among parents and teens in the South Bronx. Presented at the American Academy of Pediatrics, Future of Pediatrics Conference. Chicago, July 29–31, 2011.

[25] Rising SS, Kennedy HP, Klima CS. Redesigning prenatal care through Centering Pregnancy. J Midwifery Womens Health 2004;49(5):398–404.

[26] Mistry KB, Minkovitz CS, Riley AW, et al. A new framework for childhood health promotion: the role of policies and programs in building capacity and foundations of early childhood health. Am J Public Health 2012;102(9):1688–96.

Advances in Pediatrics 61 (2014) 271–286

ADVANCES IN PEDIATRICS

ELSEVIER
MOSBY

Management of Pediatric Mild Traumatic Brain Injury

Robert C. Caskey, MD, MSc[a], Michael L. Nance, MD[b],*

[a]Department of Surgery, University of Pennsylvania School of Medicine, 3400 Spruce Street, Philadelphia, PA 19104, USA; [b]Department of Surgery, Children's Hospital of Pennsylvania, 34th and Civic Center Boulevard, Philadelphia, PA 19104, USA

Keywords

- Mild traumatic brain injury • Concussion • Second impact syndrome
- Neuropsychological testing • Return to play protocol • Return to learn protocol

Key points

- Mild traumatic brain injury (mTBI), which includes both concussive and subconcussive injuries, is very common and underdiagnosed in the pediatric population.
- In mTBI, the primary injury results from acceleration-deceleration and/or rotational forces on the brain (not necessarily a blow to the head). The hallmark is a metabolic mismatch which, if not treated appropriately, may result in a delay in recovery or further injury to the brain.
- mTBI is a clinical diagnosis. Imaging studies are used to rule out the presence of a more significant traumatic brain injury (TBI) (eg, intracranial hemorrhage) only when suspected.
- The treatment of mTBI is centered on the prevention of secondary brain injury through both cognitive and physical rest.
- Sports-related injuries remain a significant and underdiagnosed cause of pediatric mTBI.
- There have been many important advances in mTBI since the previous article on this topic, most notably:
  o Consensus Statements of the Third and Fourth International Conferences on Concussion in Sport (2008 and 2012).
  o Validated prediction rules for cranial computed tomography following pediatric TBI.
  o Pediatric-specific (ages 5–12 years) neuropsychological testing is now available, but has yet to be thoroughly researched.
  o Adoption of Return to Learn and Return to Play algorithms.

*Corresponding author. E-mail address: nance@email.chop.edu

0065-3101/14/$ – see front matter
http://dx.doi.org/10.1016/j.yapd.2014.03.006   © 2014 Elsevier Inc. All rights reserved.

INTRODUCTION

Head injuries remain the leading cause of both morbidity and mortality in children. With more than 700,000 reported pediatric head injuries occurring annually, and many more unreported, this represents a major pediatric health problem [1,2]. Fortunately, most head injuries in children are classified as mild traumatic brain injury (mTBI). Although there is no uniformly accepted definition in the literature, mTBIs essentially encompass both concussions and subconcussive injuries. Most children (approximately 85%) recover from these injuries uneventfully when treated appropriately. However, in some patients mTBIs can be associated with significant morbidity, including developmental and psychosocial delays in addition to long-term disability. Though very rare, death has been reported with mTBIs (second impact syndrome).

As with all injuries, prevention is the most powerful tool for combating mTBI. Once a mTBI occurs, however, management is centered on the prevention of secondary damage to the brain. Several important advances in the management of mTBI have occurred in the past 10 years, perhaps most notably a heightened awareness of these injuries and the importance of appropriate care and recovery. To this end, mTBI treatment strategies currently focus on cognitive and physical rest, exemplified by the Return to Learn and Return to Play protocols. Combined with improvements in the ability to identify pediatric mTBI, these strategies should lead to a significant decrease in the morbidity associated with this prevalent pediatric disease.

PATHOPHYSIOLOGY OF TRAUMATIC BRAIN INJURIES

Traumatic brain injury (TBI) can occur any time that acceleration-deceleration and/or rotational forces are applied to the head. These forces can be applied through direct impact, such as occurs in sports-related injuries, or without direct impact, such as when rotational forces are applied to the head during a motor vehicle crash. Because of their anatomy, pediatric patients are particularly susceptible to TBI [3]. Children's heads are disproportionately larger and heavier than those of adults, and their skulls are more compliant. Children also have weaker neck muscles and, most importantly, their neurons are less myelinated. Therefore, the pediatric brain is not only more likely to sustain greater shearing forces when a force is applied but also, because of the decreased myelination, is more prone to axonal damage [3,4].

The mechanism of injury is a key factor in determining the severity of the TBI. In pediatric patients, the most common mechanism responsible for TBI occurs in an age-dependent manner. Within the age group 0 to 4 years old falls are the most common mechanism, whereas motor vehicle crashes are the most common cause of TBI in the 14- to 19-year-old group [1]. Sports-related head injuries, another common mechanism, increase with age as the child becomes old enough to participate in sports, especially contact sports, and are reported to peak in the 10- to 14-year age group. However, this may represent underreporting in athletes of high school age [4]. Finally, in any child presenting with a head injury, the possibility for abuse must always be considered, particularly in younger children and infants.

Depending on the mechanism of injury and therefore the amount of force applied, damage can occur to the neuronal tissue itself, its blood supply, or the overlying protective calvarium. This initial energy transfer is known as the primary injury. Primary injuries are further divided into extra-axial and intra-axial injuries. Extra-axial injuries do not involve the neuronal tissue and include injuries such as subarachnoid, subdural, or epidural hematomas. By contrast, intra-axial injuries involve the neuronal tissue itself and include injuries such as cerebral contusion, intracerebral hematoma, and diffuse axonal injury [5]. In severe brain injuries it is not uncommon for both intra-axial and extra-axial injuries to be present.

Following the initial injury, the brain can continue to undergo further damage in a process known as secondary injury. Secondary injury can occur at any time from immediately following the primary injury to days and even months later. This process is believed to occur as a result of complex physiologic derangements in the injured brain. Although these are poorly understood, altered cerebral blood flow and hypoxia, resulting in the production of free radicals and the release of cytokines and opiate peptides, seem to epitomize the common pathway [6]. This process can quickly lead to cerebral swelling and brain herniation. As such, secondary injury is a major cause of death following severe head injury. Strategies for the prevention of secondary injury are therefore of vital importance in the management of severe brain injury. In 2012 new evidence-based guidelines for the management of severe brain injury were published, although these fall outside the scope of this article [7].

The exact mechanisms responsible for the primary injury in mTBI have not yet been elucidated. Current evidence suggests that they are intra-axial in nature, as the proposed mechanisms all involve significant alterations in neuronal cell function; these include abrupt neuronal depolarization, changes in glucose metabolism, and decreased local autoregulation of blood flow. Historically it was assumed that there was no underlying neuronal damage following a concussion or mTBI. However, multiple animal models have now shown evidence of neuronal damage, including localized intracerebral hemorrhage and axonal injury following an induced mTBI [8,9].

Recent studies have demonstrated that, similar to more severe brain injury, a period of inflammation and secondary injury can also follow mTBI [4]. This state often occurs concurrently with a period of metabolic mismatch brought about by the increased glucose demands of the damaged neurons and the decreased supply of glucose secondary to localized vasoconstriction [4,10]. This period of metabolic mismatch has been both demonstrated in animal models and suggested clinically, and can last for up to 2 weeks [4,10,11]. During this period, those neurons that were damaged in the initial injury are particularly vulnerable to secondary insult and cell death. Therefore, any activity from exercise to cognitive stress (ie, school) that can further increase the metabolic demands of the brain during this period should be avoided; this is the guiding principle behind cognitive rest and other strategies aimed at minimizing secondary injury in patients following mTBI.

DEFINITION OF MILD TRAUMATIC BRAIN INJURY

As mentioned previously, mTBI includes both injuries classified as concussions and those classified as subconcussive. In 2012, the Fourth International Conference on Concussion in Sport published a consensus statement, which defines concussion as a "complex pathophysiological process affecting the brain, induced by biomechanical forces" [12]. This conference also concluded that concussion has many common features that may be useful in its diagnosis, namely:

1. Concussion may be caused either by a direct blow to the head, face, neck or elsewhere on the body with an 'impulsive' force transmitted to the head.
2. Concussion typically results in the rapid onset of short-lived impairment of neurologic function that resolves spontaneously. However, in some cases, symptoms and signs may evolve over a number of minutes to hours.
3. Concussion may result in neuropathological changes, but the acute clinical symptoms largely reflect a functional disturbance rather than a structural injury and, as such, no abnormality is seen on standard structural neuroimaging studies.
4. Concussion results in a graded set of clinical symptoms that may or may not involve loss of consciousness. Resolution of the clinical and cognitive symptoms typically follows a sequential course. However, it is important to note that in some cases symptoms may be prolonged [12].

In 2013, the American Academy of Neurology in their Updated Guidelines for the Evaluation and Management of Concussion in Sports also defined concussion as "a clinical syndrome of biomechanically induced alteration of brain function, typically affecting memory and orientation, which may involve loss of consciousness" [13].

Despite these definitions, however, concussion and mTBI are still often used interchangeably. Although not technically correct, this does have clinical utility in that the signs, symptoms, and management of concussion and any other form of mTBI overlap significantly.

INITIAL IDENTIFICATION AND MANAGEMENT OF MILD TRAUMATIC BRAIN INJURY

The diagnosis of mTBI is in large part based on the presence of a combination of symptoms following the injury. These symptoms can be categorized as physical, behavioral, or cognitive in nature, and are listed in Box 1. The most common symptom is headache, which is present in 71.5% of pediatric patients requiring admission following mTBI [14]. Other common symptoms are fatigue, feeling "slowed down," and memory difficulties. It should again be highlighted that brief loss of consciousness is not necessary for making the diagnosis of concussion or mTBI. Furthermore, it is also an unreliable clinical criterion, as it has been reported to be present in somewhere between less than 10% and 68.4% of patients with concussion or mTBI [14,15].

Box 1: Signs and symptoms of mTBI

Physical Symptoms

   Headaches

   Dizziness

   Insomnia

   Fatigue

   Ataxia

   Nausea

   Blurred vision

   Tinnitus

   Seizures

Behavioral Symptoms

   Excessive irritability

   Depression

   Anxiety

   Sleep disturbances

   Eating disturbances

   Emotional lability

   Personality changes

Cognitive Disturbances

   Slowed mentation

   Attention difficulties

   Concentration problems

   Memory problems (typically short term)

   Orientation problems

Patients with mTBI may access the medical system at a variety of sites. Some patients, especially those who have sustained an acute trauma (ie, motor vehicle collision) may seek immediate care through the emergency department. However, most patients with mTBI are more likely to be evaluated either by the team doctor on the sidelines immediately following the suspected injury or by their primary care physician in the hours to days following the suspected injury. In the setting of an acute trauma, patients are best evaluated using protocols established by the American College of Surgeons' Advance Trauma Life Support (ATLS) program. Such evaluation, however, is beyond the scope of this article. Although the evaluation on the sideline and that at the office may have different immediate priorities, both share the common goal of confirming the presence of mTBI.

Concussion and mTBI are clinical diagnoses and require a high index of suspicion. To begin with, a thorough history focusing on the listed symptoms of mTBI, should be taken. Sometimes, especially if loss of consciousness is involved, some history may have to be obtained from witnesses of the injury. After this a thorough concussion history, including inquiring about previous head injuries, should also be performed, particularly in athletes. After obtaining the history, a thorough physical examination with particular focus on the neurologic system should be performed. Although the history and physical examination are all that is usually needed to make the diagnosis of mTBI there are many clinical useful adjuncts that can either aid in making the diagnosis or be used to rule out more severe injuries, discussed next.

Glasgow coma scale

One of the most useful clinical tools in the management of head injuries in any setting remains the Glasgow Coma Scale (GCS) [16], because it can aid clinicians in the initial identification of a possible injury and allow the tracking of any changes in the patient's condition. The GCS is based on the assessment of 3 clinical variables: eye opening (best score 4), verbal response (best score 5), and motor response (best score 6), with 15 being the maximum score and 3 the lowest (Table 1). For assessing the verbal response in children younger than 3 years, the Children's Coma Score, which incorporates age-appropriate verbal responses,

Table 1
GCS and children's coma score

Measure	Score
Eye opening	
Spontaneous	4
To verbal stimuli	3
To painful stimuli	2
No response	1
Best motor response	
Spontaneous (follows commands)	6
Localizes pain	5
Withdraws to pain	4
Abnormal flexion to pain (decorticate posturing)	3
Abnormal extension to pain (decerebrate posturing)	2
No response	1
Best verbal response (age >3 y)	
Oriented and converses	5
Confused	4
Inappropriate words	3
Incomprehensible sounds	2
No response	1
Best verbal response (age <3 y)	
Appropriate words; coos or babbles	5
Inappropriate words; consolable crying	4
Screaming or inconsolable crying	3
Grunts or moans to painful stimuli	2
No response	1

should be used (see Table 1). In general, those patients with mTBI should have a GCS of 14 to 15 on presentation, whereas an initial GCS of 13 or lower indicates a more significant injury [4,16].

Role of neuroimaging

As mTBI is a functional abnormality rather than an anatomic injury, the role of neuroimaging is limited. However, in the acute phase imaging may occasionally be necessary to eliminate the possibility of a more serious injury. Historically it has been reported that as many as 28% of patients with significant intracranial injury can have a normal GCS at presentation [17]. Although this percentage is likely significantly lower, a normal neurologic examination and GCS by no means exclude the possibility of a significant head injury [18,19]. At present, it is estimated that approximately 50% of all children presenting to North American emergency departments with head injury receive a cranial computed tomography (CT) scan. Furthermore, it seems that most of these CT scans are ordered on children with a likely mTBI, as most are reported to have an initial GCS between 14 and 15 [18]. The practice of routinely obtaining cranial imaging has come under scrutiny, largely because of increasing concerns regarding imaging-related radiation exposure in children. Such concerns are not unfounded, as it has been suggested that a single CT examination of the head or face of a child can significantly increase his or her lifetime risk of lethal malignancy. This risk decreases with age, but is estimated to be as high as 1 in 1200 in children younger than 13 months [20].

Since the previous version of this article, 2 prospective clinical trials were performed that have provided guidelines for the use of CT scanning in pediatric patients with head injury [18,21]. These trials are well summarized in a recent article by Wing and James [5]. Of the 2 trials, the study performed by the Pediatric Emergency Care Applied Research Network (PECARN) is considered to be the more clinically useful. Not only did it include a separate algorithm for patients younger than 2 years, it also contained a validation phase [18]. Moreover, it provides the option of observation in certain patients identified as being at intermediate risk (Fig. 1). The prediction rules from the PECARN study, listed in Table 2, have remained valid in multiple separate analyses following the initial publication [5,22,23]. In the absence of any of the findings in Table 2, the published negative predictive value for a significant head injury is 100% in patients younger than 2 years and 99.95% in patients older than 2 years. The use of these prediction rules should lead to a significant decrease in the rate of CT use in mTBI without subjecting patients to the increased morbidity of a missed, more severe injury.

The use of newer imagining modalities such as functional magnetic resonance imaging, diffusion tensor imaging, and single-photon emission CT is an active area of research in mTBI. These modalities will likely become increasingly valuable diagnostic and management tools in the future for patients with a protracted course. However, there is no current evidence to recommend their use in the management of mTBI [15]. In addition, these

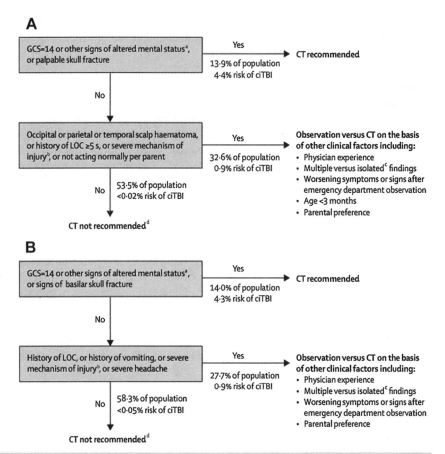

Fig. 1. Suggested CT algorithm for children younger than 2 years (A) and for those aged 2 years and older (B) with GCS scores of 14 to 15 after head trauma. [a] Other signs of altered mental status: agitation, somnolence, repetitive questioning, or slow response to verbal communication. [b] Severe mechanism of injury: motor vehicle crash with patient ejection, death of another passenger, or rollover; pedestrian or bicyclist without helmet struck by a motorized vehicle; falls of more than 0·9 m (3 feet) (or more than 1·5 m [5 feet] for panel B); or head struck by a high-impact object. [c] Patients with certain isolated findings (ie, with no other findings suggestive of traumatic brain injury), such as isolated LOC, isolated headache, isolated vomiting, and certain types of isolated scalp hematomas in infants older than 3 months [31], or have a risk of ciTBI substantially lower than 1%. [d] Risk of ciTBI exceedingly low, generally lower than risk of CT-induced malignancies; therefore, CT scans are not indicated for most patients in this group. ciTBI, clinically important traumatic brain injury; CT, computed tomography; GCS, glasgow coma scale; LOC, level of consciousness. (From Kuppermann N, Holmes JF, Dayan PS, et al, for the Pediatric Emergency Care Applied Research Network (PECARN). Identification of children at very low risk of clinically-important brain injuries after head trauma: a prospective cohort study. Lancet 2009;374:1168; with permission.)

Table 2 PECARN decision rules	
Children <2 y old	Children >2 y old
Children's Coma Score = 14 Other signs of altered mental status Palpable skull fracture	Glasgow Coma Score = 14 Other signs of altered mental status Signs of a basilar skull fracture

studies are resource intense and are not likely of value for most patients with mTBI.

Role of neuropsychological testing

Originally introduced by researchers and then clinicians in an attempt to provide an objective measure for the presence of sports-related concussion, neuropsychological tests have increasingly become an important tool in the management of mTBI. Neuropsychological testing is now largely performed as computer-based testing and is now also being used in the management of non–sports-related mTBI [24,25].

There are multiple computerized neuropsychological tests available, the most widely used of which is the Immediate Post-Concussion Assessment and Cognitive Testing (ImPACT) test (ImPACT Applications, Pittsburgh, PA). The ImPACT test is an interactive software program that incorporates concussion history, injury data, and symptom assessment in addition to neurocognitive testing in the analysis of the patient. Results can then be compared with the patient's baseline score if available (preferable; see later discussion) or age-matched and gender-matched normative values if baseline testing has not been performed [25]. Other frequently used computer-based neuropsychological tests include the Automated Neuropsychological Assessment Metrics (ANAM; Axon Sports, LLC, Wausau, WI) and Headminder (Headminder Inc, New York, NY).

In addition to the aforementioned more comprehensive neuropsychological tools, a variety of rapid screening tests is also available. These rapid tests are most commonly used in the sideline assessment of the injured athlete. The most popular of these modalities is the Sports Concussion Assessment Tool (SCAT) test, now in its third version (SCAT3). This test, created by the International Symposia on Concussion in Sport, is a brief neuropsychological test that largely assesses attention and memory function, and was specifically developed to be given on the sidelines immediately following a suspected sports-related concussion. The King-Devick test, another rapid and reliable sideline assessment tool, has also been validated for acute assessment of the injured athlete [26].

In addition to its use in sports-related concussion, neuropsychological testing may be of value in the assessment of patients presenting to the emergency department with mTBI of other origin [25]. However, although these tests have been studied in the emergency department setting and have documented significant neurocognitive deficits, the value of their routine use is not yet clear

[14,20,25,27]. The utility of formal testing in the acute setting therefore warrants further investigation before recommendations can be made for their use. At this time it is not recommended that neuropsychological testing alone be used in any setting to diagnose concussion or determine when an athlete can safely return to play [15].

Both the ImPACT and SCAT3 are readily available online. However, both require that the person giving the test be trained in how to administer it, and it must be interpreted by trained medical personnel. The ImPACT and SCAT3 are now also available as developmentally appropriate tests for children aged 5 to 12 years (the Pediatric ImPACT and Child SCAT3, respectively), but are only in the early stages of being evaluated for their use in the management of mTBI in children [28].

Further management

After significant head injury has been excluded and the diagnosis of mTBI has either been made or is being entertained, multiple decisions must be made, which will differ depending on the clinical setting. In the setting of acute trauma, the most important decision may be whether to admit the patient or not. This decision remains ultimately a clinical one, as no accepted evidence-based guidelines currently exist to help guide management. Typical indications for admission, however, are prolonged loss of consciousness (>1 minute), severe or persistent symptoms, or any patient who merits observation [12,14,29]. By contrast, on the sidelines the most critical initial decision often revolves around whether to return or remove the student athlete from play. It is currently recommended that any pediatric athlete whom is even suspected of having sustained an mTBI be removed from play [4]. In addition, 46 states now require that any pediatric athlete suspected of having a concussion be evaluated and cleared by a medical professional before being allowed to return to the game. However, for many patients the initial contact with the health care system following a suspected concussion will be at the pediatrician or general practitioner's office in the subacute period following the suspected injury. The primary goal in this setting is to correctly identify that the patient has sustained mTBI, thus allowing the clinician to initiate appropriate management centered on physical and cognitive rest.

Once a patient has been diagnosed with mTBI, clinical management centers on appropriate counseling of both the patient and family, and ensuring that the patient has appropriate follow-up care. This plan is necessary for patients with sports-related and non–sports-related concussions alike. In counseling the patient and family, it is critically important to discuss secondary injury and to provide thorough instructions regarding cognitive and physical rest. Instructions should include directions for following the Return to Learn and Return to Play protocols (see later discussion). Communicating the importance of these strategies is perhaps the most important element of post-mTBI care. Unfortunately, one recent study demonstrated that most discharge instructions fall short of communicating the importance of both cognitive and physical rest [30].

FOLLOW-UP FOLLOWING MILD TRAUMATIC BRAIN INJURY

Any patient diagnosed with mTBI should have a scheduled outpatient follow-up. Depending on the resources of the particular community, this follow-up can be performed by various health care providers. It is routinely scheduled for 2 weeks following the initial injury, but should be scheduled sooner if deemed appropriate. The importance of this visit is that it gives the health care provider the opportunity to inquire about persistent postconcussive symptoms, repeat neuropsychological testing if applicable, and refer the patient to specialists if necessary. Those patients with ongoing symptoms or those with prior neuro-psychological problems (ie, attention-deficit/hyperactivity disorder, learning difficulties) are more likely to have a prolonged course of recovery. As such, they may need further follow-up or referral to a concussion specialist.

Many patients and their families have been shown to be noncompliant with the scheduled follow-up after sustaining an mTBI [14]. This fact is unfortunate, as in the authors' series the noncompliant patients were just as likely to have sustained a more serious mTBI as determined by persistent symptoms and ImPACT testing as those who returned for follow-up [14]. This noncompliance likely occurs in large part because of the public's continued misconceptions regarding the severity of concussion and mTBI [31]. Such misconceptions are changing slowly, however, in no small part because of the recognition of the existence of chronic traumatic encephalopathy (CTE), and the extensive media attention surrounding National Football League players who have now been diagnosed with this disease.

Mild traumatic brain injury in the pediatric athlete

Sports-related mTBIs are extremely common in the pediatric age group. Much of what clinicians have learned relative to concussion management is derived from the study of concussed athletes, professional, collegiate, and recreational alike. It is currently estimated that up to 3.8 million recreational and sports-related concussions occur in the United States each year [15]. This number is almost certainly higher, as there is significant underreporting of both recreational and sports-related head injuries. Most of these injuries occur in children, as does a significant amount of the underreporting [4].

American football is responsible for the largest proportion of the sports-related injuries in children, followed closely by ice hockey [4,20]. One study estimated that approximately 15.3% of all high school football players sustain an mTBI annually. Another study reported that up to 25% of high school football players self-reported symptoms consistent with a concussion in a post-season survey [4,32]. These studies highlight both the significant number of mTBIs sustained and the degree of underreporting present in high school football alone. Largely because of American football, males are statistically more likely than females to sustain a sports-related mTBI. However, studies have shown that females are also at high risk and are potentially more likely than males to sustain an mTBI while participating in the sports of basketball, hockey, and soccer [4].

Because of the high likelihood of sustaining a sports-related mTBI, many high school and college athletic programs now perform baseline neuropsychological testing in their student athletes [33], ideally done before the playing season starts. The baseline results are then available for comparison if the student athlete is suspected of sustaining an mTBI. If baseline preinjury data is not available, the results of the neuropsychological testing can be compared with normative age-matched and gender-matched data. However, this must be done with caution because normative data may not account for any baseline neuropsychological problems the patient may have [4]. Again, it must be stressed that neuropsychological testing and the rapid screening tests should not be used to diagnose concussion or to make decisions regarding safe return to play. Instead they should be used to increase the detection of mTBI even in athletes who are otherwise asymptomatic [34,35].

Prevention of secondary injury

In the adult patient, care following mTBI is frequently centered on a safe return to work. In the pediatric patient, the focus must be on the safe return to the cognitive activities of school and, subsequently, sporting activities and exercise. Pediatric patients with mTBI are much more susceptible to the multiple dangers associated with the premature return to cognitive of physical activities, including prolongation of postconcussive symptoms, increased incidence of recurrent concussion (possible lower threshold), and, in very rare cases, death [4,20]. Increasing evidence also suggests that younger patients may take longer to recover from mTBI [4,20]. For example, high school athletes have been shown to have a slower return to baseline than college and professional athletes [22]. Therefore, to ensure a safe recovery it is critical to protect the pediatric brain from any further damage brought about by metabolic mismatch discussed earlier. To accomplish this, all activities that significantly increase the metabolic demands of the brain must be minimized or avoided altogether.

Cognitive rest: return to learn

Although much attention has been placed on student athletes recovering from mTBI before returning to play, cognitive rest is equally important to athletes and nonathletes alike. Some general guidelines for cognitive rest are listed in Box 2. Although again there are no accepted evidence-based guidelines,

Box 2: Cognitive rest
- No school (initially)
- No homework
- No reading
- No video games, computers, cell phones
- No television
- Minimized travel
- Increased time for rest and sleep

many experts recommend that pediatric patients have a minimum of 1 to 3 days of cognitive rest following the injury [36]. During this time avoidance of "screen time," including televisions, cellular telephones, computers, video games, and tablets, is crucial. Before returning to school, patients should be asymptomatic at rest and be able to perform an academic task for at least 30 minutes without increasing symptoms. The academic workload and time at school can then be gradually increased in coordination with the patient's teachers, counselors, and the clinician [36]. Recently, these and other cognitive rest guidelines were developed into a Return to Learn protocol, which is shown in Table 3 [37]. It is now recommended that any pediatric patient should completely work through this protocol before engaging in physical activities, including the Return to Play protocol [37].

Physical rest: return to play

Once the Return to Learn pathway has been completed, the pediatric athlete can then work through the Return to Play protocol. The currently recommended protocol, as recommended by the consensus statement of the Fouth International Conference on Concussion in Sport, is shown in Table 4 [12].

Current recommendations require that the athlete should spend a minimum of 24 hours at each step of the pathway. Therefore, it should take the athlete a minimum of 1 week to progress through the Return to Play protocol. If symptoms recur at any step the patient should return to the previous asymptomatic step, and only attempt to progress again after remaining asymptomatic for 24 hours at this previous step [12]. It should be noted that most research in this field to date has been performed in high school and college-age athletes.

Table 3		
Stage	Activity	Objective
No activity	Complete cognitive rest: no school, no homework, no reading, no screen time	Allow for recovery
Reintroduction of cognitive activities	Introduce cognitive activities for 5–15 min. Relaxation of previous restrictions	Controlled increase in cognitive activities
Homework at home before return to school	Homework for longer periods of time (20–30 min)	Increase cognitive stamina with self-paced cognitive activities
Return to school	Return to school for partial day after tolerating 1–2 cumulative hours of homework at home	Restart school with accommodations to permit for controlled increase in cognitive load
Gradual reintegration into school	Gradually increase to full school day	Accommodations decrease as cognitive stamina further increases
Resumption of full cognitive load	May take tests, may make up missed essential work	Full return to school, may begin return to play protocol if applicable

Table 4

Stage	Activity	Objective
No activity	Complete physical rest	Allow for recovery
Light aerobic exercise	Walking, swimming, stationary bike up to 70% of maximum predicted heart rate; no resistance training	Increase heart rate
Sport-specific exercise	Sport-specific exercise such as running in soccer, skating in ice hockey; no head impacts	Add movement
Noncontact training drills	Gradually reintroduce complex drills and resistance training	Exercise, coordination and cognitive load
Full contact practice	Normal practice after final medical clearance	Restore confidence, allow for assessment of motor skills by coaches
Return to play	Normal game play	Return to play

Therefore, an even more prolonged progression through the Return to Play protocol should be considered for younger children, especially those younger than 11 years [12]. Lastly, mention must be made of the difficult decision to temporarily or even permanently retire the student athlete from the offending sport(s). Patients with multiple or recurrent mTBI in one season, severe or persistent symptoms following even one concussion, or with baseline neuropsychological problems may benefit from such retirement [4,15]. This decision should optimally be made in consultation with a concussion specialist.

SUMMARY

mTBI is a very common and underdiagnosed problem in the pediatric population. While most children who receive appropriate management recover uneventfully (80%–90%), referral to a concussion specialist is necessary for those with a complicated course. Fortunately, further improvements in identifying those children who have sustained an mTBI, coupled with strict adherence to the Return to Learn and Return to Play protocols, will ultimately lead to better long-term outcomes.

References

[1] Faul M, Xu L, Wald MM, et al. Traumatic brain injury in the United States: emergency department visits, hospitalizations, and deaths. Atlanta (GA): National Center for Injury Prevention and Control; Centers for Disease Control and Prevention; 2010. Available at: http://www.cdc.gov/traumatic%20braininjury/pdf/blue_book.pdf. Accessed November 1, 2013.

[2] Schneier AJ, Shields BJ, Hostetler SG, et al. Incidence of pediatric traumatic brain injury and associated hospital resource utilization in the United States. Pediatrics 2006;118(2): 483–92.

[3] Pinto PS, Poretti A, Meoded A. The Unique features of traumatic brain injury in children. Review of the characteristics of the pediatric skull and brain, mechanisms of trauma, patterns of injury, complications and their imaging findings—part 1. J Neuroimaging 2012;22: e1–17.

[4] Grady MF. Concussion in the adolescent athlete. Curr Probl Pediatr Adolesc Health Care 2010;40:154–69.

[5] Wing R, James C. Pediatric head injury and concussion. Emerg Med Clin North Am 2013;31:653–75.

[6] Savitsky EA, Votey SR. Current controversies in the management of minor pediatric head injuries. Am J Emerg Med 2000;18:96–101.

[7] Kochanek PM, Carney N, Adelson PD, et al. Guidelines for the acute medical management of severe traumatic brain injury in infants, children, and adolescents-second edition. Pediatr Crit Care Med 2012;13(Suppl 1):S1–82.

[8] Gurkoff GG, Giza CC, Hovda DA. Lateral fluid percussion injury in the developing rat causes an acute, mild behavioral dysfunction in the absence of significant cell death. Brain Res 2006;1077(1):24–36.

[9] Yuen TJ, Browne KD, Iwata A, et al. Sodium channelopathy induced by mild axonal trauma worsens outcome after a repeat injury. J Neurosci Res 2009;87(16):3620–5.

[10] Lovell M. The neurophysiology and assessment of sports-related head injuries. Neurol Clin 2008;26:45–62.

[11] Dick RW. Is there a gender difference in concussion incidence and outcomes? Br J Sports Med 2009;43(Suppl 1):i46–50.

[12] McCrory P, Meeuwisse WH, Aubry M, et al. Consensus statement on concussion in sport: The 4th International Conference on Concussion in Sport held in Zurich, November 2012. Br J Sports Med 2013;47:250–8.

[13] Giza CC, Kutcher JS, Ashwal S, et al. Summary of evidence-based guideline update: evaluation and management of concussion in sports: report of the Guideline Development Subcommittee of the American Academy of Neurology. Neurology 2013;80:2250–7.

[14] Blinman TA, Houseknecht E, Snyder C, et al. Postconcussive symptoms in hospitalized pediatric patients after mild traumatic brain injury. J Pediatr Surg 2009;44:1223–8.

[15] Halstead ME, Walter KD, Council on Sports Medicine and Fitness, et al. American Academy of Pediatrics. Clinical report—sport-related concussion in children and adolescents. Pediatrics 2010;126:597–615.

[16] Cicero MX, Cross KP. Predictive value of initial Glasgow coma scale score in pediatric trauma patients. Pediatr Emerg Care 2013;29(1):43–8.

[17] Dietrich AM, Bowman MJ, Ginn-Pease ME, et al. Pediatric head injuries: can clinical factors reliably predict an abnormality on computed tomography? Ann Emerg Med 1993;22:535–40.

[18] Kupperman N, Homes JF, Dayan JD, et al. Identification of children at very low risk of clinically-important brain injuries after head trauma: a prospective cohort study. Lancet 2009;374:1160–70.

[19] Hamilton M, Mrazik M, Johnson DW. Incidence of delayed intracranial hemorrhage in children after uncomplicated minor head injuries. Pediatrics 2010;126(1):e33–9.

[20] Atabaki SM. Updates in the general approach to pediatric head trauma and concussion. Pediatr Clin North Am 2013;60:1107–22.

[21] Osmond MH, Klassen TP, Wells GA, et al. CATCH: a clinical decision rule for the use of computed tomography in children with minor head injury. CMAJ 2010;182:341–8.

[22] Nigrovic LE, Lee LK, Hoyle J, et al. Prevalence of clinically important traumatic brain injuries in children with minor blunt head trauma and isolated severe injury mechanisms. Arch Pediatr Adolesc Med 2012;166(4):356–61.

[23] Nigrovic LE, Lillis K, Atabaki SM, et al. The prevalence of traumatic brain injuries after minor blunt head trauma in children with ventricular shunts. Ann Emerg Med 2013;61(4):389–93.

[24] Atabaki S, Gioia G, Zuckerbraun N, et al. Practice patterns in emergency department management and follow-up of pediatric mild traumatic brain injury. Accepted abstracts from the International Brain Injury Association's eighth world congress on brain injuries. Brain Inj 2010;24:335.

[25] Wiebe DJ, Collins MW, Nance ML. Identification and validation of prognostic criteria for persistence of mild traumatic brain injury related impairment in the pediatric patient. Pediatr Emerg Care 2012;28:498–502.

[26] Galetta KM, Brandes LE, Maki K, et al. The King-Devick test and sports-related concussion: study of a rapid visual screening tool in a collegiate cohort. J Neurol Sci 2011;309(1–2): 34–9.

[27] Zemek R, Osmond MH, Barrowman N, et al. Predicting and preventing postconcussive problems in paediatrics (5P) study: protocol for a prospective multicentre clinical prediction rule derivation study in children with concussion. BMJ Open 2013;3:pii:e003550.

[28] Newman JB, Reesman JH, Vaughan CG, et al. Assessment of processing speed in children with mild TBI: a "first look" at the validity of pediatric ImPACT. Clin Neuropsychol 2013;27(5):779–93.

[29] Simma B, Lütschg J, Callahan JM. Mild head injury in pediatrics: algorithms for management in the ED and in young athletes. Am J Emerg Med 2013;31(7):1133–8.

[30] Sarsfield MJ, Morley EJ, Callahan JM, et al. Evaluation of emergency medicine discharge instructions in pediatric head injury. Pediatr Emerg Care 2013;29(8):884–7.

[31] Guilmette TJ, Paglia MF. The public's misconception about traumatic brain injury: a follow-up survey. Arch Clin Neuropsychol 2004;19:183–9.

[32] McCrea M, Hammeke T, Olsen G, et al. Unreported concussion in high school football players: implications for prevention. Clin J Sport Med 2004;14:13–7.

[33] Pardini J, Collins M. Creating a successful concussion management program at the high school level. In: Echemendia RJ, editor. Sports neuropsychology: assessment and management of traumatic brain injury. New York: Guilford Press; 2006. p. 36–42.

[34] Van Kampen DA, Lovell MR, Pardini JE, et al. The "value added" of neurocognitive testing after sports-related concussion. Am J Sports Med 2006;34:1630–5.

[35] Broglio SP, Macciocchi SN, Ferrara MS. Neurocognitive performance of concussed athletes when symptom free. J Athl Train 2007;42(4):504–8.

[36] Grady MF, Master CL, Gioia GA. Concussion pathophysiology: rationale for physical and cognitive rest. Pediatr Ann 2012;41(9):377–82.

[37] Master CL, Gioia GA, Leddy JJ, et al. Importance of 'return-to-learn' in pediatric and adolescent concussion. Pediatr Ann 2012;41(9):1–6.

Advances in Pediatrics 61 (2014) 287–312

ADVANCES IN PEDIATRICS

ELSEVIER
MOSBY

Foodborne Illnesses

Sabah Kalyoussef, DO,
Kristina N. Feja, MD, MPH*

Division of Allergy, Immunology and Infectious Diseases, The Children's Hospital at Saint Peter's University Hospital, 254 Easton Avenue, New Brunswick, NJ 08901, USA

Keywords

- Foodborne pathogens • Food safety • Foodborne infections in children
- Preventive measures • High-risk populations

Key points

- Foodborne illness should be part of the differential diagnosis for all children presenting with gastroenteritis.
- Globalization of the food supply has led to novel food items being implicated in foodborne illnesses.
- Children are affected frequently, and sometimes severely, by foodborne infections.
- Special instructions on foodborne illness prevention should be given to patients in immunocompromised states whether acquired or congenital and in other special populations.
- Education and prevention are key to reducing the incidence of foodborne illnesses.

INTRODUCTION

Information regarding food exposure is an important part of a sick patient's history. Food products that can potentially transmit foodborne illnesses increase annually with each novel food item associated with an outbreak. Foodborne illness, otherwise known as foodborne infection or foodborne disease, is a preventable entity caused by a variety of agents that a person ingests via a contaminated food or beverage. Foodborne disease outbreak occurs when 2 or more people develop similar illnesses after ingestion of a common food item. There

Disclosures: None.

*Corresponding author. MOB 3110, 254 Easton Avenue, New Brunswick, NJ 08901.
E-mail address: kfeja@saintpetersuh.com

0065-3101/14/$ – see front matter
http://dx.doi.org/10.1016/j.yapd.2014.04.003   © 2014 Elsevier Inc. All rights reserved.

are more than 250 different foodborne diseases described and 1 in 6 Americans is estimated to have a foodborne illness each year [1,2]. The ingestion of poisonous toxins or chemicals can lead to foodborne disease; however, most of the illnesses are infections caused by bacteria, viruses, or parasites. This article reviews changes in food supply and the epidemiology, method of transmission, clinical symptoms, diagnosis, treatment, as well as prevention of the most important foodborne infections. The focus is on pediatric data where available.

FOOD SUPPLY

The characteristics of the human food supply have changed dramatically over the past century. In the early nineteenth century food was grown locally and purchased in a local food store. Over time, food was transported farther and farther from its place of origin, leading to globalization of the food supply. The advantage of this is that people have a more diverse food selection to choose from and availability year round [2,3]. Food imports have increased 10% annually and this diversification continues to increase [3]. Food imports of produce and seafood alone have increased from $41 billion in 1998 to $78 billion in 2007 [4]. Furthermore, the farm-to-table continuum, which consists of food production, processing, storage of food product, and transport to a retail venue, has become more complex. Food production and processing facilities are more centralized and are larger (ie, large farms and animal production facilities) and, because of the longer distances travelled by food products, storage and transport are also more complicated. These phenomena have led to the spread of foodborne pathogens and have provided new challenges in identifying source agents and providing adequate regulation.

Practices involving food preparation have dramatically changed as well. Because of mass production, meals are no longer only prepared in the home [2,5,6]. Most Americans dine out on a weekly basis, a practice that increases their risk of foodborne illnesses [6]. Food is also no longer primarily cooked on stoves but is heated in microwaves. Microwave food cooking produces uneven temperatures, which in turn affects killing time of potential pathogens [2].

METHODS OF CONTAMINATION AND TRANSMISSION

There are multiple means by which food and water may be contaminated with pathogens. Contamination can occur during any part of the farm-to-table continuum. Means of contamination include use of inappropriate organic fertilizers or inadequately composted manure; planting of fields where animals have grazed; soil contamination; or contamination during transport (open vehicles), processing (cutting, slicing), packing (improper packaging, contaminated packing equipment), distribution, or at retail markets [7]. Both direct human contact after improper hand hygiene as well as the process by which animals are slaughtered can lead to contamination of fruits, vegetables, and nuts that may be grown nearby [5].

Some foodborne illnesses are related to foods that were exposed to contaminated water. There are multiple methods by which this can occur, because water is an important part of food production, processing, and preparation. These methods include the use of untreated water or sewage for irrigation and the use of contaminated water for washing, food preparation, and ice preparation. Clean water is not readily available in some parts of the world, so these types of illnesses may be more prevalent in travelers to these affected areas [3]. Foodborne pathogens are listed here according to the most likely mode of transmission.

1. Foodborne (ingestion of contaminated food products):
   a. *Campylobacter, Listeria, Escherichia coli, Salmonella, Botulism, Bacillus cereus, Shigella, Cyclospora, Staphylococcus aureus, Toxoplasma, Amebiasis, Yersinia,* and Norovirus
2. Waterborne (ingestion of contaminated water):
   a. *Cryptosporidium, Cyclospora, Giardia, Toxoplasma,* Norovirus, *E coli, Amebiasis,* and *Shigella*

EPIDEMIOLOGY
Foodborne illness surveillance
Foodborne illness is an important preventable public health problem, surveillance is needed to track trends and determine preventive efforts. The national reporting of foodborne pathogens, as listed in Box 1, is an important first step in the surveillance of foodborne illnesses. The United States has multiple surveillance systems that monitor foodborne diseases. One of the most important is the Foodborne Diseases Active Surveillance Network, or FoodNet, which is

---

Box 1: Required reporting of foodborne illnesses to US Centers for Disease Control and Prevention (CDC)/Department of Health

Listeriosis

Typhoid fever

Cyclosporiasis

Trichinellosis

Hemolytic uremic syndrome (postdiarrheal)

Vibriosis

Shiga toxin–producing *E coli* (STEC)

Giardiasis

Foodborne botulism

Salmonellosis

Shigellosis

Data from McEntire J. Foodborne disease: the global movement of food and people. Infect Dis Clin North Am 2013;27(3):687–93; and Adams DA, Gallagher KM, Jajosky RA, et al. Summary of Notifiable Diseases - United States, 2011. MMWR Morb Mortal Wkly Rep 2013;60(53):1–117.

an active population-based surveillance system located at 10 different US sites that monitors laboratory-confirmed infections of *Campylobacter, Cryptosporidium, Cyclospora, Listeria, Salmonella,* Shiga toxin–producing *E coli* (STEC) O157 and non-O157, *Shigella, Vibrio,* and *Yersinia* [8]. This collaborative program between the US Centers for Disease Control and Prevention (CDC), 10 state health departments, the US Department of Agriculture (USDA) Food Safety and Infection Service (FSIS), and the US Food and Drug Administration (FDA) is also responsible for the active surveillance of hemolytic uremic syndrome (HUS) in children less than 18 years old. This collaboration also provides a means of monitoring STEC infection and the effectiveness of preventive measures [5,8,9]. This network accounts for about 15% of the population or 48 million persons.

PulseNet is a national molecular subtyping network of 80 laboratories for foodborne disease surveillance and outbreak detection coordinated by CDC, USDA, and the FDA [10]. The use of PulseNet has led to increased molecular typing of bacterial foodborne pathogens leading to increased detection of foodborne outbreaks. Other surveillance networks that can identify trends in foodborne illnesses include the National Notifiable Diseases Surveillance System (NNDSS), Cholera and other *Vibrio* Illness Surveillance (COVIS), and the Foodborne Disease Outbreak Surveillance System (FDOSS). In addition, a new Web-based database and analytical tool called PATRN (pathogen-annotated tracking resource network system) has been developed to aid the global food safety community in the investigation of foodborne disease pathogens and outbreaks with the intent of improving detection and response to foodborne illnesses on national and global levels [11].

FoodNet surveillance data from 2012 identified a total of 19,531 laboratory-confirmed infections, 4563 hospitalizations, and 68 deaths associated with foodborne illness. The incidence of most infections (*Campylobacter, Cryptosporidium, Salmonella,* STEC O157 and non-O157, *Shigella,* and *Yersinia*) were highest in children younger than 5 years of age, whereas the hospitalizations and deaths were more common among the elderly (>65 years old). The incidence of *Campylobacter* and *Vibrio* increased compared with 2006 to 2008 data; however, the incidence of the other pathogens remained stable [8]. FoodNet also reported 627 physician-diagnosed HUS cases between the years 2000 and 2007 with 66% occurring in children less than 5 years old [9].

More than a thousand foodborne outbreaks are reported each year [12,13]. Outbreaks occur nationally as reported on an almost monthly basis with causes ranging from contaminated lettuce to tomatoes at large chains [14]. However, most illness does not occur in a known outbreak setting. Because of underdiagnosis and underreporting of foodborne illnesses, the true incidence is thought to be much higher than reported. The CDC estimates that 31 major pathogens caused 9.4 million episodes of foodborne illness annually [15]. Viruses caused most cases (59%), followed by bacteria (39%) and parasites (2%). Among specific pathogens, norovirus was responsible for an estimated 5.5 million cases a year, accounting for 58% of all foodborne illness cases [16].

The 31 major pathogens are estimated to account for almost 56,000 hospitalizations annually. Although viruses such as norovirus caused most of the disease, bacteria caused 64% of the hospitalizations; among them *Salmonella* species (35%) and *Campylobacter* spp (15%) together accounting for half of all cases. Of the estimated 1351 deaths yearly, most (64%) were caused by bacteria, with nontyphoidal *Salmonella* species (28%) and *Listeria monocytogenes* (19%) being the most common [15]. An additional 38 million episodes of gastroenteritis, 71,000 hospitalizations, and almost 1700 deaths each year are estimated to be caused by unspecified agents [17]. Some causal agents, such as group A *Streptococcus*, are not thought to be transmitted by food, although an outbreak of group A streptococcal pharyngitis associated with pasta at a high school banquet was reported recently [18].

Foodborne outbreaks during the years 1998 to 2008 had a known cause in 7998 outbreaks. Viruses and bacteria each caused 45% of outbreaks and the rest were caused by chemical and toxic agents [12]. The overall annual national rate of foodborne disease was 4.2 outbreaks per 1 million people [5]. The 2 most common pathogens in outbreaks of foodborne illnesses are Norovirus (43% of outbreaks) and *Salmonella enteritidis* (18% of outbreaks). When outbreaks crossed state lines, 53% were caused by *Salmonella* and 29% by STEC O157 [12]. Of the national foodborne outbreaks, 68% of contaminated food was prepared in a restaurant or deli setting. An updated list of foodborne disease outbreaks reported to the CDC can be found at http://wwwn.cdc.gov/foodborneoutbreaks/Default.aspx. Recent data from 2012 regarding the most common foodborne pathogens reported to FoodNet are listed in Box 2.

Box 2: Common foodborne pathogens in order of decreasing incidence from 2012 FoodNet

1. *Salmonella*
2. *Campylobacter*
3. *Shigella*
4. *Cryptosporidium*
5. STEC non-O157
6. STEC O157
7. *Vibrio*
8. *Yersinia*
9. *Listeria*
10. *Cyclospora*

From Center for Disease Control and Prevention. Incidence and trends of infection with pathogens transmitted commonly through food - foodborne diseases active surveillance network, 10 U.S. sites, 1996–2012. MMWR Morb Mortal Wkly Rep 2013;62(15):283–7.

Food vehicles

Identifying the contaminated ingredient that is causing a foodborne illness can be challenging for more than one reason. First, people may not remember exactly what they ate, especially when the causative ingredient may have been ingested days to weeks ago. Another reason is that some foods contain many different ingredients from multiple sources. In addition, it is possible that not all persons ingesting a product will show signs and symptoms of illness. Once the causative food vehicle is identified and removed from the food chain, then the source of contamination that may occur at any point along the farm-to-table continuum needs to be identified and rectified.

The list of specific foods identified as causing foodborne illnesses continues to expand as new items are continuously discovered. Table 1 lists food products that have been associated with certain foodborne illnesses. Surveillance data for foodborne outbreaks from 1998 to 2008 indicate that a food vehicle was identified in 60% of outbreaks. The most commonly implicated food products in outbreaks were poultry and fish, followed by beef. However, the food commodities associated with the largest number of outbreak-related illnesses were poultry (17%), leafy vegetables (13%), beef (12%), and fruits/nuts (11%) [12]. The most common pathogen pairs noted in outbreak-related illness were Norovirus and leafy vegetables followed by *Clostridium perfringens* and poultry, *Salmonella* and vine-stalk vegetables, and *C perfringens* and beef [12].

Leafy green vegetables, including spinach and lettuce in ready-to-eat salads, are an increasingly important source of the foodborne illness burden, causing an increased number of outbreaks during recent decades [7]. Fresh salsa and guacamole, food items that are growing more popular, have also emerged as an important source of foodborne infections [19].

Table 1
Food products and associated foodborne pathogens

Type of food	Associated pathogens
Apple cider	*E coli, Cryptosporidium*
Unpasteurized milk and cheeses	*Yersinia, Salmonella, Campylobacter, Cryptosporidium*
Beef	*E coli, Salmonella, Listeria, Toxoplasma, Clostridium perfringens*
Pork	*Yersinia, Salmonella, Toxoplasma*
Chicken	*Salmonella, Campylobacter, Listeria, Toxoplasma, C perfringens*
Seafood	*V parahaemolyticus, Campylobacter,* Norovirus
Kimchi	*E coli, Staphylococcus aureus, Listeria, Salmonella*
Fresh produce	*Salmonella,* STEC, *Shigella, Listeria, Campylobacter, Cryptosporidium*
Leafy vegetables	Norovirus, STEC
Game meat	*Toxoplasma, Trichinella*
Canned food	*Clostridium botulinum*
Infant formula	*Salmonella*
Contaminated water	*Shigella, Cryptosporidium, Cyclospora, Giardia,* STEC, *Toxoplasmosis,* Amebiasis, Norovirus, *Yersinia* (well water)

Foods with low water activity, defined as foods and food ingredients naturally low in moisture or produced from high-moisture foods that are deliberately dried, have become an increasingly common vehicle for pathogens and more of a problem than previously thought [20]. Some examples of low-water-activity foods are cereals, peanut butter, powders, spices, nuts, seeds, and dried formula [20]. Contamination of spices with bacterial pathogens was identified as a cause of at least 14 foodborne outbreaks in 10 countries in a recent review. The most common bacterial pathogens associated with spice-related outbreaks were *Salmonella* and *Bacillus* spp. Children less than 14 years of age were most affected in 5 of the 14 reported spice-related outbreaks [21]. New food vehicles have been noted recently such as bagged spinach, peppers, pine nuts, and peanut butter, which leads to the question of what is safe to eat [6].

Specific foodborne disease agents

Foodborne illness should always be part of the differential diagnosis of a patient with gastroenteritis. Symptoms often include nausea, vomiting, abdominal pain, and diarrhea. However, people may develop serious complications such as bacteremia, meningitis, joint infections, hemorrhagic colitis, renal failure, or paralysis [5]. As with every patient, history is important in the diagnosis of foodborne illnesses and includes a food and water exposure history. Important questions for clinicians to ask when formulating the differential diagnosis in identifying the specific foodborne diseases are listed here.

1. What food product and water exposure is suspected?
2. When did the exposure occur?
3. With what type of symptoms did the patient present?
4. Is this an immunocompromised host?
5. Are there any other ill persons who have been exposed to the same food product?

Salmonella

Salmonella is a gram-negative rod and one of the most common pathogens in foodborne illnesses. A review of FoodNet data from 2012 found 7800 cases of salmonellosis out of a total of 19,531 foodborne illness cases [8].

Salmonellosis is transmitted via the fecal-oral route or ingestion of contaminated food products. Reservoirs of the organism include poultry, livestock, reptiles, and pets. The foodborne salmonellosis is most often of animal origin: poultry, beef, egg, and dairy products [22]. However, other food vehicles have also been found to carry *Salmonella*, such as peanut butter, frozen pot pies, powdered infant formula, fruits, peppers, cereal, and bakery products [4,6,23,24].

Nontyphoidal *Salmonella* species are known to cause symptoms ranging from asymptomatic gastric carriage and gastroenteritis to bacteremia, meningitis, and osteomyelitis. The clinical spectrum seen with *Salmonella typhi* is known as typhoid fever, whereas other serotypes (*Salmonella* Newport, 9%; *Salmonella*

Enteritidis, 39%) cause enteric fever. Patients may present with classic symptoms that include fever, headache, anorexia, abdominal pain, hepatomegaly, splenomegaly, rose spots, or change in mental status. However, symptoms may also present as a nonspecific febrile illness in an otherwise well-appearing child [23]. *Salmonella* can be isolated from stool, blood, cerebrospinal fluid, and urine by routine bacterial culture methods. The incubation period for enteric fever is 7 to 14 days (range, 3–60 days) and for nontyphoidal *Salmonella* gastroenteritis it is 12 to 36 hours (range, 6–72 hours) [23].

Most noninvasive infections with nontyphi *Salmonella* resolve without the use of antibiotics. Antimicrobial treatment does not alter the duration of infection; therefore, most uncomplicated cases do not require antibiotics. Nontyphoidal gastroenteritis may be treated in high-risk groups such as infants less than 3 months old, children with human immunodeficiency virus (HIV), chronic gastrointestinal tract disease, malignancies, hemoglobinopathies, and immunosuppressive conditions. In patients with invasive disease caused by *Salmonella typhi*, ceftriaxone remains the initial drug of choice. Therapy can be changed to an oral agent active against intracellular organisms to complete 10 to 14 days for enteric fever and 4 to 6 weeks for osteomyelitis, abscess, or meningitis [23].

A trend in increasing antibiotic resistance among *Salmonella* isolates has led to public health concerns and treatment challenges. The use of antibiotics in animals before slaughter is thought to have led to increased antibiotic resistance patterns in meat products. A recent study by White and colleagues [25] of the prevalence of *Salmonella* in retail ground meats found increased antibiotic resistance. Surveillance by the CDC shows increase in ceftriaxone resistance and decrease in efficacy of ciprofloxacin in some human nontyphi *Salmonella* strains that is thought to be caused by the use of antimicrobials in animals [26].

Diapered and incontinent children should be on contact precautions for the duration of their illness. Children with typhoid fever should continue on contact precautions until 3 consecutive stool samples obtained 2 days after completion of antimicrobial therapy are negative.

Families with reptiles should be encouraged to make sure children wash their hands before eating. Breastfeeding has been found to be protective [27]. Prevention of salmonellosis also includes the use of typhoid vaccine in children older than 2 years when traveling to an area of increased risk of exposure, such as the Indian subcontinent, Latin America, Asia, the Middle East, and Africa [23].

E coli

One of the most serious infections in humans, especially in children, is enterohemorrhagic *E coli* (EHEC) or STEC, which includes *E coli* O157:H7. In 2012, 1081 laboratory-confirmed cases of STEC were reported to FoodNet [8]. A decline of *E coli* foodborne outbreaks was found in 2010 compared with the 2006 to 2008 period [5]. PulseNet has been partly responsible for the decline, allowing molecular subtyping on a nationwide basis leading to earlier detection of outbreaks. Further decline is caused by improved food safety regulations implemented on meat, eggs, and produce [2].

Beef cattle are thought to be reservoirs of *E coli* O157 and non-O157 STEC [28], thus outbreaks have been associated with hamburger meat [29–31] and contaminated vegetables [14,22]. Other recent food items and beverages associated with *E coli* infections are meat, apple cider, spinach, contaminated water, unpasteurized milk, fresh produce, kimchi, and salami [6,16,32–34].

STEC has an infectious dose of 100 to 1000 organisms and can cause diarrhea, vomiting, and fever in 50% of children or acute bloody diarrhea after a short incubation period of 3 to 4 days (range, 1–8 days) [3,33,35–37]. It is also the most common organism associated with HUS, which predominantly affects infants and young children and is the most common cause of acute renal failure in this population [36,38]. HUS is distinguished by the triad of microangiopathic hemolytic anemia, thrombocytopenia, and acute renal dysfunction [37] and can develop up to 3 weeks after onset of diarrhea. Stool culture using sorbitol-enriched MacConkey agar is the diagnostic test of choice for detection of *E coli.* Latex agglutination testing for the O157:H7 serotype is routinely performed in most laboratories.

Primary treatment is supportive, including rehydration and monitoring of complete blood count and basic metabolic panel for signs of HUS. If an isolate other than EHEC or STEC is identified, consideration may be given for treatment, based on culture results. Children should be on contact isolation for the duration of their diarrheal illness. In addition, they should wait 2 weeks before returning to water activities and have 2 negative stool cultures for return to daycare [37].

Shigella

Shigellosis is caused by the gram-negative rod *Shigella sonnei* (most commonly), *Shigella flexneri*, or *Shigella dysenteriae* [39]. More than 2100 cases were reported to FoodNet in 2012 [8]. Shigellosis is transmitted via the fecal-oral route or via ingestion of contaminated food or water. Humans are the natural reservoir for the organism. Most foodborne infections and 58% of reported outbreaks from *Shigella* occur because of contamination of food by a food worker with poor hand hygiene [40]. Food associated with *Shigella* foodborne infections include tomatoes, raw carrots, ground beef, raw oysters, and bean salad [41–45]. *Shigella* is a hardy organism that can survive in refrigerated foods. Seven percent of recent foodborne outbreaks associated with fresh salsa and guacamole in restaurants were caused by *Shigella* [19].

Shigella has a low infectious dose: 500 organisms for *S sonnei* and 10 organisms for *S dysenteriae*, thus it is very contagious [46]. The incubation period is usually 1 to 3 days (but may be up to 7 days) [39]. Shigellosis may present with symptoms ranging from watery stools with mild constitutional symptoms to high fever (dysentery), or abdominal cramps, and painful, mucoid stools with or without blood (severe colitis). *S dysenteriae* is associated with complications such as pseudomembranous colitis, toxic megacolon, intestinal perforation, septicemia, HUS, and seizures in children. Reactive arthritis is a complication that can occur weeks to months after initial infection [47]. Stool culture is the diagnostic test of choice and the presence of fecal leukocytes indicates invasive colitis.

Infection is usually self-limited, lasting 2 to 3 days; however, *Shigella* is one of the bacterial gastroenteritides in which antimicrobial therapy has been shown to be beneficial in decreasing the duration of illness and shedding. Treatment is recommended in immunosuppressed patients, or in children with severe disease. Forty-six percent of *Shigella* isolates in 2009 were resistant to ampicillin [39]. Treatment options are azithromycin for 3 days, ceftriaxone for 5 days, or ciprofloxacin for 3 days. The use of antidiarrheal agents should be avoided. If a malnourished child is undergoing treatment of shigellosis, vitamin A and zinc supplementation is recommended [39].

Contact isolation measures are recommended for the duration of illness. Return to daycare or school depends on local health authorities, which may require at least one negative stool culture. Avoidance of water activities should continue for 1 week after symptoms resolve.

Listeria

Listeria is a gram-positive bacillus that can survive for many months in soil and 20 to 30 days in tap water. Listeriosis occurs in 1 in every 22,000 pregnancies and 1 in 8000 pregnancies of Hispanic decent [48]; however, only 121 cases of foodborne listeriosis was reported to FoodNet in 2012 [8]. The overall incidence of listeriosis has decreased 24% from 1996 to 2003, which is thought to be caused by preventive, regulatory (including the zero-tolerance policy of the FDA and USDA-FSIS), and educational measures [49–51]. *Listeria* is a foodborne pathogen commonly found in soft cheeses, ready-to-eat foods, deli meat, raw vegetables, hot dogs, unpasteurized milk, chicken, beef, and recently in cantaloupes [10,48,52–54].

In a recent *Morbidity and Mortality Weekly Report*, 74% of patients with invasive listeriosis had the following comorbidities (in order of decreasing frequency): immunosuppression (caused by chemotherapy, steroids, radiation, and recently infliximab), malignancy, diabetes mellitus, liver disease, renal failure, and HIV/ acquired immunodeficiency syndrome [55–57]. Other high-risk populations include the elderly, pregnant women, and people of Hispanic descent [48,53,58].

Listeriosis can lead to clinical presentations of gastroenteritis, bacteremia, and meningitis. In pregnant women, infection can be asymptomatic or an influenzalike illness with fever, malaise, headache, back pain, and gastrointestinal symptoms [59]. Diagnosis can be made from blood culture or enriched culture media with horse or rabbit blood from other sterile sites. *Listeria* can be misdiagnosed as a contaminant because of its diphtheroid morphology [59]. Treatment consists of ampicillin and gentamicin for severe infections; in normal hosts, ampicillin may be given alone. Trimethoprim-sulfamethoxazole is an alternative drug because cephalosporins are inactive against *Listeria*.

Listeriosis is a preventable disease. Deli meats, hot dogs, and soft cheeses are foods that should be avoided in pregnancy and immunocompromised children [48]. In addition to the routine prevention measures discussed later, the *Red*

Book recommends that high-risk patients avoid goat milk, raw or unpasteurized milk, dairy products, refrigerated pâtés and other meat spreads, and inappropriately smoked seafood that has not been reheated properly [59]. Deli meat should be eaten within 3 to 5 days after opening the packaging and hot dogs within 1 week.

Toxoplasma

Toxoplasmosis is an intracellular parasitic infection caused by the protozoan *Toxoplasma gondii* through ingestion of oocytes. Cats are definitive hosts for the parasite *T gondii* and excrete contagious fecal oocytes [60]. Humans can become infected by ingestion of contaminated water or vegetables grown in contaminated soil or from contaminated meat. Food items associated with the transmission of toxoplasmosis include undercooked meat, pork, lamb, wild game meat, food contaminated with cat feces, and unpasteurized goat milk [61]. Game meat that may be infected with *Toxoplasma* includes venison, elk, moose, wild pig, and bear. In addition, the organism has also been isolated from cured, dried, or smoked meat; clams; and mussels [62]. New consumer demands for organic food and chicken may lead to an increase in toxoplasmosis [63,64]. Up to 50% of infected people do not have identifiable risk factors or symptoms with toxoplasmosis [65].

Infected children may have symptoms of sore throat, arthralgia, and myalgia. Immunocompromised patients (usually infants) may present with intracranial calcifications, chorioretinitis or encephalitis, pneumonitis, or fever of unknown origin. Toxoplasmosis has an incubation period of approximately 7 days with a range of 4 to 21 days [65]. Diagnosis is through serologic testing and polymerase chain reaction (PCR) of body fluids. The Palo Alto Medical Foundation Toxoplasma Serology Laboratory (www.pamf.org/serology) can be used to assist with diagnosis, especially in the setting of possible congenital infection. Treatment is only indicated if the symptoms are severe or persistent, and includes pyrimethamine and sulfadiazine with leucovorin. Consultation with an infectious disease consultant is recommended for further assistance. Routine standard precautions are recommended.

Prevention of toxoplasmosis should include isolation of cats from areas where animals or vegetables are located that are destined for human consumption to prevent accidental contamination [60]. Cat litter should be disposed of in garbage to prevent leakage to the water supply. *T gondii* is highly resistant to freezing and disinfectants. Microwaves do not kill the parasite reliably, therefore stove-top cooking of food and water is preferred [63]. Freezing meat to an internal temperature of $-12°C$ has been shown to kill the tissue cysts as well as irradiation [62]. Other tips include covering children's sandboxes when not in use, and the avoidance of raw oysters, clams, and unpasteurized goat's milk.

Campylobacter

Campylobacter is a comma-shaped motile gram-negative rod known to cause acute gastroenteritis. *Campylobacter jejuni* and *Campylobacter coli* are the most common species implicated in foodborne infections, whereas *Campylobacter fetus* usually causes systemic infections [66]. *C jejuni* was identified in 66% of outbreaks from 1997 to 2008, whereas *C coli* and *C fetus* were each identified in only 2% [67]. More than 6700 cases of campylobacter infections were identified in FoodNet in 2012 [8]. The organism lives in the gastrointestinal tract of domestic and wild birds, farm animals, and pets such as dogs, cats, and hamsters, especially young animals [68]. The transmission of *Campylobacter* occurs by the fecal-oral route and 80% of transmission occurs through food [69]. Food items associated with transmission have included dairy products (29%) such as unpasteurized milk, unpasteurized cheeses, and ice cream; produce (10%); seafood (5%); and poultry (4% of outbreak cases) [67,70,71].

The infectious dose can be as low at 500 organisms [68]. The incubation time usually varies between 2 and 5 days, but is sometimes longer. Children usually present with acute diarrhea, abdominal cramps, nausea, and fever. Stools can have frank or occult blood. Abdominal pain may mimic appendicitis or intussusception [68]. Bacteremia may occur, as well as a relapsing form of campylobacteriosis. Immunocompromised children are at higher risk of prolonged severe illness [68]. Potential complications associated with *Campylobacter* are Guillain-Barré syndrome, reactive arthritis, and meningitis [47,69,72,73]. *Campylobacter* spp is usually identified in the stool in selective media at 42°C incubation. Stool enzyme immunoassay studies (EIA) are also available commercially. Children usually do not require antibiotic therapy because patients improve with rehydration alone. Azithromycin or erythromycin given for 3 days may shorten the duration of illness if given early [68]. Contact isolation is recommended for diapered and incontinent children for the duration of illness. Children should be kept out of daycare until diarrheal illness has resolved. Freezing meat has been shown to decrease the colony-forming units of *Campylobacter*, thereby decreasing the risk of foodborne illness [74].

Other bacterial pathogens

Clostridium spp are spore-forming, anaerobic, gram-positive rods. *C perfringens* is responsible for 10% of foodborne illnesses overall [15]. It is estimated to causes 1 million foodborne illnesses each year [75]. *Clostridium* is usually found in food that has been left at room temperature or warm outdoor temperatures for several hours [75]. The most commonly found food product associated with clostridial infection was beef cooked in a restaurant during the holiday months [76].

Foodborne botulism caused by ingestion of preformed toxin from *Clostridium botulinum* is an uncommon cause of foodborne illnesses. Botulism occurs when spores contaminate food that is then anaerobically stored, allowing production of toxin. The spores of *C botulinum*, if present in a canned product, are usually removed with heating. Therefore, illness is often associated with improper canning methods or improper heating. The FDA instituted mandated temperatures for cooking food before canning, which has decreased the rates of botulism overall [77]. *C botulinum* was associated for the first time in a national outbreak with a commercial canned hot dog chili sauce [78]. The lack of proper sterilization allowed the spores to survive the canning process in the chili sauce factory. Honey may contain spores of *C botulinum*, therefore it should not be given to infants less than 1 year of age [79].

Incubation time can vary from 12 to 48 hours, with a range of 6 hours to 8 days [79]. Symptoms of botulism include dysphagia, blurred vision, slurred speech, muscle weakness, and descending flaccid paralysis. Children usually present with diarrhea and abdominal pain. Diagnosis is through stool and serum testing. Foodborne botulism is a self-limited illness and antibiotics should be avoided [80]. Treatment of botulism consists of heptavalent botulinum antitoxin, which is available at the CDC and state health departments [79].

To prevent foodborne botulism, several measures can be taken. Foods should be cooked in a pressure cooker and to an internal temperature of 85°C for 10 minutes to destroy any toxin that may be present [79]. Any canned products that may be bulging or contain gas should be discarded. The preparation of home canned food should follow proper sterile technique and garlic in oil products should be refrigerated [81].

B cereus and *S Aureus* foodborne illnesses both occur after ingestion of heat-stable enterotoxins. *S aureus* food poisoning is associated with homemade products and pork dishes, whereas fried rice and poultry are most commonly associated with *B cereus* foodborne illness [76]. The incubation time is 4 hours for *S aureus* and 5 hours in *B cereus* foodborne outbreaks. Children with either infection can present with vomiting and diarrhea. Recovery of *Bacillus* spp or *S Aureus* is possible from stool culture or from the contaminated food product [76]. Supportive care is recommended in both foodborne illnesses, and tracing back to the suspected food and notification of the Department of Health. Standard isolation is used for these patients in a hospital setting.

Yersinia enterocolitica is a gram-negative bacillus that colonizes the pharynx of pigs. There were 155 cases reported to FoodNet in 2012 [8]. Transmission is thought to occur through ingestion of contaminated food products, uncooked pork or pork intestines, unpasteurized milk, and contaminated well water. Yersiniosis is commonly associated with the ingestion of pork chitterlings (raw pork intestines), most frequently in African American households in the southern United States and by Asian families [82]. Transmission to children usually occurs from the adult caregivers. Young children less than 5 years of age had the highest incidence of infections [82]. A decline in incidence occurred in black children less than 5 years old, from 41.5 to 3.5 per 100,000 persons from 1996 to 2009 [82]. Educational campaigns are thought to contribute to the decrease in overall incidence. In the Asian community, children less than 5 years of age were also disproportionally affected, which is thought to be because of the use of pig intestines. Children with excess iron states and immunocompromised children are at higher risk because excess iron aids in the growth of *Yersinia* [83].

The incubation period is from 4 to 6 days. Children usually present with fever, diarrhea (at times bloody), and a pseudoappendicitis syndrome, but bacteremia may occur. Clinical features may mimic those of Kawasaki disease, as noted in Japan [84]. *Yersinia* can be isolated from routine stool and blood culture. Treatment with cefotaxime or trimethoprim-sulfamethoxazole is usually reserved for children with bacteremia. No treatment benefit has been found with children with acute gastroenteritis caused by *Yersinia* [83]. Children should be placed on contact isolation for the duration of their diarrheal illness.

Vibrio

Vibrio spp are anaerobic gram-negative bacilli that cause acute gastroenteritis, bacteremia, and wound infections. The most common species associated with foodborne infection, in order of frequency, are *Vibrio parahaemolyticus, Vibrio vulnificus* and *Vibrio alginolyticus. Vibrio* spp caused 193 laboratory-confirmed cases in 2012 according to FoodNet data [8]. A recent review of FoodNet and COVIS found an increase in the incidence of vibriosis [85]. Most recent data from FoodNet shows the highest incidence of vibriosis in children ages 5 to 9 year old [8]. Children with low gastric acidity (eg, on chronic proton pump inhibitors), immunodeficiencies, and those with liver disease are at increased risk of infection. The organism is found in seawater and brackish water, likely explaining the higher incidence in the Gulf Coast states. Foodborne illnesses caused by *Vibrio* spp have been associated with undercooked seafood such as clams, oysters, crabs, and shrimps. Children most commonly present with acute onset of watery diarrhea and crampy abdominal pain, but they may also present with fever, chills, headache, and vomiting. The incubation period for gastroenteritis is 23 hours, with a range of 5 to 92 hours [86]. *Vibrio* spp can be isolated from stool specimens, but laboratories should be notified to check for *Vibrio*. The illness is self-limited; however, antimicrobials like doxycycline and a third-generation cephalosporin may be given to patients with suspected sepsis. Contact precautions should be implemented for the course of diarrheal illness.

Norovirus

Overall, viruses account for 59% of foodborne illnesses, with norovirus (previously called Norwalk virus) causing most illnesses and about 11% of hospitalizations [12,15]. Norovirus is a common cause of foodborne outbreaks because of its highly contagious properties [87]. It is known to have a low infectious inoculum of as low as 18 viral particles and remains infectious on surfaces for 2 weeks and in water for more than 2 months [88]. In addition, norovirus is resistant to many disinfectants including hand sanitizers, therefore hand washing with soap and water is preferred [35,89,90]. Transmission often occurs from a household member via the fecal-oral route, ingestion of aerosolized vomitus, contact with fomites, or ingestion of contaminated food or water [91]. Patients continue to shed the virus for as long as 3 weeks [87].

Food can easily be contaminated along the food processing pathway from farm to table. Because of these highly contagious properties, outbreaks are common, especially on cruise ships and in schools and nursing homes and occur more commonly in the winter months [91]. Norovirus caused 39% of all confirmed single-cause outbreaks between 1998 and 2008 [12]. Leafy vegetables contaminated with norovirus were responsible for most outbreak-related illnesses (more than 4000 illnesses) in the same 10-year period [12]. Other food items implicated in outbreaks include strawberries, oysters (water contaminated with human waste), and other ready-to-eat foods (sandwiches, fresh salsa, and guacamole) [13,19,91].

Symptoms in children usually include abrupt onset of vomiting, nausea, abdominal pain, headache, and nonbloody watery diarrhea that can last from 1 to 3 days [13,87]. Symptoms may be prolonged and more severe in immunocompromised patients [89]. The median incubation period is more than 24 hours in an outbreak setting but can range from 12 to 48 hours in acute gastroenteritis [13,87]. The diagnostic test of choice is reverse transcription PCR, which is available through the CDC and some commercial laboratories. A norovirus EIA is also commercially available for diagnostic testing. Treatment is supportive care for symptomatic patients. Patients should be on contact isolation until 2 days after resolution of symptoms [87]. Children should not return to school for at least 24 to 72 hours after recovery from illness.

Parasites

Parasites are generally uncommon foodborne pathogens in the United States. This article focuses on the most common pathogens such as *Giardia*, amebiasis, *Cyclospora*, and *Cryptosporidium*. Less common parasites such as *Angiostrongylus cantonensis*, *Gnathostoma spinigerum* (dog and cat roundworm), and *Baylisascaris procyonis* (raccoon roundworm) can cause eosinophilic meningitis if raw fish, frog, bird, snake meat, snails, or slugs are eaten. This practice is more common in Asian countries. A useful resource is a recent review by Steiner [92] on treating foodborne illnesses.

Giardia

Giardia is a protozoa that leads to diarrhea after ingestion of contaminated water or contaminated food from an infected food handler [93]. The incubation period is between 1 and 14 days with symptoms lasting up to 3 weeks [94]. Stools may be greasy and foul smelling. Diagnosis is usually made with stool antigen (EIA) testing or microscopic evaluation. Treatment of giardiasis is with either 5 days of metronidazole or 3 days of nitazoxanide [95]. Contact isolation during the course of diarrheal illness is also recommended. Children may return to daycare when their symptoms resolve. Swimming and water-related activities should be avoided for 2 weeks after diarrhea has resolved [96].

Amebiasis

Entamoeba histolytica is protozoa pathogenic in humans, but *Entamoeba dispar* and *Entamoeba moshkovskii* are thought to be nonpathogens. Transmission of the protozoa may be acquired through ingestion of food or water contaminated with cysts. The incubation period is between 2 and 4 weeks. Most cases are asymptomatic or have self-limited disease, with only 1% of cases developing a liver abscess [97]. Treatment of patients with gastrointestinal tract symptoms or liver abscess is with a 5-day course of metronidazole followed by paromomycin (luminal amebicide) [97]. Children should be placed on contact isolation for the duration of diarrheal symptoms. Water activities should also be restricted until therapy is completed to prevent transmission to other contacts.

Cyclospora

Cyclospora cayetanensis, a coccidian parasite, causes acute gastroenteritis or cyclosporiasis. Children between the ages of 10 and 19 years have the highest incidence of cyclosporiasis in children overall [98]. The parasite is transmitted through contaminated food or water and humans are the only host. *Cyclospora* has been found in fresh produce such as raspberries, lettuce, basil, and snow peas and has led to multistate outbreaks [98–100]. The incubation period varies from 2 to 14 days [98]. Patients present with watery diarrhea, weight loss, abdominal pain, and prolonged fatigue. Diagnosis is made by obtaining stool for ova and parasite; however, these studies may have a low yield because of low-level shedding of *Cyclospora*. PCR testing is available at the CDC. Treatment is usually supportive, but trimethoprim-sulfamethoxazole or ciprofloxacin (if allergic) may be given to those with severe symptoms because some patients have a remitting-relapsing infectious course of cyclosporiasis [92].

Cryptosporidium

Cryptosporidium is a coccidian protozoan that caused more than 1200 laboratory-confirmed cases in 2012 [8]. *Cryptosporidium parvum* and *Cryptosporidium hominis* are the most common human pathogens [101]. *C parvum* infects humans, cattle, and other mammals and is the most common source of human infections. It most commonly affects children less than 9 years of age, with children aged 1 to 4 years reported as having the highest number of cases [102,103]. The incidence rate of cryptosporidiosis in children less than 5 years old in 2012 Food-Net was reported as 3.68 per 100,000 population [8]. Cryptosporidiosis in children peaks in summer months because of increased use of recreational water venues. The parasite is very contagious (chlorine treatment resistant) and can infect children with low inoculums (reportedly <10 oocytes) [46,94].

Children acquire the infection through contact with animals, the fecal-oral route, or ingestion of contaminated water. Foodborne illnesses have been associated with contaminated apple cider, unpasteurized milk, chicken salad, and raw produce [94]. Immunocompromised children (ie, HIV, immunodeficiencies, transplants, the malnourished) and very young children are at increased risk of infection [101].

Children are likely to present earlier than adults with symptoms of acute gastroenteritis, consisting of watery diarrhea that may last up to 10 days, although patients can also be asymptomatic. Children may also present with abdominal pain, weight loss, fever, fatigue, vomiting, and anorexia. The presentation of diarrhea may be acute or chronic (lasting more than 14 days); the chronic condition is more common in developing nations [94]. The incubation period is 1 week.

Antigen testing of the stool and stool microscopy are helpful in diagnosis. Stool studies should be obtained on 3 occasions from separate days to increase the yield of recovery [103]. Treatment with nitazoxanide is given in immunocompromised hosts, otherwise the illness is self-limited. Contact precautions should be for the duration of the illness. Hand washing is recommended because *Cryptosporidium* oocytes are not effectively inactivated by alcohol-based hand sanitizers [103].

Special high-risk populations

This population is delicate and requires anticipatory guidance and constant counseling to avoid foodborne infection [76,104,105]. The at-risk pediatric patient population, which has grown over time, includes pregnant teenagers; solid organ and stem cell transplant recipients; oncology patients; those with inflammatory bowel disease (IBD); diabetics; infants; patients with HIV; and those on long-term steroids, monoclonal antibodies, chronic proton pump inhibitors (PPI), immunosuppressive medications, and anti–tumor necrosis factor drugs [106]. Malnutrition should also be included because children often have poor diet based on their economic status or food insecurity.

Pregnant women had an increased relative risk of listeriosis compared with nonpregnant women in a recent study [58]. This is due to changes in their cellular immune function that lead to increased susceptibility to intracellular infections with *Toxoplasma* and *Listeria*. A decrease in foodborne toxoplasmosis and listeriosis among immunosuppressed children has likely occurred because of the routine prophylaxis with trimethoprim-sulfamethoxazole given to prevent *Pneumocystis jiroveci* infections [104,107]. Patients with HIV are at risk for foodborne pathogens such as *Salmonella, Listeria, Giardia, Shigella, Campylobacter, Cryptosporidium, Isospora,* and *Cyclospora* [108]. Patients with IBD are also at increased risk of *Salmonella, Listeria,* and *Toxoplasma* because of their immunosuppressive regimens [104].

PREVENTIVE FOOD MEASURES

Food safety

The government has a responsibility to ensure food safety through various programs and organizations; however, there are also measures that individuals can take to prevent foodborne illnesses. The FDA, CDC, USDA/FSIS mandate practices that encourage the safety of animals and water during food production, and monitor the food processing techniques such as pasteurization, canning, and irradiation.

The FDA is responsible for setting standards for food safety in the United States. However, it is unable to monitor all the food processing plants that exist domestically let alone screen all the imported food products. An example of a recent FDA regulation pertains to eggs. The FDA has mandated that egg producers apply proper preventive measures during egg production and refrigeration during storage and transport [109]. Since these changes, there has been a decrease in salmonellosis.

The CDC is another government entity that contributes to food safety by running surveillance systems, performing outbreak investigations, carrying out education campaigns such as Clean, Separate, Cook, and Chill, and making recommendations regarding processes such as food irradiation and pasteurization [57,110]. Irradiation of foods is a good method to kill the microbes that are most commonly isolated in meats and has been proposed for all high-risk food products because it has been shown to decrease bacterial load in the food products [77,111]. The CDC estimates a reduction of 900,000 cases of food-borne illness and 352 deaths if only 50% of meat and poultry were irradiated [77]. Irradiation of meat was implemented in 1997 and of iceberg lettuce and spinach in 2008 [6]. Pasteurization of milk, a process recommended by the CDC since the 1920s, has led to the decrease of *Listeria, Salmonella,* bovine tuberculosis, *Campylobacter,* and *E coli* [77]. Only 1 state, Pennsylvania, allows the sale of unpasteurized milk, which has become the source of a multistate *Campylobacter* outbreak [70].

Policy
In 2011, President Obama passed the Food Safety Modernization Act (FMSA), the first reform in more than 70 years in food safety to shift the focus from re-action to prevention of foodborne illnesses. The act allows the FDA to (1) require food facilities to have prevention measures in place to avoid contami-nation, (2) hold businesses accountable for their actions, and (3) set evidence-based standards for the safe production and harvesting of fruits and vegetables [112].

Under FMSA, imported food is also monitored and verified to ensure its safety for human consumption. The FDA under FMSA is able to require veri-fication of measures used by international companies to ensure food safety of their products sold in the United States. The importance of the FMSA should not be underestimated because the global supply of food can lead to pandemic outbreaks without careful monitoring [55]. An estimated 15% of the US food supply is imported, including 60% of fresh fruits and vegetables and 80% of seafood [5,110,112,113]. Furthermore, the FDA has been given the authority to order, if necessary, a mandatory recall of food products, because facilities currently are expected to voluntarily comply with a food recall.

Important preventive measures that individuals should follow pertain to good hand hygiene, food preparation techniques, cooking food to proper inter-nal temperatures, and appropriate food storage. The use of appropriate hand hygiene is the most important factor in preventing all infections, and foodborne infections are no exception. Strict hand hygiene should be encouraged to pre-vent accidental ingestion of bacteria when:

- Preparing food or formula for infants
- Before eating
- After using the bathroom
- After visiting petting zoos
- After gardening or contact with soil
- After handling fruits, vegetables, and raw meat or seafood

Appropriate food storage is another important preventive measure that can occur through multiple measures such as keeping cold food cold and hot food hot. Food should be chilled and refrigerated quickly in order to keep food temperatures out of the danger zone in which pathogens tend to replicate. Remind parents to avoid cluttering the fridge to ensure adequate air circulation and cooling [114]. Use of a refrigerator thermometer to ensure adequate cooling temperatures of 4°C (40°F) or lower and freezing temperatures of −18°C (0°F) or lower is also recommended [59]. Meat should be frozen to −12°C (10°F) for 24 hours to kill foodborne pathogens and should be refrigerated during food transport and processed in a clean manner [74]. If spills occur in refrigerators, the units, including walls and shelves, should be cleaned with hot soapy water. In addition, keeping fruits and vegetables at the appropriate temperatures helps preserve them and prevent mold growth. Thaw foods in the refrigerator, microwave, or cold water [115]. Mixed infant formula and marinades should be stored in the refrigerator [104,114].

Families should be educated about the peak of foodborne infections noted in summer months. During this time, people spend more time outdoors with picnics and barbeques, which are venues where electricity for cooling is not always available. Food and milk products should not be left out for more than 1 hour in 32°C (90°F) weather. Clean water should be available for all to use during a meal.

The recommendation to keep shallow leftovers under tight seals for only 4 days may be supported by a new smartphone application called Leftovers. This is part of the 4-Day Throw Away campaign to help families with small children in the Midwest determine when specific types of food should be thrown out [116]. Parents should also ensure that children's school lunches are kept at appropriate temperatures, because most are not [117]. Preventive measures pertaining to food preparation are as follows [10,65,114,115]:

- Wash fruits and vegetables before ingestion.
- Prevent contamination of food with raw or undercooked meat or with soil.
- Separate meat from vegetables; have separate cutting boards for vegetables and meat. Boards and utensils used for raw animal products should be washed in hot soapy water to prevent cross-contamination.
- Clean surfaces often with hot soapy water to avoid accidental cross-contamination.
- Cook food to appropriate temperatures as per Table 2.
- Water from a possibly unsafe source should be treated or boiled for 1 minute.

Table 2
Appropriate internal food temperature

Food type	Internal temperature (°C)
Poultry	74
Meat (whole cuts)[a]	66 (minimum of 63)
Ground meat and wild game meat	71
Seafood	Steaming hot
Egg dishes or casseroles	71
Food leftovers	74

[a]Measure temperature in thickest part of meat; allow 3-minute rest time before cutting meat [118].

Preventive measures specific to infant formula preparation are as follows. Infant bottles should be cleaned and treated in boiled water. Formula should be reconstituted in hot boiled water and cooled before feeding the infant. Attention should be given to potential recalls because formula has been recalled for contamination with *Cronobacter sakazakii* and *Salmonella* in the past [119].

The following foods and beverages should be avoided, especially by high-risk individuals [10,38,65,114,115]:

1. Raw or undercooked meat (pork, lamb, venison, beef)
2. Raw shellfish: oysters, clams, mussels
3. Smoked or cured meat in brine
4. Untreated water, or ice made from such water
5. Unpasteurized milk and dairy products
6. Unwashed green leafy vegetables
7. Accidental ingestion of lake/pool water (recreational use)

In conclusion, physicians should remain vigilant in learning about novel foodborne illnesses, outbreaks, and the ever-changing food items associated with these outbreaks. Advances are required in highlighting the need to regulate antibiotic use in animal products destined for human consumption so as not to further increase the antibiotic resistant patterns of foodborne pathogens [25]. In addition, continued collaboration is needed between public health officials, physicians, and animal health experts, as in the One Health initiative, if optimal health is to be attained for people, animals, and the environment [120,121].

IMPORTANT WEB SITES FOR REFERENCE
1. PulseNet: http://www.cdc.gov/pulsenet
2. Food safety from the CDC: http://www.cdc.gov/winnablebattles/foodsafety/index.html
3. President's Food Safety Working Group: http://www.foodsafetyworkinggroup.gov
4. Food safety; Gateway to Food Safety Information provided by government agencies: http://www.foodsafety.gov
5. Partnership for Food Safety Education: http://www.fightbac.org/
6. Think-Eat-Save Reduce your Foodprint Web site with explanation of expiration dates: http://thinkeatsave.org/index.php/new-nrdc-report-food-expiration-date-confusion-causing-up-to-90-of-americans-to-waste-food-wed-sep-18-2013
7. USDA/FSIS fact sheet for at-risk populations: http://www.fsis.usda.gov/wps/portal/fsis/topics/food-safety-education/get-answers/food-safety-fact-sheets/at-risk-populations
8. USDA/FSIS: mold fact sheet: http://www.fsis.usda.gov/wps/portal/fsis/topics/food-safety-education/get-answers/food-safety-fact-sheets/safe-food-handling/molds-on-food-are-they-dangerous_/
9. USDA Meat and Poultry Hotline 1-800-674-6854 for specific questions
10. Food Safety Automated Response System available 24/7 to ask questions about food safety: www.AskKaren.gov, www.PregunteleaKaren.gov (for Spanish speakers), m.askkaren.gov for mobile use.

Acknowledgments

The authors acknowledge Dr Robert W. Tolan Jr (posthumously) for his mentorship and guidance.

References

[1] Tauxe RV. Emerging foodborne pathogens. Int J Food Microbiol 2002;78(1–2):31–41.

[2] Braden CR, Tauxe RV. Emerging trends in foodborne diseases. Infect Dis Clin North Am 2013;27(3):517–33.

[3] McEntire J. Foodborne disease: the global movement of food and people. Infect Dis Clin North Am 2013;27(3):687–93.

[4] Center for Disease Control and Prevention. CDC research shows outbreaks linked to imported foods increasing. Vol 2013: Center for Disease Control and Prevention 2012. Available at: http://www.cdc.gov/media/releases/2012/p0314_foodborne.html.

[5] Center for Disease Control and Prevention. Vital signs: incidence and trends of infection with pathogens transmitted commonly through food–foodborne diseases active surveillance network, 10 U.S. sites, 1996-2010. MMWR Morb Mortal Wkly Rep 2011;60(22): 749–55.

[6] Maki DG. Coming to grips with foodborne infection–peanut butter, peppers, and nationwide salmonella outbreaks. N Engl J Med 2009;360(10):949–53.

[7] Mercanoglu Taban B, Halkman AK. Do leafy green vegetables and their ready-to-eat [RTE] salads carry a risk of foodborne pathogens? Anaerobe 2011;17(6):286–7.

[8] Center for Disease Control and Prevention. Incidence and trends of infection with pathogens transmitted commonly through food - foodborne diseases active surveillance network, 10 U.S. sites, 1996-2012. MMWR Morb Mortal Wkly Rep 2013;62(15):283–7.

[9] Ong KL, Apostal M, Comstock N, et al. Strategies for surveillance of pediatric hemolytic uremic syndrome: Foodborne Diseases Active Surveillance Network (FoodNet), 2000-2007. Clin Infect Dis 2012;54(Suppl 5):S424–31.

[10] McCollum JT, Cronquist AB, Silk BJ, et al. Multistate outbreak of listeriosis associated with cantaloupe. N Engl J Med 2013;369(10):944–53.

[11] Gopinath G, Hari K, Jain R, et al. The Pathogen-annotated Tracking Resource Network (PATRN) system: a web-based resource to aid food safety, regulatory science, and investigations of foodborne pathogens and disease. Food Microbiol 2013;34(2):303–18.

[12] Gould LH, Walsh KA, Vieira AR, et al. Surveillance for foodborne disease outbreaks - United States, 1998-2008. MMWR Surveill Summ 2013;62(2):1–34.

[13] Widdowson MA, Sulka A, Bulens SN, et al. Norovirus and foodborne disease, United States, 1991-2000. Emerg Infect Dis 2005;11(1):95–102.

[14] Taylor EV, Nguyen TA, Machesky KD, et al. Multistate outbreak of *Escherichia coli* O145 infections associated with romaine lettuce consumption, 2010. J Food Prot 2013;76(6): 939–44.

[15] Scallan E, Hoekstra RM, Angulo FJ, et al. Foodborne illness acquired in the United States–major pathogens. Emerg Infect Dis 2011;17:7–15. Available at: http://www.ncbi.nlm.nih.gov/pubmed/21192848.

[16] Inatsu Y, Bari ML, Kawasaki S, et al. Survival of *Escherichia coli* O157:H7, *Salmonella enteritidis*, *Staphylococcus aureus*, and *Listeria monocytogenes* in Kimchi. J Food Prot 2004;67(7):1497–500.

[17] Scallan E, Griffin PM, Angulo FJ, et al. Foodborne illness acquired in the United States–unspecified agents. Emerg Infect Dis 2011;17(1):16–22.

[18] Kemble SK, Westbrook A, Lynfield R, et al. Foodborne outbreak of group A *Streptococcus* pharyngitis associated with a high school dance team banquet–Minnesota, 2012. Clin Infect Dis 2013;57(5):648–54.

[19] Kendall ME, Mody RK, Mahon BE, et al. Emergence of salsa and guacamole as frequent vehicles of foodborne disease outbreaks in the United States, 1973-2008. Foodborne Pathog Dis 2013;10(4):316–22.

[20] Beuchat LR, Komitopoulou E, Beckers H, et al. Low-water activity foods: increased concern as vehicles of foodborne pathogens. J Food Prot 2013;76(1):150–72.

[21] Van Doren JM, Neil KP, Parish M, et al. Foodborne illness outbreaks from microbial contaminants in spices, 1973-2010. Food Microbiol 2013;36(2):456–64.

[22] Trevejo RT, Barr MC, Robinson RA. Important emerging bacterial zoonotic infections affecting the immunocompromised. Vet Res 2005;36(3):493–506.

[23] American Academy of Pediatrics, editor. *Salmonella* 2012. Elk Grove Village (IL): American Academy of Pediatrics; 2012.

[24] Gieraltowski L, Julian E, Pringle J, et al. Nationwide outbreak of *Salmonella* Montevideo infections associated with contaminated imported black and red pepper: warehouse membership cards provide critical clues to identify the source. Epidemiol Infect 2013;141(6): 1244–52.

[25] White DG, Zhao S, Sudler R, et al. The isolation of antibiotic-resistant *Salmonella* from retail ground meats. N Engl J Med 2001;345(16):1147–54.

[26] Medalla F, Hoekstra RM, Whichard JM, et al. Increase in resistance to ceftriaxone and non-susceptibility to ciprofloxacin and decrease in multidrug resistance among *Salmonella* strains, United States, 1996-2009. Foodborne Pathog Dis 2013;10(4):302–9.

[27] Rowe SY, Rocourt JR, Shiferaw B, et al. Breast-feeding decreases the risk of sporadic salmonellosis among infants in FoodNet sites. Clin Infect Dis 2004;38(Suppl 3):S262–70.

[28] Hussein HS. Prevalence and pathogenicity of Shiga toxin-producing *Escherichia coli* in beef cattle and their products. J Anim Sci 2007;85(Suppl 13):E63–72.

[29] Tuttle J, Gomez T, Doyle MP, et al. Lessons from a large outbreak of *Escherichia coli* O157:H7 infections: insights into the infectious dose and method of widespread contamination of hamburger patties. Epidemiol Infect 1999;122(2):185–92.

[30] Slutsker L, Ries AA, Maloney K, et al. A nationwide case-control study of *Escherichia coli* O157:H7 infection in the United States. J Infect Dis 1998;177(4):962–6.

[31] Cieslak PR, Noble SJ, Maxson DJ, et al. Hamburger-associated *Escherichia coli* O157:H7 infection in Las Vegas: a hidden epidemic. Am J Public Health 1997;87(2): 176–80.

[32] Besser RE, Lett SM, Weber JT, et al. An outbreak of diarrhea and hemolytic uremic syndrome from *Escherichia coli* O157:H7 in fresh-pressed apple cider. JAMA 1993;269(17): 2217–20.

[33] Tilden J Jr, Young W, McNamara AM, et al. A new route of transmission for *Escherichia coli*: infection from dry fermented salami. Am J Public Health 1996;86(8):1142–5.

[34] Cho SH, Kim J, Oh KH, et al. Outbreak of enterotoxigenic *Escherichia coli* O169 enteritis in schoolchildren associated with consumption of kimchi, Republic of Korea, 2012. Epidemiol Infect 2014;142:616–23.

[35] Cheesbrough JS, Green J, Gallimore CI, et al. Widespread environmental contamination with Norwalk-like viruses (NLV) detected in a prolonged hotel outbreak of gastroenteritis. Epidemiol Infect 2000;125(1):93–8.

[36] Su C, Brandt LJ. *Escherichia coli* O157:H7 infection in humans. Ann Intern Med 1995;123(9):698–714.

[37] American Academy of Pediatrics. *Escherichia coli* diarrhea (including hemolytic-uremic syndrome). In: Pickering LK, Baker CJ, Kimberlin DW, et al, editors. Red book: 2012 report of the Committee of Infectious Diseases. Elk Grove Village (IL): American Academy of Pediatrics; 2012. p. 324–8.

[38] Page AV, Liles WC. Enterohemorrhagic *Escherichia coli* infections and the hemolytic-uremic syndrome. Med Clin North Am 2013;97(4):681–95, xi.

[39] American Academy of Pediatrics. *Shigella* infections. In: Pickering LK, Baker CJ, Kimberlin DW, et al, editors. Red book: 2012 report of the Committee of Infectious Diseases. Elk Grove Village (IL): American Academy of Pediatrics; 2012. p. 645–7.

[40] Nygren BL, Schilling KA, Blanton EM, et al. Foodborne outbreaks of shigellosis in the USA, 1998-2008. Epidemiol Infect 2013;141:233–41.

[41] Agle ME, Martin SE, Blaschek HP. Survival of *Shigella boydii* 18 in bean salad. J Food Prot 2005;68(4):838–40.

[42] Warren BR, Yuk HG, Schneider KR. Survival of *Shigella sonnei* on smooth tomato surfaces, in potato salad and in raw ground beef. Int J Food Microbiol 2007;116(3):400–4.

[43] Gaynor K, Park SY, Kanenaka R, et al. International foodborne outbreak of *Shigella sonnei* infection in airline passengers. Epidemiol Infect 2009;137(3):335–41.

[44] Warren BR, Parish ME, Schneider KR. Shigella as a foodborne pathogen and current methods for detection in food. Crit Rev Food Sci Nutr 2006;46(7):551–67.

[45] Terajima J, Tamura K, Hirose K, et al. A multi-prefectural outbreak of *Shigella sonnei* infections associated with eating oysters in Japan. Microbiol Immunol 2004;48(1):49–52.

[46] Kothary MH, Babu US. Infective dose of foodborne pathogens in volunteers: a review. J Food Saf 2001;21(1):49–73.

[47] Batz MB, Henke E, Kowalcyk B. Long-term consequences of foodborne infections. Infect Dis Clin North Am 2013;27(3):599–616.

[48] Silk BJ, Date KA, Jackson KA, et al. Invasive listeriosis in the Foodborne Diseases Active Surveillance Network (FoodNet), 2004-2009: further targeted prevention needed for higher-risk groups. Clin Infect Dis 2012;54(Suppl 5):S396–404.

[49] Tappero JW, Schuchat A, Deaver KA, et al. Reduction in the incidence of human listeriosis in the United States. Effectiveness of prevention efforts? The Listeriosis Study Group. JAMA 1995;273(14):1118–22.

[50] Mead PS, Slutsker L, Dietz V, et al. Food-related illness and death in the United States. Emerg Infect Dis 1999;5(5):607–25.

[51] Voetsch AC, Angulo FJ, Jones TF, et al. Reduction in the incidence of invasive listeriosis in foodborne diseases active surveillance network sites, 1996-2003. Clin Infect Dis 2007;44(4):513–20.

[52] Olsen SJ, Patrick M, Hunter SB, et al. Multistate outbreak of *Listeria monocytogenes* infection linked to delicatessen turkey meat. Clin Infect Dis 2005;40(7):962–7.

[53] Posfay-Barbe KM, Wald ER. Listeriosis. Semin Fetal Neonatal Med 2009;14(4):228–33.

[54] Cartwright EJ, Jackson KA, Johnson SD, et al. Listeriosis outbreaks and associated food vehicles, United States, 1998-2008. Emerg Infect Dis 2013;19(1):1–9 [quiz: 184].

[55] Kelesidis T, Salhotra A, Fleisher J, et al. *Listeria* endocarditis in a patient with psoriatic arthritis on infliximab: are biologic agents as treatment for inflammatory arthritis increasing the incidence of *Listeria* infections? J Infect 2010;60(5):386–96.

[56] Williams G, Khan AA, Schweiger F. *Listeria* meningitis complicating infliximab treatment for Crohn's disease. Can J Infect Dis Med Microbiol 2005;16(5):289–92.

[57] Center for Disease Control and Prevention. Vital signs: listeria illnesses, deaths, and outbreaks–United States, 2009-2011. MMWR Morb Mortal Wkly Rep 2013;62(22):448–52.

[58] Pouillot R, Hoelzer K, Jackson KA, et al. Relative risk of listeriosis in Foodborne Diseases Active Surveillance Network (FoodNet) sites according to age, pregnancy, and ethnicity. Clin Infect Dis 2012;54(Suppl 5):S405–10.

[59] American Academy of Pediatrics. *Listeria monocytogenes* infections (listeriosis). In: Pickering LK, Baker CJ, Kimberlin DW, et al, editors. Red book: 2012 report of the Committee of Infectious Diseases. Elk Grove Village (IL): American Academy of Pediatrics; 2012. p. 471–4.

[60] Dabritz HA, Conrad PA. Cats and *Toxoplasma*: implications for public health. Zoonoses Public Health 2010;57(1):34–52.

[61] Dubey JP, Hill DE, Jones JL, et al. Prevalence of viable *Toxoplasma gondii* in beef, chicken, and pork from retail meat stores in the United States: risk assessment to consumers. J Parasitol 2005;91(5):1082–93.

[62] Jones JL, Dargelas V, Roberts J, et al. Risk factors for *Toxoplasma gondii* infection in the United States. Clin Infect Dis 2009;49(6):878–84.

[63] Jones JL, Dubey JP. Foodborne toxoplasmosis. Clin Infect Dis 2012;55(6):845–51.

[64] Dubey JP. *Toxoplasma gondii* infections in chickens (*Gallus domesticus*): prevalence, clinical disease, diagnosis and public health significance. Zoonoses Public Health 2010;57(1):60–73.

[65] American Academy of Pediatrics. *Toxoplasma gondii* infections (toxoplasmosis). In: Pickering LK, Baker CJ, Kimberlin DW, et al, editors. Red book: 2012 report of the Committee of Infectious Diseases. Elk Grove Village (IL): American Academy of Pediatrics; 2012. p. 720–8.

[66] Schlenker C, Surawicz CM. Emerging infections of the gastrointestinal tract. Best Pract Res Clin Gastroenterol 2009;23(1):89–99.

[67] Taylor EV, Herman KM, Ailes EC, et al. Common source outbreaks of *Campylobacter* infection in the USA, 1997-2008. Epidemiol Infect 2013;141(5):987–96.

[68] American Academy of Pediatrics. *Campylobacter* infections. In: Pickering LK, Baker CJ, Kimberlin DW, et al, editors. Red book: report of the Committee of Infectious Diseases. Elk Grove Village (IL): American Academy of Pediatrics; 2012. p. 262–4.

[69] DuPont HL. Clinical practice. Bacterial diarrhea. N Engl J Med 2009;361(16):1560–9.

[70] Longenberger AH, Palumbo AJ, Chu AK, et al. *Campylobacter jejuni* infections associated with unpasteurized milk–multiple States, 2012. Clin Infect Dis 2013;57(2):263–6.

[71] Friedman CR, Hoekstra RM, Samuel M, et al. Risk factors for sporadic *Campylobacter* infection in the United States: a case-control study in FoodNet sites. Clin Infect Dis 2004;38(Suppl 3):S285–96.

[72] Barzegar M, Alizadeh A, Toopchizadeh V, et al. Association of *Campylobacter jejuni* infection and GuillainBarre syndrome: a cohort study in the northwest of Iran. Turk J Pediatr 2008;50(5):443–8.

[73] Mishu B, Ilyas AA, Koski CL, et al. Serologic evidence of previous *Campylobacter jejuni* infection in patients with the Guillain-Barre syndrome. Ann Intern Med 1993;118(12):947–53.

[74] Maziero MT, de Oliveira TC. Effect of refrigeration and frozen storage on the *Campylobacter jejuni* recovery from naturally contaminated broiler carcasses. Braz J Microbiol 2010;41(2):501–5.

[75] Grass JE, Gould LH, Mahon BE. Epidemiology of foodborne disease outbreaks caused by *Clostridium perfringens*, United States, 1998-2010. Foodborne Pathog Dis 2013;10(2): 131–6.

[76] Bennett SD, Walsh KA, Gould LH. Foodborne disease outbreaks caused by *Bacillus cereus*, *Clostridium perfringens*, and *Staphylococcus aureus*–United States, 1998-2008. Clin Infect Dis 2013;57(3):425–33.

[77] Tauxe RV. Food safety and irradiation: protecting the public from foodborne infections. Emerg Infect Dis 2001;7(Suppl 3):516–21.

[78] Juliao PC, Maslanka S, Dykes J, et al. National outbreak of type a foodborne botulism associated with a widely distributed commercially canned hot dog chili sauce. Clin Infect Dis 2013;56(3):376–82.

[79] American Academy of Pediatrics. Botulism and infant botulism. In: Pickering LK, Baker CJ, Kimberlin DW, et al, editors. Red book: 2012 report of the Committee of Infectious Diseases. Elk Grove Village (IL): American Academy of Pediatrics; 2012. p. 281–4.

[80] American Academy of Pediatrics. *Clostridium perfringens* food poisoning. In: Pickering LK, Baker CJ, Kimberlin DW, et al, editors. Red book: 2012 report of the Committee of Infectious Diseases. Elk Grove Village (IL): American Academy of Pediatrics; 2012. p. 288–9.

[81] National Center for Emerging and Zoonotic Infectious Diseases. Botulism 2011; National Center for Emerging and Zoonotic Infectious Diseases. Available at: http://www.cdc.gov/nczved/divisions/dfbmd/diseases/botulism/. Accessed December 5, 2013.

[82] Ong KL, Gould LH, Chen DL, et al. Changing epidemiology of *Yersinia enterocolitica* infections: markedly decreased rates in young black children, Foodborne Diseases Active Surveillance Network (FoodNet), 1996-2009. Clin Infect Dis 2012;54(Suppl 5):S385–90.

[83] Abdel-Haq NM, Asmar BI, Abuhammour WM, et al. *Yersinia enterocolitica* infection in children. Pediatr Infect Dis J 2000;19(10):954–8.

[84] Vincent P, Salo E, Skurnik M, et al. Similarities of Kawasaki disease and *Yersinia pseudo-tuberculosis* infection epidemiology. Pediatr Infect Dis J 2007;26(7):629–31.

[85] Newton A, Kendall M, Vugia DJ, et al. Increasing rates of vibriosis in the United States, 1996-2010: review of surveillance data from 2 systems. Clin Infect Dis 2012;54(Suppl 5):S391–5.

[86] American Academy of Pediatrics. Other *Vibrio* infections. In: Pickering LK, Baker CJ, Kimberlin DW, et al, editors. Red book: 2012 report of the Committee of Infectious Diseases. Elk Grove Village (IL): American Academy of Pediatrics; 2012. p. 791–2.

[87] American Academy of Pediatrics. Human calicivirus infections (norovirus and sapovirus). In: Pickering LK, Baker CJ, Kimberlin DW, et al, editors. Red book: 2012 report of the Committee of Infectious Diseases. Elk Grove Village (IL): American Academy of Pediatrics; 2012. p. 261–2.

[88] Teunis PF, Moe CL, Liu P, et al. Norwalk virus: how infectious is it? J Med Virol 2008;80(8):1468–76.

[89] Dicaprio E, Ma Y, Hughes J, et al. Epidemiology, prevention, and control of the number one foodborne illness: human norovirus. Infect Dis Clin North Am 2013;27(3):651–74.

[90] Cheesbrough JS, Barkess-Jones L, Brown DW. Possible prolonged environmental survival of small round structured viruses. J Hosp Infect 1997;35(4):325–6.

[91] Hall AJ, Eisenbart VG, Etingue AL, et al. Epidemiology of foodborne norovirus outbreaks, United States, 2001-2008. Emerg Infect Dis 2012;18(10):1566–73.

[92] Steiner T. Treating foodborne illness. Infect Dis Clin North Am 2013;27(3):555–76.

[93] Yoder JS, Gargano JW, Wallace RM, et al. Giardiasis surveillance–United States, 2009-2010. MMWR Surveill Summ 2012;61(5):13–23.

[94] Huang DB, White AC. An updated review on *Cryptosporidium* and *Giardia*. Gastroenterol Clin North Am 2006;35(2):291–314, viii.

[95] Rossignol JF. *Cryptosporidium* and *Giardia*: treatment options and prospects for new drugs. Exp Parasitol 2010;124(1):45–53.

[96] American Academy of Pediatrics. *Giardia intestinalis* (formerly *Giardia lamblia* and *Giardia duodenalis*) infections. In: Pickering LK, Baker CJ, Kimberlin DW, et al, editors. Red book: 2012 report of the Committee of Infectious Diseases. Elk Grove Village (IL): American Academy of Pediatrics; 2012. p. 333–5.

[97] Pritt BS, Clark CG. Amebiasis. Mayo Clin Proc 2008;83(10):1154–9 [quiz: 1159–60].

[98] Hall RL, Jones JL, Hurd S, et al. Population-based active surveillance for *Cyclospora* infection–United States, Foodborne Diseases Active Surveillance Network (FoodNet), 1997-2009. Clin Infect Dis 2012;54(Suppl 5):S411–7.

[99] Center for Disease Control and Prevention. Notes from the field: outbreaks of cyclosporiasis - United States, June-August 2013. MMWR Morb Mortal Wkly Rep 2013;62(43):862.

[100] Purayidathil FW, Ibrahim J. A summary of health outcomes: multistate foodborne disease outbreaks in the U.S., 1998-2007. J Environ Health 2012;75(4):8–13.

[101] Huang DB, Chappell C, Okhuysen PC. Cryptosporidiosis in children. Semin Pediatr Infect Dis 2004;15(4):253–9.

[102] Barry MA, Weatherhead JE, Hotez PJ, et al. Childhood parasitic infections endemic to the United States. Pediatr Clin North Am 2013;60(2):471–85.

[103] Yoder JS, Wallace RM, Collier SA, et al. Cryptosporidiosis surveillance–United States, 2009-2010. MMWR Surveill Summ 2012;61(5):1–12.

[104] Lund BM, O'Brien SJ. The occurrence and prevention of foodborne disease in vulnerable people. Foodborne Pathog Dis 2011;8(9):961–73.

[105] Makkuni D, Kent R, Watts R, et al. Two cases of serious food-borne infection in patients treated with anti-TNF-alpha. Are we doing enough to reduce the risk? Rheumatology (Oxford) 2006;45(2):237–8.

[106] Acheson D, McEntire J, Thorpe CM. Foodborne illness: latest threats and emerging issues. Preface. Infect Dis Clin North Am 2013;27(3):xiii–xiv.

[107] Morris JG Jr, Potter M. Emergence of new pathogens as a function of changes in host susceptibility. Emerg Infect Dis 1997;3(4):433–41.

[108] Sax PE. Opportunistic infections in HIV disease: down but not out. Infect Dis Clin North Am 2001;15(2):433–55.

[109] Food and Drug Administration. Egg safety final rule. 2013. Available at: http://www.fda.gov/Food/GuidanceRegulation/GuidanceDocumentsRegulatoryInformation/Eggs/ucm170615.htm. Accessed December 10, 2013.

[110] Foodsafety.gov. Check Your steps. 2013. Available at: www.foodsafety.gov/keep/basics. Accessed November 15, 2013.

[111] Osterholm MT, Norgan AP. The role of irradiation in food safety. N Engl J Med 2004;350(18):1898–901.

[112] Food and Drug Administration. Food safety legislation key facts. 2013. Available at: http://www.fda.gov/Food/GuidanceRegulation/FSMA/ucm237934.htm. Accessed October 16, 2013.

[113] Foodsafety.gov. Food Safety Modernization Act: putting the focus on prevention. Available at: http://www.foodsafety.gov/news/fsma.html. Accessed October 9, 2013.

[114] United States Department of Agriculture Food Safety and Inspection Service. *Campylobacter* questions and answers. 2013. Available at: http://www.fsis.usda.gov/wps/portal/fsis/topics/food-safety-education/get-answers/food-safety-fact-sheets/foodborne-illness-and-disease/campylobacter-questions-and-answers/. Accessed September 25, 2013.

[115] Acheson D. Iatrogenic high-risk populations and foodborne disease. Infect Dis Clin North Am 2013;27(3):617–29.

[116] Albrecht JA, Larvick C, Litchfield RE, et al. Leftovers and other food safety information for iPhone/iPad application ("smartphone" technology). J Nutr Educ Behav 2012;44(5):469–71.

[117] Almansour FD, Sweitzer SJ, Magness AA, et al. Temperature of foods sent by parents of preschool-aged children. Pediatrics 2011;128(3):519–23.

[118] United States Department of Agriculture Food Safety and Inspection Service. Foodborne illness: what consumers need to know. 2013. Available at: http://www.fsis.usda.gov/wps/portal/fsis/topics/food-safety-education/get-answers/food-safety-fact-sheets/foodborne-illness-and-disease/foodborne-illness-what-consumers-need-to-know/ct_index. Accessed October 30, 2013.

[119] Norberg S, Stanton C, Ross RP, et al. *Cronobacter* spp. in powdered infant formula. J Food Prot 2012;75(3):607–20.

[120] Institute of Medicine (US). Improving food safety through a One Health approach: workshop summary. Washington, DC: National Academies Press (US); 2012.

[121] Ross AG, Olds GR, Cripps AW, et al. Enteropathogens and chronic illness in returning travelers. N Engl J Med 2013;368(19):1817–25.

Advances in Pediatrics 61 (2014) 313–333

ADVANCES IN PEDIATRICS

ELSEVIER
MOSBY

Lead Poisoning in Children

Heda Dapul, MD[a,b,*], Danielle Laraque, MD[b,c]

[a]Pediatric Critical Care Medicine, 4802 Tenth Avenue, Brooklyn, NY 11219, USA; [b]Maimonides Medical Center, Infants and Children's Hospital of Brooklyn, 4802 Tenth Avenue, Brooklyn, NY 11219, USA; [c]New York University School of Medicine, 550 First Avenue, New York City, NY 10016, USA

Keywords
- Blood lead level • Primary prevention • Chelation • Neuro-developmental

Key points
- Lead is ubiquitous. It comes from a variety of sources and can be ingested or inhaled.
- There is no safe lead level. The presence of any amount of lead in the blood can lead to neuro-developmental deficits, and in larger amounts lead can cause multiorgan damage and even death.
- "Treatment" of lead poisoning should be geared toward primary prevention, targeting environmental hazards, particularly that of lead-based paint used in pre-1978 housing.

BACKGROUND

Lead poisoning in children is a persistent worldwide problem. According to the World Health Organization, it accounts for about 0.6% of the global burden of disease [1]. Although recent data have shown a decline in the prevalence of elevated blood lead levels (BLLs) in children in the developed world, lead remains a well-known environmental health threat.

WHAT IS LEAD?

Lead is a naturally occurring, bluish-grey metal that exists in both organic and inorganic forms. It is soft, pliable, and resistant to corrosion. It does not conduct electricity and is effective in shielding against radiation. It has been used by humans for thousands of years in a variety of ways and is still widely used today [2].

*Corresponding author. Pediatric Critical Care Medicine, Maimonides Medical Center, Infants and Children's Hospital of Brooklyn, 949 48th Street, Brooklyn, NY 11219. *E-mail address:* HDapul@maimonidesmed.org

0065-3101/14/$ – see front matter
http://dx.doi.org/10.1016/j.yapd.2014.04.004 © 2014 Elsevier Inc. All rights reserved.

HISTORY

The earliest record of lead mining dates back to as far 6500 BC in Turkey; decorative lead beads were found in a tomb in the ancient city of Anatolia [3]. The effects of lead *toxicity* have been documented as early as 2000 BC. Even back then, lead was readily available, inexpensive, and durable. Because of its low melting point, it is easily malleable and therefore its widespread use in civilized societies led to chronic low-level exposure that has been described by various philosophers and historians over the years. Hippocrates (460–370 BC) wrote about a man mining lead that had loss of appetite, colic, weight loss, pallor, fatigue, and irritability [4], all consistent with symptoms of lead poisoning that we see today.

During the Roman period, lead was used extensively in the building of the aqueducts. It also was used as a pigment in paint, face powders (ie, "rouge"), and mascaras. Lead sugar, or lead (II) acetate, was used to sweeten wine and preserve fruit. Because of its diverse uses and widespread availability, the Romans minimized the hazards of lead use and this was theorized to be the cause of the fall of the Roman Empire [5]. Although this belief has since been refuted, the mental instability described in many Roman rulers, the sterility of many aristocratic men, and the infertility in many aristocratic women were thought to be caused by their daily low-level exposure to the metal [4].

In the Renaissance period, alchemists used lead in their attempts to turn metals into gold, and painters used lead-based colors for their work. It also was used as a slow-acting poison by Lucrezia Borgia and Catherine De Medici in the 1400s [6]. In 1621, lead found its way to the New World, when the earliest colonists settling in Virginia began lead mining and smelting.

The Industrial Revolution saw an increase in the number of workers who exhibited symptoms of metal intoxication and prompted scientists and physicians to study these symptoms and identify a cause [7]. In the late 1800s, the first form of legislation was passed in the United Kingdom to minimize workers' exposure to harmful metals in the workplace (Factories' Prevention of Lead Poisoning Act of 1883).

In the United States, it was not until the early twentieth century that the occupational and environmental toxicity of lead was acknowledged. In 1914, a Baltimore boy died of lead poisoning from ingesting white lead paint from his crib [8]. In the 1920s, the discovery of tetraethyl lead as an antiknock, fuel-efficient gasoline additive boosted the American automotive industry. This compound was later linked to the development of mental illness and, eventually, the death of 15 factory workers in New Jersey and Ohio. In May 1925, the production and sale of leaded gasoline was suspended temporarily while the Surgeon General appointed a panel of experts to investigate the cause of these deaths. This panel was largely composed of industry representatives and in 1926, their report said that there was not enough time or sufficient evidence to prove a link between exposure to triethyl lead and the symptoms of chronic disease [6].

Throughout the world war II and postwar era, there continued to be no regulations on leaded gasoline or on lead-based paint, which were the major sources of lead exposure at the time. Deaths from acute lead poisoning continued to be common. In the 1940s, BLLs of 40 μg/dL (1.9 μmol/L) were considered within "expected" limits, and the absence of symptoms was reassuring [8]. In 1965, geochemist Clair Patterson published that the high environmental lead levels in developed countries were from industrial sources. But industry scientist Robert Kehoe challenged his findings and denied the link between environmental lead and public health issues [9].

Over the next few decades, many more studies revealed that severe behavioral and learning deficits resulted from chronic exposure to lead. In 1972, 4 workers developed tetraethyl-lead lead poisoning after cleaning a tank of lead petrol. Their BLLs were between 64.2 and 92.5 μg/dL [10]. In 1974, Herbert Needleman, in an article in *Nature*, established the use of deciduous teeth to establish lead levels. Then in 1979, he published the seminal findings detailing an inverse relationship between dentine lead and intelligent quotient. He noted the frequency of nonadaptive classroom behavior increased in a dose-related fashion to dentine lead level. Further, he noted that lead exposure, at doses below those producing symptoms leading to a diagnosis, were associated with neuropsychological deficits that might interfere with classroom performance [11,12].

But it was not until 1975 that the US Environmental Protection Agency (EPA) was given the authority to regulate leaded gasoline. In 1977, the US Consumer Product Safety Commission banned the use of lead-based paint in residential housing. By 1985, the primary phase-out of leaded gas in the United States was complete. Blood lead levels declined by almost 80% from 1978 to 1991 during the phase-out [9].

In 1994, the United Nations Commission on Sustainable Development called on all governments to eliminate lead from gasoline, and on January 1, 2000, the European Union banned leaded gasoline as a public health hazard [13].

In 2011, an independent study from California State University estimated that the global phase-out of lead from gasoline resulted in considerable health, social, and economic benefits. More than 1 million deaths per year (of which 125,000 were children) were prevented and an estimated $2.4 trillion (4% of global GDP) costs were saved per year. Previous research had shown that children with elevated lead levels were more likely to be aggressive, violent, and delinquent. Since the global phase-out of leaded gas, there have been higher intelligence quotients (IQs) and lower crime rates (58 million fewer crime cases reported) [14,15].

EPIDEMIOLOGY

- There has been a precipitous decline in BLLs in the pediatric population since the 1970s. A compilation of the National Health and Nutrition Examination Survey (NHANES) results from the periods of 1976 to 1980, 1991 to 1994, 1999 to 2002, and 2007 to 2010 are shown in Table 1. The mean BLLs during these periods are shown in Table 2 [16].
- In 1991, the Centers for Disease Control and Prevention (CDC) identified a BLL of 10 μg/dL or higher as the "level of concern" for children aged 1 to 5 years.

Table 1
Decrease in the prevalence of BLL greater than 10 µg/dL in children aged 1 to 5 years

NHANES survey	Children aged 1–5 y with BLL >10 µg/dL, %
1976–1980	88.0
1991–1994	4.4
1999–2002	1.6
2007–2010	0.8

Abbreviations: BLL, blood lead level; NHANES, National Health and Nutrition Examination Survey.

- In 2012, the CDC replaced the term "level of concern" with an upper reference interval value defined as the 97.5th percentile of BLLs in US children aged 1 to 5 years from 2 consecutive cycles of NHANES (2007–2008 and 2009–2010). This reference value was calculated as 5 µg/dL (0.24 µmol/L) [16].
- Based on the 2007 to 2010 NHANES data, the percentage of children aged 1 to 5 with BLLs greater than 5 µg/dL was 2.6%, indicating an estimate of 535,000 children [16].
- Mean BLLs are higher in younger children, those that belong to low-income families, and/or those who are enrolled in Medicaid. Those who live in homes built before 1970 also have higher BLLs. Race and ethnicity also are predictive of high lead levels, with the greatest risk being in the non-Hispanic black population [16].
- Although the disparity in risk for BLLs greater than or equal to 10 µg/dL by income and race are no longer statistically significant, disparities by race/ethnicity and income still persist at lower BLLs [17].
- Children who live in certain areas identified to have the highest prevalence of lead levels also are at risk. National and state-specific surveillance data from 1997 to 2012 that identify these zip codes is available at http://www.cdc.gov/nceh/lead/data/national.htm.

EXPOSURE AND SOURCES

Lead is ubiquitous, especially in industrialized societies, and exposure to lead can happen in a variety of ways. Ingestion or inhalation are the primary modes by which toxicity occurs; however, prenatal and dermal exposure have also been reported. Lead is absorbed through the respiratory and digestive tracts,

Table 2
Decline in estimated GM BLLs of children aged 1 to 5 years

NHANES survey	GM BLL, µg/dL	95% CI
1976–1980	15.0	14.2–15.8
1988–1991	3.6	3.3–4.0
1999–2002	1.9	1.8–2.1
2007–2010	1.3	1.3–1.4

Abbreviations: BLL, blood lead level; CI, confidence interval; GM, geometric mean; NHANES, National Health and Nutrition Examination Survey.

enters the bloodstream, and is distributed to all tissues throughout the body. The toxic effects of lead are related to its concentration in the blood. Children are at risk of lead poisoning by ingestion because of their propensity for chewing on things and placing objects in their mouths. Also, lead makes things taste sweet, further attracting ingestion by children. Adults are more likely to be exposed occupationally to lead through inhalation of lead dust and vapor.

Ingestion
Lead-based paint
Before the 1950s, white house paint was 50% lead, which is why old houses are high risk for lead exposure. In 1971, federal law reduced the maximum allowable lead content in paint to 1%, and by 1977 it was down to 0.06%. Although most homes have since been repainted with nonleaded paint, lead may still be released into the home during renovations or if paint is peeled, chipped, or cracked. Once believed to be due to ingested paint chips, lead toxicity has now been linked more so to household dust containing lead, which may be inhaled or ingested during a child's hand-to-mouth and toy-to-mouth activity [8,18].

Water
Drinking water can be contaminated by the lead solder that is used to hold copper pipes together. Municipal water supplies are usually regulated to prevent contamination at the source, but when older fixtures are corroded, lead can leach into the water supply that is delivered to homes. In 1991, the EPA published the Lead and Copper Rule to control the amount of lead and copper in drinking water. The EPA "action level" of lead in water is 15 parts per billion. This is unlikely to cause clinically significant elevation of BLL in adults; however, children may be more susceptible to lead poisoning because of their relatively smaller body size and specifics of their metabolism and storage of lead. In January 2011, Congress enacted the Reduction of Lead in Drinking Water Act to amend Section 1417 of the Safe Drinking Water Act regarding the use and introduction into commerce of lead pipes, plumbing fittings or fixtures, solder, and flux [19,20].

Soil
Lead released from combustion of leaded gasoline, deterioration of lead-based paint, factory and smelter emissions, and other industrial sources can become airborne and eventually settle onto the surrounding soil. The accepted safety standard for soil in residential areas is 400 parts per million (ppm) in play areas and 1200 ppm for nonplay areas [21,22].

Food
Lead makes its way into food products during its production, handling, packaging, preparation, and/or storage. As mentioned previously, lead from the air settles onto soil and results in the contamination of any produce that is grown on it. If lead solder is used during the canning process, this too makes its way into food once the can is opened and oxidation occurs. Imported spices from other countries that are not tested for lead content also can contaminate food during its preparation. Food stored, prepared, or served in lead crystal,

lead-glazed pottery, or porcelain can be contaminated as well. Lead also has been found in some candies imported from Mexico, particularly some candy ingredients, such as chili powder and tamarind [23].

Leaded objects, including children's toys, cosmetics, and other recreational items
Children's toys, jewelry, and or furniture may contain lead-based paint. Many lipsticks are manufactured using lead. Topical exposure or contact with these objects presents a low risk of contamination; however, ingestion of these products (chewing and/or swallowing) may cause lead poisoning. Since 2008, the federal government has banned lead greater than 100 ppm in weight in most children's products [23,24].

Alternative medicine or "folk remedies"
Hispanic traditional remedies called *Greta* and *Azarcon* are used to treat an upset stomach, diarrhea, and vomiting. These are fine orange powders that may have as much as 90% lead content. *Ba-baw-san* is a Chinese herbal remedy used to treat colic pain or to pacify young children, and *Ghasard* is a brown powder used as a tonic in India. These have both been found to contain lead. *Daw Tway* is a folk remedy from Thailand and Myanmar (Burma) used to aid digestion that has been found to contain extremely high levels of lead and arsenic [25].

Inhalation
Leaded gasoline
Before the 1970s, leaded gasoline was responsible for most lead exposure through inhalation. More recently, lead-based paint in older housing has become the most important source of lead toxicity in vulnerable populations, particularly children. The use of lead in gasoline was gradually phased out from the United States from 1975 to 1986, and from Europe in the 1990s.

Occupational hazards
Lead dust is created through occupational means and can be extremely hazardous to the exposed workers and those who live with them. It settles on skin, hair, and clothes and can be brought home where family members are exposed [26]. Increased risk of occupational exposure occurs in the following:

- Battery manufacturing and recycling plants
- Demolition, remodeling, and renovation projects
- Rubber and plastic industries
- Ammunition manufacturing
- Automotive/radiator repair
- Lead soldering (ie, electronic manufacturing) and welding
- Painting
- Plumbing

Artificial turf
Artificial turf used as playing fields are made of nylon or nylon/polyethylene blend fibers that may contain lead. With frequent use, wear, and tear, lead dust is released into the air where it may be inhaled or even ingested. The

amount of exposure, BLLs, and/or extent of lead poisoning from this source has not yet been determined [27].

Prenatal exposure and breastfeeding

In utero lead poisoning occurs when lead enters the maternal bloodstream during environmental exposure or from mobilization of bone lead stores accumulated from past exposure. This prenatal exposure to lead has been linked to neurodevelopmental delays after birth, although a threshold level for toxicity has yet to be identified. Lead crosses the placenta readily, hence the presence of any lead in maternal blood should be a cause for concern [28]. Additionally, studies have estimated a direct relationship between maternal blood levels at 1 month postpartum and the BLLs of their breastfed infants [29].

Dermal exposure

Skin absorption is not considered a significant mode of exposure among the general population. Organic lead is more likely to be absorbed through the skin than inorganic lead, and mostly occurs among people who work closely with it [2].

Additional sources of lead can be found on the following Web site: www.cdc.gov/nceh/lead/CaseManagement/caseManage_appendixes.htm.

PATHOGENESIS

Lead exerts its effects by binding to the sulfhydryl group of proteins, making it particularly toxic to multiple enzyme systems. Much of its toxicity also results from its binding to calcium-activated proteins with much higher affinity than calcium, interfering with various calcium-dependent cellular functions. It interferes with heme production by inhibiting the enzyme delta-aminolevulinic acid dehydratase and by preventing the incorporation of iron into the protoporphyrin molecule via the enzyme ferrochelatase; the result is a hypochromic, microcytic anemia.

The half-life of lead is approximately 30 to 40 days in the blood of adult men, but in children and pregnant women this may be longer. It then diffuses into the soft tissues (including the kidneys, brain, liver, and bone marrow), where it may stay for several months. In the liver, lead interferes with the cytochrome P450 enzymes. In the kidneys, vitamin D synthesis also is impaired. Lead then enters bone and is stored there for as long as several years. Lead in the bones, teeth, hair, and nails is bound tightly and not available to other tissues, and is generally thought not to be harmful [30]. Compared with 94% in adults, only 70% of absorbed lead is deposited in the bones in children, which may partially explain why children are more susceptible to the clinical effects of lead toxicity [31]. This also means that the BLL is not an accurate reflection of the total body lead burden.

CLINICAL PRESENTATION

Today, most lead-exposed children are asymptomatic at the time of screening. When present, the early symptoms of lead poisoning may be vague and nonspecific (eg, anorexia, abdominal pain, irritability). With continued exposure, these symptoms may worsen and develop into a spectrum of multi-organ dysfunction, as described in the following sections.

Nervous system
The neurologic effects of lead poisoning range from subtle developmental delays to frank encephalopathy. At high levels (BLL >100–150 µg/dL [4.8–7.2 µmol/L]), lead can cause acute symptoms, such as ataxia, stupor, coma, convulsions, hyperirritability, and death. Lower levels (BLL >10 µg/dL [0.48 µmol/L]) have been linked to the development of behavioral changes and neurocognitive decline [32,33].

Lead affects brain development and results in loss of milestones, reduced IQ, shortened attention span, increased antisocial behavior, and reduced educational attainment. Effects on learning behavior have been found to be associated with the degree of exposure to lead between the ages of 12 and 36 months [34].

Hematologic system
Anemia associated with lead poisoning may be due to either disruption of heme synthesis or hemolysis. At BLLs of 40 µg/dL (1.9 µmol/L), lead interferes with heme biosynthesis and results in decreased hemoglobin production [35]. A hypochromic microcytic anemia results and symptoms of weakness and fatigue develop. At higher levels (BLL >70 µg/dL [3.4 µmol/L]) acute hemolysis occurs and the anemia may be normocytic [2].

Renal system
Even at a blood level lower than 10 µg/dL, lead poisoning can result in impairment of proximal tubular function, manifested by aminoaciduria, glycosuria, and hyperphosphaturia [36]. Chronic exposure results in lead nephropathy, seen histologically as an interstitial nephritis that is often irreversible. In addition, lead in the kidney interferes with activation of vitamin D 1,2-dihydroxy cholecalciferol, which has an important role in calcium metabolism.

Other effects
Gastrointestinal effects of lead poisoning include anorexia, vomiting, constipation, and abdominal pain. Lead poisoning has been linked to the development of hypertension and its sequelae. Reproductive studies in men have revealed that chronic lead exposure may diminish sperm concentrations, total sperm counts, and total sperm motility. Effects on actual fertility are unclear. Developmental studies suggest that low-level exposure may lead to premature births and low birth weights. There is no evidence to suggest the development of major congenital anomalies, although learning disabilities have been reported in children whose parents were previously exposed to lead [2].

PREVENTION
The Lead Contamination Control Act of 1988 led to the creation of the CDC Childhood Lead Poisoning Prevention Program for the purpose of eliminating childhood lead poisoning in the United States. The CDC has helped state and local governments to develop and implement lead poisoning prevention

programs, which include public health education, policy development, screening protocols, and case management guidelines. The CDC has provided funding and research support to enhance lead poisoning prevention at the federal, state, and local levels. This included the creation of a Childhood Blood Lead Surveillance System that allows states to report data to the CDC. In 2010, the Advisory Committee on Childhood Lead Poisoning Prevention convened a Work Group to reconsider the approach, terminology, and strategy for elevated BLLs in children [37].

Primary prevention
Health management: the role of the clinician
The task of educating families about lead exposure prevention should fall on the primary care physician. Anticipatory guidance should include information regarding in-home exposures to lead, unsafe renovation practices, and potential exposure from parental occupations and hobbies. Effective prevention requires the identification of populations that are at high risk because of their physical and social environment. Non-Hispanic black individuals have the highest prevalence of elevated BLLs. Furthermore, the clinician should recognize a higher risk of exposure in specific immigrant populations, refugees, and children from foreign countries [37]. The CDC provides fact sheets for prospective parents who wish to adopt children from other countries, as well as toolkits for newly arrived refugee children that give guidance on lead exposure screening and prevention.

Personal lead risk assessment questionnaires. Lead risk questionnaires are useful in identifying children who should be screened for elevated BLLs. This assessment should be performed annually for all children aged 6 months to 6 years. The tool varies in every state and for each health department, but should include questions based on current public health guidelines. Box 1 lists some common questions included in a risk assessment questionnaire.

Nutritional assessment. Lead absorption is enhanced by high fat intake and/or calcium and iron deficiency. A careful assessment of the patient's nutritional status should be done and parents should be advised to serve foods that are rich in calcium, iron, and vitamin C. Supplementation should be started if necessary.

Occupationally exposed adults. When evaluating lead exposure in children, their parents also should be questioned for lead exposure at work. The Occupational Safety and Health Administration is responsible for issuing standards and regulations for workplace exposure to lead.

Pregnant and breastfeeding women. Since 2010, the CDC has recommended follow-up activities and interventions beginning at BLLs of 5 μg/dL in pregnant women. Their Guidelines for the Identification and Management of Lead Exposure in Pregnant and Lactating Women includes advice on preventing lead exposure, assessment and lead level testing during pregnancy, and strategies to reduce fetal exposure to lead. It also includes guidance for breastfeeding, as well as follow-up of infants and children exposed to lead in utero [28].

Box 1: Lead risk assessment questions

1. Does your child live in or regularly visit an older home/building with peeling or chipping paint, or with recent or ongoing renovation or remodeling?

2. Has your child spent any time outside the United States in the past year?

3. Does your child have a brother/sister, housemate/playmate being followed or treated for lead poisoning?

4. Does your child eat nonfood items (pica)? Does your child often put things in his/her mouth, such as toys, jewelry, or keys?

5. Does your child often come in contact with an adult whose job or hobby involves exposure to lead?

6. Does your family use traditional medicine, health remedies, cosmetics, powders, spices, or food from other countries?

7. Does your family cook, store, or serve food in leaded crystal, pewter, or pottery from Asia or Latin America?

Adapted from New York State Department of Health. Available at: www.health.ny.gov/publications/2501/#questions. Accessed January 27, 2014.

Removal of lead from the environment

The environment should be assessed thoroughly and repeatedly to identify and mitigate lead hazards before children demonstrate BLLs at or higher than the reference value. Each state and local health department should develop prevention strategies to reduce environmental lead exposures in soil, dust, paint, and water before children are exposed [38]. Fig. 1 illustrates how correct public policy and aggressive implementation over the past several decades have resulted in a drastic decline in BLLs from the 1970s.

No single discipline or profession is responsible for the elimination of lead hazards, which involves housing, public health, and environmental dimensions. The Healthy People Initiative is a collaborative health promotion and disease prevention effort dedicated to improving the health of the nation over the course of a decade. "Healthy People 2020" was launched in December 2010, and one of their goals included the elimination of childhood lead poisoning as a public health problem. The CDC, EPA, Department of Housing and Urban Development, and other agencies have developed a federal interagency strategy to achieve this goal by 2020. More information can be found on www.healthypeople.gov.

Removal of lead in the home

Title X of the 1992 Housing and Community Development Act, also known as the Residential Lead-Based Paint Hazard Reduction Act (Public Law 102–550), mandated the creation of an infrastructure that would correct lead paint hazards in housing. Depending on the level of suspicion, a lead hazard screen, risk assessment, or inspection can be done, preferably by a certified risk lead inspector or risk assessor, to determine the presence of lead risk hazards and how they should be addressed. The risk assessor may then recommend either *interim controls* (ie, short-term or temporary actions and recommendations) or long-term or permanent

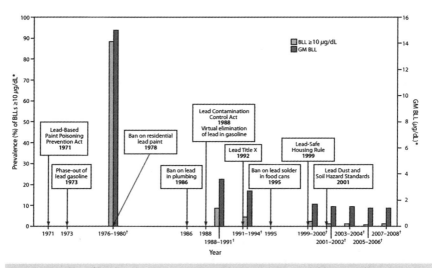

Fig. 1. Timeline of lead poisoning prevention policies and BLLs in children aged 1 to 5 years, by year: National Health and Nutrition Examination Survey, United States, 1971–2008. * National estimates for GM BLLs and prevalence of BLLs ≥10 µg/dL, by NHANES survey period and sample size of children aged 1–5 years: 1976–1980: N = 2,372; 1988–1991: N = 2,232; 1991–1994: N = 2,392; 1999–2000: N = 723; 2001–2002: N = 898; 2003–2004: N = 911; 2005–2006: N = 968; 2007–2008: N = 817. † NHANES survey period. (*From* Brown MJ, Margolis S. Lead in drinking water and human blood lead levels in the United States. MMWR Surveill Summ 2012;61(Suppl):3.)

interventions to remove lead or *abatement.* The EPA recommends hiring a certified lead-based paint professional to perform the abatement if a child residing in the house has a blood-lead level of 20 µg/dL or higher for a single venous test (or 15–19 µg/dL in 2 consecutive tests taken 3–4 months apart) (Table 3) [39].

Table 3	
Evaluation of lead in the home	
Lead hazard screen	A *lead hazard screen* is a limited version of a risk assessment for houses with a low chance of lead risks. The outcome is either a conclusion that lead-based paint hazards are probably not present or a recommendation that a full risk assessment be conducted to determine if such hazards are present.
Risk assessment	A *risk assessment* is an on-site investigation to determine the presence, type, severity, and location of lead-based paint hazards. The presence of deteriorated lead-based paint or high levels of lead in dust or soil pose potential hazards to children who may ingest lead inside or while playing outside
Lead-based paint inspection	A lead-based paint *inspection* is a surface-by-surface investigation to determine whether there is lead-based paint in the home and where it is located. An inspection may be particularly useful before renovation, repainting, or paint removal.

Adapted from EPA. Testing your home for lead in paint, dust, and soil. 2002. Available at: www.epa.gov.

Secondary prevention: lead screening

The presence of any amount of lead in blood is no longer acceptable, because even lower levels have been associated with subtle neurobehavioral deficits. Because most children with lead poisoning are asymptomatic, screening criteria should be based on risk of exposure, rather than the presence of signs and symptoms. In 1991, the CDC called for *universal screening* of all children ages 1 and 2 years. In 1997, because of the declining lead levels in the United States, the CDC and the American Academy of Pediatrics (AAP) recommend *targeted screening* of all children deemed to be at risk based on their age, ethnicity, housing age, high-risk zip code, and/or enrollment in Medicaid.

Screening should be done in children who live in areas where at least 27% of houses were built before 1950 and in places where the prevalence of elevated blood levels in children ages 1 to 2 years is greater than 12%. BLL testing is required at ages 1 and 2 years for all Medicaid-enrolled children, and if they have not been screened by the age of 6 years, they should be tested at presentation. If a personal risk questionnaire elicits a positive response to at least 1 or more of the items, then they should be screened as well. All foreign-born children (ie, refugees, immigrants, and international adoptees) should be screened immediately on arrival to the United States and again 3 to 6 months later if they are 6 months to 6 years of age. Each state or local health department should develop their own guidelines for lead screening based on local BLL prevalence and data on housing age, but in the absence of such information, universal screening should still be done (Table 4) [40,41].

Screening may done with a capillary or venous blood sample, but if a capillary lead level is elevated (greater than the reference level of 5 µg/dL), it should be confirmed with a venous lead level. Guidelines for confirmatory testing (if the initial lead test is performed using a capillary blood sample) and recommendations on a follow-up schedule may vary among states (Table 5).

Table 4
Standard surveillance definitions and classifications

Screening test	A blood lead test for a child age <72 mo who previously did not have a confirmed elevated BLL. (NOTE: A child may be screened in multiple years or even multiple times within a given year, but would be counted only once for each year.)
Elevated BLL	A single blood lead test (capillary or venous) at or above the reference range value of 5 µg/dL established in 2012.
Confirmed elevated BLL ≥5 µg/dL	A child with 1 venous blood specimen ≥5 µg/dL, or 2 capillary blood specimens ≥5 µg/dL drawn within 12 wk of each other.
Unconfirmed elevated BLL ≥5 µg/dL	A single capillary blood lead test ≥5 µg/dL, or 2 capillary tests ≥5 µg/dL drawn more than 12 wk apart.

Abbreviation: BLL, blood lead level.
Adapted from the Centers for Disease Control and Prevention. Available at: www.cdc.gov/nceh/lead/data/definitions.htm.

Table 5
Recommended schedule for obtaining a confirmatory venous sample

Blood, µg/dL	Time to confirmation testing
≥5–9	1–3 mo
10–44	1 wk–1 mo*
45–59	48 h
60–69	24 h
≥70	Urgently as emergency test

*The higher the BLL on the screening test, the more urgent the need for confirmatory testing.
  Adapted from the Advisory Committee on Childhood Lead Poisoning Prevention of the Centers for Disease Control and Prevention. Low level lead exposure harms children: a renewed call for primary prevention. Atlanta: CDC; 2012.

The CDC used the term "blood level of concern" to indicate the reference value by which children are identified as having been exposed to lead and thereby require intervention. Since 1960, the BLL of concern has been lowered incrementally from greater than 60 µg/dL (2.9 µmol/L) to 10 µg/dL by 1991. In 2012, the CDC replaced the term "level of concern" with a reference value of greater than 5 µg/dL (0.24 µmol/L) [37]. This change allows earlier detection of children who have been exposed to lead and thus results in earlier action to prevent further exposure, rather than simply treating those who have already been exposed.

For example, in New York City, all BLLs higher than the reference value of 5 µg/dL are reported to the Department of Health and Mental Hygiene (DOHMH). If a child is found to have a BLL of 5 to 14 µg/dL, the DOHMH contacts their families and medical providers to ensure timely follow-up and suggest strategies for lead exposure reduction. Educational materials are sent, including a brochure on tenant rights. The threshold for environmental intervention and care coordination is a BLL of 15 µg/dL. If a child younger than 18 is found to have a BLL of 15 µg/dL or greater, an inspection of the home is performed. More recently, home inspection has been recommended for children younger than 3 with even lower BLLs (5–9 µg/dL) [42,43].

For adults, the reference BLL is 10 µg/dL, according to the National Institute for Occupational Safety and Health [44]. The US national BLL geometric mean among adults was 1.2 µg/dL in 2009–2010 [45]. The current biologic exposure index (a level that should not be exceeded) for lead-exposed workers in the United States is 30 µg/dL in a random blood specimen.

EVALUATION OF THE PATIENT WITH SUSPECTED LEAD EXPOSURE AND POISONING

History and physical examination

A careful history should be obtained from the families of all children suspected of lead toxicity. The onset and duration of each symptom should be characterized, and dietary history should be obtained as well. History of pica, ingestion of nonfood substances after the age of 18 months, any recent travel to endemic areas, and a history of lead exposure in any family member are also relevant. Preventive screening questionnaires should be used to identify potential environmental sources [37].

This should be followed by a complete physical examination, paying particular attention to the systems most likely to be affected by lead toxicity. The neurologic examination should include an assessment of language and behavior. Developmental milestones should be evaluated and documented. Blood pressure should be checked for hypertension. A purplish line on the gums (lead line) is rarely seen in children nowadays, but if present indicates prolonged exposure to lead [2,37].

Diagnostic tests
BLL
A venous BLL is the most useful screening and diagnostic test for lead exposure. Initial screening may be performed using a fingerstick capillary sample. However, a poorly collected capillary sample may be contaminated with environmental lead and could be falsely positive. Levels greater than 10 µg/dL must be confirmed with a venous sample [40]. BLLs reflect recent or current lead exposure, but not necessarily the total body lead burden, as lead may be stored in bones.

Free erythrocyte protoporphyrin level
Lead interferes with heme synthesis by inhibiting the enzyme ferrochelatase in mitochondria. This results in the accumulation of free erythrocyte protoporphyrin (FEP). FEP levels have a high threshold for detection; its sensitivity decreases below BLLs less than 35 µg/dL. In light of the lower criterion for BLL used to prompt action, FEP alone is no longer used as a screening tool for lead poisoning. When used in conjunction with BLL, FEP levels are useful to discriminate between acute and chronic lead exposure. If FEP is normal in the setting of high BLLs, the exposure is more likely acute; if both are elevated, the exposure is more likely chronic.

Complete blood count
A complete blood count can reveal *hypochromic microcytic anemia*. Basophilic stippling, although pathognomonic for lead poisoning, is uncommon in children.

Hair samples
Analysis of hair samples has been used to measure environmental exposure to some heavy metals; however, this is not as sensitive as BLLs. This has been used for screening in other countries, but is not currently used in lead surveillance in the United States.

Imaging
Abdominal radiographs may show radiopaque foreign bodies in the gastrointestinal tract and is helpful in cases of acute ingestion (Fig. 2). Long-bone radiographs may demonstrate radiodensities found at the distal end of long bones called "lead lines" (Fig. 3) and indicate chronic lead exposure.

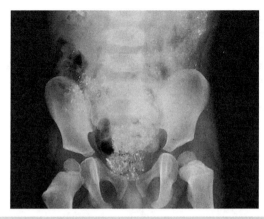

Fig. 2. Plain abdominal radiograph in a 3-year-old patient showing multiple metallic particles due to ingested flakes of lead paint. (Image reprinted with permission *from* Medscape Reference (http://emedicine.medscape.com/), 2014. Available at: http://emedicine.medscape.com/article/410113-overview.)

MANAGEMENT OF THE PATIENT WITH LEAD POISONING

The management of patients with lead exposure involves not only the pharmacologic management of toxicity, but also strategies for intervention and prevention of further exposure. Once an elevated lead level is found, the local health department should be notified and a home risk assessment should be

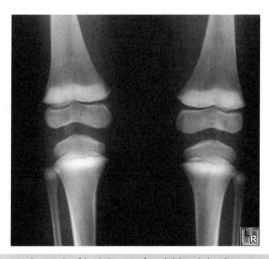

Fig. 3. Long-bone radiograph of both knees of a child with lead poisoning showing dense metaphyseal bands involving the distal femurs, proximal tibias and proximal fibulas. (*From* LearningRadiology.com; and *Courtesy of* William Herring, MD, FACR; with permission. Available at: http://www.learningradiology.com/notes/bonenotes/leadpoisonpage.htm. Accessed February 14, 2014.)

performed to determine the need for abatement strategies. With the gradual lowering of the "BLL of concern" by the CDC, the threshold for action has decreased as well. The Pediatric Environmental Health Specialty Unit Network has made recommendations on further evaluation and/or intervention based on the BLL, as outlined in Table 6 [46].

Decontamination

There is no benefit to using activated charcoal for lead ingestion, as it binds lead poorly. Gastric lavage may be performed; however, the American Academy of Clinical Toxicology stated that there is no evidence to show that its use improves clinical outcomes. Whole bowel irrigation has a theoretical benefit for decontamination of heavy metal ingestions; however, there are insufficient data to support or exclude its use.

Chelating agents

Chelation is recommended for BLLs of 45 μg/dL or higher. Before starting therapy, the level must be repeated immediately for confirmation. The patient must be admitted to a hospital that has proficiency with chelation therapy or an expert in the field should be consulted. The decision on which agent should be used will depend on the blood lead concentration, the patient's symptoms, and the environmental lead burden. The chelating agents available for use are as follows:

2,3 dimercaptosuccinic acid (DMSA, succimer)

Succimer is the water-soluble analog of dimercaprol. It has a wider therapeutic index than dimercaprol and edetate calcium disodium ($CaNa_2EDTA$); hence, it is recommended by the AAP for initial management of children with blood levels greater than 45 μg/dL and less than 70 μg/dL. It can rapidly decrease lead levels and repletes sulfhydryl-dependent enzymes. The most common adverse effects are abdominal distress, transient rash, elevated hepatocellular enzyme levels, and neutropenia [41]. Studies have shown that despite being able to lower blood lead concentrations, succimer does not reverse or diminish the cognitive impairment or other behavioral or neuropsychologic effects of lead in children with lower lead levels; hence, it is not recommended for levels less than 45 μg/dL [47,48].

Dimercaprol, or British anti-Lewisite

British anti-Lewisite forms a nonpolar compound with lead that is excreted in bile and urine. Its ability to rapidly cross the blood-brain barrier makes it the drug of choice in patients with acute lead encephalopathy. However, it has a narrow therapeutic range and is recommended for use (in combination with $CaNa_2EDTA$) only in children whose BLLs are greater than 70 μg/dL or in children with lead encephalopathy [41].

$CaNa_2EDTA$

$CaNa_2EDTA$ is an intravenous medication used in combination with dimercaprol in children whose BLLs are greater than 70 μg/dL or in children with lead encephalopathy. It may also be used an alternative initial treatment for

Table 6
Management of childhood lead exposure and poisoning

Blood lead concentration	Recommendation
<5 µg/dL	1. Review laboratory results with family. For reference, the geometric mean BLL for children 1–5 y is <2 µg/dL. 2. Repeat the BLL in 6–12 mo if the child is at high risk or risk changes during the time frame. Ensure levels are done at 1 and 2 y of age. 3. For children screened at age <12 mo, consider retesting in 3–6 mo, as lead exposure may increase as mobility increases. 4. Perform ROUTINE HEALTH MAINTENANCE, including assessment of nutrition, physical and mental development, and iron deficiency risk factors. 5. Provide ANTICIPATORY GUIDANCE on common sources of environmental lead exposure: paint in homes built before 1978, soil near roadways or other sources of lead, take-home exposures related to adult occupations, imported spices, cosmetics, folk remedies, and cookware.
5–14 µg/dL	1. Perform steps as described previously for levels <5 µg/dL. 2. Retest venous BLL within 1–3 mo to ensure the lead level is not rising. If it is stable or decreasing, retest the BLL in 3 mo. Refer patient to local health authorities if such resources are available. Most states require that elevated BLLs are reported to the state health department. Contact the CDC at 800-CDC-INFO (800-232-4636) or the National Lead Information Center at 800-424-LEAD (5323) for resources regarding lead poisoning prevention and local childhood lead poisoning prevention programs. 3. EDUCATION: Take a careful environmental history to identify potential sources of exposures (see recommendation 5 described previously for levels <5 µg/dL) and provide preliminary advice about REDUCING/ELIMINATING exposures. Take care to consider other children who may be exposed. 4. Provide NUTRITIONAL COUNSELING related to calcium and iron. In addition, recommend having a fruit at every meal, as iron absorption quadruples when taken with foods that contain vitamin C. Encourage the consumption of iron-enriched foods (eg, cereals, meats). 5. IRON STATUS: Ensure iron sufficiency with adequate laboratory testing (CBC, Ferritin, CRP) and treatment per AAP guidelines. Consider starting a multivitamin with iron. 6. NEURODEVELOPMENTAL MONITORING: Perform structured developmental screening evaluations at child health maintenance visits, as lead's effect on development may manifest over years.
15–44 µg/dL	1. Perform steps as described previously for levels of 5–14 µg/dL. 2. Confirm the blood lead level with repeat venous sample within 1–4 wk. 3. IMAGING: Specific evaluation of the child, such as abdominal radiograph should be considered based on the environmental investigation and history (eg, pica for paint chips, mouthing behaviors). Gut decontamination may be considered if leaded foreign bodies are visualized on radiographs. 4. TREATMENT: Any treatment for BLLs in this range should be done in consultation with an expert. Contact local PEHSU or PCC for guidance.

(continued on next page)

Table 6
continued

Blood lead concentration	Recommendation
>44 µg/dL	1. Follow guidance for BLL 15–44 µg/dL as listed previously. 2. Confirm the BLL with repeat venous lead level within 48 h. 3. Consider HOSPITALIZATION and/or CHELATION therapy (managed with the assistance of an experienced provider). Safety of the home with respect to lead hazards, isolation of the lead source, family social situation, and chronicity of the exposure are factors that may influence management. Contact your regional PEHSU or PCC for assistance.

Abbreviations: AAP, American Academy of Pediatrics; BLL, blood lead level; CBC, complete blood count; CDC, Centers for Disease Control and Prevention; CRP, C-reactive protein; PCC, Poison Control Center; PEHSU, Pediatric Environmental Health Specialty Unit.

Adapted from Newman N, Binns HJ, Karwowski M, et al. Recommendations on Medical Management of Childhood Lead Exposure and Poisoning. Pediatric Environmental Health Specialty Unit (PEHSU) Network. June 2013 update; with permission. Available at: http://aoec.org/pehsu/facts.html.

BLL greater than 45 µg/dL if the child is allergic to succimer. It decreases blood lead concentration, reverses the hematologic effects of lead, and forms nonionizing soluble complexes with lead, thereby enhancing its excretion in the urine. However, if used alone, it may aggravate symptoms in patients with very high BLLs. It is contraindicated for use in pregnancy or during breastfeeding.

D-penicillamine
D-penicillamine has been used since 1957 for the treatment of lead poisoning and was the only oral chelator for lead until the availability of DMSA. Its sulfhydryl group combines with lead to form ring compounds to facilitate elimination. However, it is not approved by the Food and Drug Administration for use in the United States.

Supportive therapy
Airway protection may be necessary in the event of acute encephalopathy. Benzodiazepines and/or barbiturates may be useful for seizures. For prolonged seizures, intracranial hypertension is likely and must be addressed accordingly (eg, hyperosmolar therapy).

Discharge criteria
Medical management of lead poisoning always should be accompanied by aggressive environmental interventions, and the patient should not be returned to the same home and/or workplace until it is deemed lead free.

SUMMARY
There is no safe lead level in children. Primary prevention is the most effective way to bring about the complete removal of lead from the environment and

eliminate lead poisoning as a public health concern. The National Lead Information Center can be reached via the Internet at www.epa.gov/lead and www.hud.gov/lead, or via phone at 1-800-424-LEAD (5323).

References

[1] WHO Lead Working Group. Childhood lead poisoning. Switzerland (Geneva): World Health Organization; 2010. Available at: http://www.who.int/ceh/publications/leadguidance.pdf.

[2] Tarragó O, Demers R. Case studies in environmental medicine: lead toxicity. Atlanta (GA): Agency for Toxic Substances and Disease Registry (ATSDR); 2010. Available at: http://www.atsdr.cdc.gov/csem/lead/docs/lead.pdf.

[3] Needleman HL. History of Lead Poisoning in the World. International Conference on lead Poisoning Prevention and Treatment. Bangalore, February 8–10, 1999.

[4] Lessler MA. Lead and lead poisoning from antiquity to modern times. Ohio J Science 1988;88(3):78–84.

[5] Scarborough J. The myth of lead poisoning among the Romans: an essay review. J Hist Med Allied Sci 1984;39(4):469–75.

[6] Lewis J. Lead poisoning: an historical perspective. EPA J 1985. Available at: http://www2.epa.gov/aboutepa/lead-poisoning-historical-perspective.

[7] Riva MA, Lafranconi A, D'Orso MI, et al. Lead poisoning: historical aspects of a paradigmatic "occupational and environmental disease". Safe Health Work 2012;3(1):11–6.

[8] Laraque D, Trasande L. Lead poisoning: successes and 21st century challenges. Pediatrics Review 2005;26(12):432–43.

[9] Kovarik W. How a classic occupational disease became an International Public Health Disaster. Int J Occup Environ Health 2005;11:384–97.

[10] Beattie AD, Moore MR, Goldberg A. Tetraethyl-lead poisoning. Lancet 1972;300(7766): 12–5.

[11] Needleman HL, Gunnoe C, Leviton A, et al. Deficits in psychologic and classroom performance of children with elevated dentine lead levels. N Engl J Med 1979;300(13): 689–95 [Erratum appears in N Engl J Med 1994;331(9):616–7].

[12] Needleman HL, Tuncay OC, Shapiro IM. Lead levels in deciduous teeth of urban and suburban American children. Nature 1972;235(5333):111–2.

[13] Special Timeline: Leaded Gasoline. Sept. 3, 2012. Available at: www.environmental history.org. Accessed October 4, 2013.

[14] Hatfield T, Tsai P. Global benefits from the phaseout of leaded fuel. J Environ Health 2011;74(5):8–14.

[15] United Nations Environment Programme (UNEP) News Centre. Multi-Trillion Dollar Benefits of Phasing Out Lead Petrol Spotlighted in New Report. October 2011. Available at: www.unep.org/newscentre. Phase Out: Eliminating Lead thru Partnership. 2014. Available at: http://rio20.ipieca.org/.

[16] Centers for Disease Control and Prevention. Blood levels in children aged 1–5 years—United States. MMWR Morb Mortal Wkly Rep 2012;62(13):245–8.

[17] Jones R, Homa D, Meyer P, et al. Trends in blood lead levels and blood lead testing among U. S. children aged 1 to 5 years: 1998-2004. Pediatrics 2009;123:e376–85.

[18] Lanphear P, Hornung R, Ho M, et al. Environmental lead exposure during early childhood. J Pediatr 2002;140(1):40–7.

[19] Centers for Disease Control and Prevention. Available at: http://www.cdc.gov/nceh/lead/tips/water.htm.

[20] U.S. Environmental Protection Agency. Available at: http://water.epa.gov/drink/info/lead/index.cfm.

[21] U.S. Department of Housing and Urban Development - Office of Healthy Homes and Lead Hazard Control. Guidelines for the evaluation and control of lead-based paint hazards in housing. 2nd edition. Washington, DC: HUD; 2012.

[22] U.S. Environmental Protection Agency. Available at: http://www2.epa.gov/lead/protect-your-family#soil.

[23] Lee D, Hurwitz R. Childhood lead poisoning: exposure and prevention. 2013. Available at: www.uptodate.com.

[24] US Environmental Protection Agency. Available at: http://www2.epa.gov/lead/protect-your-family#products.

[25] Centers for Disease Control and Prevention. Available at: http://www.cdc.gov/nceh/lead/tips/folkmedicine.htm.

[26] Kansas Department of Health and Environment. Available at: http://www.kdheks.gov/ables/occupation.html.

[27] Centers for Disease Control and Prevention. Available at: http://www.cdc.gov/nceh/lead/tips/artificialturf.htm.

[28] Ettinger AS, Gurthrie Wengrovitz A, editors. Guidelines for the identification and management of lead exposure in pregnant and lactating women. Atlanta (GA): National Center for Environmental Health/Agency for Toxic Substances and Disease Registry, Centers for Disease Control and Prevention; 2010.

[29] Ettinger AS, Tellez-Rojo MM, Amarasiriwardena C, et al. Effect of breast milk lead on infant blood lead levels at 1 month of age. Environ Health Perspect 2004;112(14): 1381–5.

[30] Rubin R, Strayer DS, editors. Environmental and nutritional pathology. Rubin's pathology: clinicopathologic foundations of medicine. 5th edition. Philadelphia: Lippincott Williams & Wilkins; 2008. p. 266.

[31] Barbosa F Jr, Tanus-Santos JE, Gerlach RF, et al. A critical review of biomarkers used for monitoring human exposure to lead: advantages, limitations, and future needs. Environ Health Perspect 2005;113(12):1669–74.

[32] Mendelsohn AL, Dreyer BP, Fierman AH, et al. Low-level lead exposure and behavior in early childhood. Pediatrics 1998;101(3):E10.

[33] Baghurst PA, McMichael AJ, Wigg NR, et al. Environmental exposure to lead and children's intelligence at the age of seven years. The Port Pirie Cohort Study. N Engl J Med 1992;327(18):1279.

[34] Bellinger DC, Stiles KM, Needleman HL. Low-level lead exposure, intelligence, and academic achievement: a long-term follow-up study. Pediatrics 1992;90:855–61.

[35] Lubran MM. Lead toxicity and heme biosynthesis. Ann Clin Lab Sci 1980;10(5):402.

[36] Loghman-Adham M. Aminoaciduria and glycosuria following severe childhood lead poisoning. Pediatr Nephrol 1998;12:218–21.

[37] CDC Advisory Committee on Childhood Lead Poisoning Prevention. Low level lead exposure harms children: a renewed call for primary prevention. Report of the Advisory Committee on Childhood Lead Poisoning Prevention of the Centers for Disease Control and Prevention. Atlanta, January 4, 2012.

[38] CDC response to Advisory Committee on Childhood Lead Poisoning Prevention Recommendations in "Low level lead exposure harms children: a renewed call of primary prevention." Available at: www.cdc.gov. Accessed October 1, 2013.

[39] U.S. Environmental Protection Agency. Testing your home for lead in paint dust, and soil, EPA 747-K-00–001, July 2000. Available at: www.epa.gov.

[40] AAP Committee on Environmental Health. Screening for elevated lead levels. Pediatrics 1998;101:1072.

[41] AAP Committee on Environmental Health. Lead exposure in children: prevention, detection, and management. Pediatrics 2005;116(4):1036–46.

[42] New York City Department of Health and Mental Hygiene. Report to the New York City Council on progress in preventing childhood lead poisoning in New York City. Available at: www.nyc.gov. Accessed February 1, 2014.

[43] New York City Department of Health and Mental Hygiene. Lead poisoning: prevention, identification, and management in children. Available at: www.nyc.gov.

[44] CDC. NIOSH Adult Blood Lead Epidemiology & Surveillance (ABLES) program description. Cincinnati (OH): US Department of Health and Human Services, CDC, National Institute for Occupational Safety and Health; 2013.

[45] CDC. Fourth National Report on Human Exposure to Environmental Chemicals Updated Tables, September 2012. Atlanta (GA): US Department of Health and Human Services, CDC; 2012.

[46] Newman N, Binns HJ, Karwowski M, et al. Fact sheet: recommendations on medical management of childhood lead exposure and poisoning. Pediatric Environmental Health Specialty Unit (PEHSU) Network. June 2013 update. Available at: http://aoec.org/pehsu/facts.html.

[47] Rogan WJ, Dietrich KN, Ware JH, et al. The effect of chelation therapy with succimer on neuropsychological development in children exposed to lead. N Engl J Med 2001;344: 1421–6.

[48] Badawy MK, Conners GP, et al. Pediatric lead toxicity. June 26, 2013. Available at: www.medscape.com.

Advances in Pediatrics 61 (2014) 335–356

ADVANCES IN PEDIATRICS

ELSEVIER
MOSBY

Atypical Hemolytic Uremic Syndrome

Larry A. Greenbaum, MD, PhD

Department of Pediatrics, Emory University and Children's Healthcare of Atlanta, 2015 Uppergate Drive NE, Atlanta, GA 30322, USA

Keywords
- Atypical hemolytic uremic syndrome • Complement • Acute kidney injury
- Thrombocytopenia

Key points

- The classic triad of hemolytic uremic syndrome (HUS) is a microangiopathic hemolytic anemia, thrombocytopenia, and acute kidney injury, but ischemic injury can occur in any organ.
- HUS in children is most commonly due to *Escherichia coli* infection, but may be caused by defects in the complement system (atypical HUS).
- Atypical HUS is a hereditary disorder or acquired disorder that may present at any age and has a high risk of causing permanent kidney failure.
- Treatment options for atypical HUS include plasmapheresis and liver transplantation, but the complement inhibitor eculizumab has emerged as the preferred treatment for many patients.

INTRODUCTION

Atypical hemolytic uremic syndrome (aHUS) is a rare, life-threatening disease caused by uncontrolled activation of the alternative pathway of complement. Clinically, patients usually have the classic triad of microangiopathic hemolytic anemia, thrombocytopenia, and acute kidney injury (AKI), although almost any organ in the body is susceptible to injury. An increasing number of genes encoding complement regulatory proteins have been identified where mutations make patients susceptible to the development of aHUS. Supportive

Disclosures: L.A. Greenbaum has received research support and consulting income from Alexion Pharmaceuticals. He serves on the advisory board of the Alexion-sponsored International Registry of Atypical HUS.

E-mail address: Lgreen6@emory.edu

0065-3101/14/$ – see front matter
http://dx.doi.org/10.1016/j.yapd.2014.04.001 © 2014 Elsevier Inc. All rights reserved.

care, including blood transfusions and dialysis when indicated, is the initial focus of treatment. A subset of patients respond to plasma infusion or plasmapheresis, which may transiently correct the underlying defect in the regulation of complement. Liver transplantation has been used to repair the underlying genetic defect in a small number of patients with aHUS. More recently, eculizumab (Soliris), a monoclonal antibody that binds to the terminal complement component C5, has been shown to be an effective short-term and long-term treatment for aHUS.

TERMINOLOGY AND DIFFERENTIAL DIAGNOSIS

aHUS is a thrombotic microangiopathy (TMA). As illustrated in Box 1, there are many different causes of TMA, which was classically divided into 2 major groups: HUS and thrombotic thrombocytopenic purpura (TTP). The most common cause of HUS in children is infection with shiga-toxin producing *Escherichia coli* [1]. In addition, there are rare cases of other shiga-toxin–producing organisms (eg, Shigella) triggering HUS. Because most cases of HUS due to shiga-toxin–producing *E coli* are preceded by bloody diarrhea,

---

Box 1: Thrombotic microangiopathies

Hemolytic Uremic Syndrome (HUS)

    Shiga and Shigalike toxin–producing bacteria

        Escherichia coli

        Shigella dysenteriae

    Streptococcus pneumoniae

    Defect in cobalamin metabolism

    Atypical HUS

        Disorders of complement regulation

        Disorders of coagulation

Thrombotic thrombocytopenic purpura (ADAMTS13 deficiency)

    Acquired (autoantibody)

    Congenital (recessive inheritance)

Secondary

    HIV infection

    Pregnancy

    Antiphospholipid antibody syndrome

    Malignancy

    Medications (chemotherapy, calcineurin inhibitors)

    Radiation

    Transplantation

    Severe hypertension

the term "diarrhea-positive," or D^+, HUS has been applied to these cases. However, this is misleading because some patients with HUS secondary to shiga-toxin–producing $E\ coli$ do not have a preceding diarrheal illness. More importantly, a diarrheal illness is a common trigger for an initial episode of aHUS [2–4]. Thus, shiga-toxin–producing $E\ coli$ hemolytic uremic syndrome (STEC-HUS) is a more precise term. This terminology also eliminates the vague term "diarrhea-negative," or D^-, HUS, which suggests all patients without a diarrheal illness, but also has been used interchangeably with aHUS.

$Streptococcus\ pneumoniae$ infection may also cause HUS [5]. This form of HUS is most commonly seen in young children, and is believed to be due to the effect of a neuraminidase produced by the $S\ pneumoniae$ that cleaves sialic acid residues, exposing the Thomsen-Friedrich antigen (T-antigen) on the surface of red blood cells and endothelial cells. HUS may be caused by a genetic defect in cobalamin metabolism. This autosomal recessive disorder usually presents during infancy, although late-onset cases may occur [6,7].

TTP is the most common cause of TMA in adults, and it is usually due to the development of autoantibodies to the von Willebrand factor cleaving protease, ADAMTS13 [8]. TTP is generally characterized by more neurologic involvement than renal involvement, although AKI, frequently mild, is fairly common. Congenital TTP (Upshaw-Schulman syndrome) is a rare autosomal recessive disorder that leads to the absence or a decrease of functional ADAMTS13. It classically presents in neonates or young children, although adult-onset cases, often triggered by pregnancy, also occur [9–11]. Because of its young age of onset, congenital deficiency of ADAMTS13 is commonly considered a form of HUS, but it more closely resembles TTP, based on its pathophysiology. There are a variety of secondary causes of TMA, and whether to consider these entities HUS or TTP is somewhat arbitrary, frequently dictated by the age of the patient, the presence of renal involvement, and the subspecialty of the treating physician.

Along with TMA, a number of other conditions may cause anemia, thrombocytopenia, and AKI. Lupus is a particular concern, especially in teenage girls and young women, because TMA may be mimicked by anemia (chronic disease or autoimmune), autoimmune thrombocytopenia, and AKI due to lupus nephritis. Sepsis, with concomitant disseminated intravascular coagulation (DIC), is another cause of thrombocytopenia, anemia, and AKI.

The term aHUS has been applied broadly or narrowed to varying degrees. An improvement in our understanding of pathophysiology with simultaneous increased diagnostic capability has enabled a mechanistic classification to replace a broader descriptive classification system based on clinical presentation. The availability of targeted therapy (see later in this article) demands diagnostic specificity. The broadest definition of aHUS included any patient with TMA and the absence of STEC-HUS or acquired TTP. Most experts would exclude patients with $S\ pneumoniae$ HUS and the secondary forms of TMA. In addition, congenital TTP and defects in cobalamin metabolism are no longer considered a form of aHUS.

Until recently, this left a narrow, mechanistic definition of aHUS: a disorder of complement regulation. The recent discovery of aHUS due to mutations in *DGKE* [12], which encodes diacylglycerol kinase-ε (DGKE-ε), has led to a broader definition of aHUS, as DGKE-ε does not appear to have a role in complement regulation; rather, it is part of the coagulation pathway and deficiency results in a prothrombotic state that causes TMA. Moreover, mutations in *PLG*, the gene for plasminogen, also are associated with aHUS and presumably contribute to TMA without a direct effect on the complement system, although patients with *PLG* mutations and aHUS frequently also have mutations in genes regulating the alternative pathway of complement [13]. A role for complement and the coagulation pathway in the pathogenesis of aHUS is further supported by the observation that mutations in *THBD*, the gene for thrombomodulin, are associated with aHUS [14]. Thrombomodulin has a role in regulating coagulation and the complement system [14,15].

PATHOPHYSIOLOGY

aHUS can occur in patients with loss-of-function gene mutations, gain-of-function gene mutations, or in patients who develop autoantibodies (Box 2). Most patients with aHUS have impaired regulation of the alternative pathway of complement on the surface of endothelial cells. The activation of the alternative pathway of complement on the surface of bacteria leads to bacterial lysis and recruitment of additional inflammatory molecules and cells. However, complement activation can occur on the surface of endothelial cells, where it has deleterious consequences. Consequently, there is a system in place for protecting endothelial cell surfaces from activation of the alternative pathway of complement. The archetypal protein for protecting cell surfaces from activation of the alternative pathway of complement is complement factor H (CFH), a plasma protein that can adhere to endothelial cells. CFH binds to C3b, competing with factor B binding, and thus preventing formation of the C3

Box 2: Mechanisms of atypical HUS

Loss-of-function mutations
   Complement factor H
   Membrane cofactor protein
   Complement factor I
   Thrombomodulin
   Diacylglycerol kinase ε
Gain-of-function mutations
   Complement factor B
   C3
Complement factor H autoantibodies

convertase. Moreover, CFH binds to C3b on the surface of endothelial cells and serves as a cofactor for complement factor I (CFI), which cleaves C3b into inactive fragments. This is called "cofactor activity." In addition, CFH has "decay-accelerating activity"; it binds to the C3 convertase and facilitates its cleavage into Bb and C3b, which can then be inactivated. A number of other proteins also participate in the regulation of the alternative pathway of complement and hence protect endothelial cells from injury. The specific complement regulatory proteins where gene mutations have been associated with the development of aHUS and their mechanism of action are discussed in the remainder of this section.

Uncontrolled complement activation leads to platelet activation, neutrophil activation, and endothelial cell injury. This creates a milieu that promotes microthrombi formation within small blood vessels. These microthrombi include platelets, leading to thrombocytopenia. The microthrombi also create jagged vessel surfaces, with consequent damage to red blood cells as they transit the blood vessels. This is the mechanism of the microangiopathic hemolytic anemia and schistocytes that are classic features of aHUS. Mechanical damage and destruction of platelets also occurs. Ultimately, microthrombi lead to tissue ischemia. The renal vasculature is particularly susceptible, and this explains the high rate of AKI in aHUS. However, all vessels may be affected, which explains the protean clinical manifestations of aHUS.

CFH

CFH was the first protein in which gene mutations were shown to predispose patients to develop aHUS [16]. As mentioned previously, CFH has cofactor activity and decay-accelerating activity. *CFH* mutations are the most common cause of aHUS, with approximately 25% of patients with aHUS having *CFH* mutations [2,17,18]. Mutations are generally heterozygous, with rare exceptions, and thus inheritance is autosomal dominant, but with a penetrance of only about 50% [2,17]. A variety of mutations have been reported, but most cluster in the C terminus of the protein and impair the complement regulatory functions of CFH [2,19]. Serum CFH levels are normal in approximately 50% of patients because only protein function is impaired [17]. C3 is low in approximately 50% of patients.

The *CFH* gene is adjacent to the genes for CFH-related protein 1 (*CFHR1*) and CFH-related protein 3 (*CFHR3*). In some patients with aHUS, nonhomologous allelic recombination between *CFH* and *CFHR3* generates a fusion protein that is deficient in regulating complement [18,20]. In other instances, a hybrid gene has been created via microhomology-mediated end joining, also resulting in a protein with loss of complement regulatory function [21].

CFI

CFI is a protease that cleaves and inactivates C3b, and thus has an important role in controlling complement activation on the surface of endothelial cells. Mutations in the gene for factor I are heterozygous, but penetrance is approximately 50% [2]. Fewer than 10% of patients with aHUS have mutations in factor I [2,17,18]. C3 is low in approximately 50% of patients.

Membrane cofactor protein

Membrane cofactor protein (MCP) is a transmembrane protein. It has cofactor activity, and thus binds C3b and facilitates its cleavage by CFI. Most mutations are heterozygous, but homozygous or compound heterozygous mutations also occur [17]. Mutations may lead to decreased synthesis or impair function, with the later mutations usually located in the extracellular domain [2]. *MCP* mutations occur in 6% to 9% of patients with aHUS [2,17,18]. Patients with *MCP* mutations have a high rate of relapses, but have a better prognosis, with relatively lower rates of developing permanent kidney failure [17]. There is also a low risk of recurrence after transplantation when renal failure does occur [22].

Decreased expression of MCP is present in most patients, permitting diagnosis of this abnormality by measuring cell surface expression of MCP. However, levels are normal in some patients with *MCP* mutations. C3 may be low, but is usually normal in patients with *MCP* mutations.

Thrombomodulin

Thrombomodulin, via binding to C3b and CFH, accelerates inactivation of C3b by CFI. It also activates procarboxypeptidase B, which inactivates C3a and C5a. In addition, thrombomodulin has an important role in the anticoagulant pathway [15], and thus decreased functional thrombomodulin presumably mediates aHUS via complement dysregulation and the creation of a procoagulant state.

Heterozygous inactivating mutations in the gene for thrombomodulin (*THBD*) occur in fewer than 5% of patients with aHUS [14,17,18]. C3 is low in approximately half of the patients [14]. Most patients with thrombomodulin mutations presented during childhood. Permanent kidney failure and death among affected family members was relatively common in the initial report [14].

C3

Mutations in the gene for C3 are heterozygous, and result in a gain of function [2]. Host cells are normally protected from complement activation by the binding of C3b by CFH or MCP. The mutations decrease the affinity of this binding and thus decrease C3b inactivation. Approximately 75% of these patients have low levels of C3 [2]. *C3* mutations were present in approximately 8% of patients with aHUS in European studies, although they were less common in an American cohort [2,17,18].

Factor B

Complement factor B (CFB) gene mutations that cause aHUS are heterozygous and result in gain of function [23–25]. CFB combines with C3 to form the C3 convertase. The described mutations enhance the formation of the C3 convertase, decrease the inactivation of the C3 convertase, or possibly enhance the ability of the C3 convertase to cleave C3 [23,24].

C3 is frequently low [25]. Fewer than 5% of patients with aHUS have *CFB* mutations [2,17,18].

Factor H autoantibodies

A distinct form of aHUS is secondary to the development of autoantibodies to CFH [26–28]. These autoantibodies bind to the C-terminus of CFH, and interfere with its ability to bind to cell surfaces and regulate complement activity [29,30]. CFH autoantibodies cause approximately 5% to 15% of cases of aHUS, and most cases present during childhood, but a significant number of patients initially present as adults [27,29,31,32]. Gastrointestinal symptoms, including diarrhea, are common at presentation, and there is a high rate of extrarenal complications, including seizures, myocardial dysfunction, pancreatitis, and elevated liver enzymes [27,33]. A positive antinuclear antibody test was found in 24% of tested patients in a large case series, and this could be a potential source of diagnostic confusion [27].

Almost all patients with autoantibodies to CFH have homozygous deletions of the genes for CFH-related protein 1 (*CFHR1*) and CFH-related protein 3 (*CFHR3*) [32,34], although some patients have isolated deficiency of functional CFHR1 and this may be the required predisposing defect [35]. The mechanism whereby these gene deletions predispose to CFH autoantibodies is unknown, and it important to note that the homozygous deletions of *CFHR1* and *CFHR3* are fairly common in the general population. Hence, the gene deletions appear necessary for the development of autoantibodies, but do not lead to autoantibodies in most carriers.

Measurement of factor H autoantibody levels is the definitive diagnostic test and permits monitoring of response to treatment for patients treated with plasmapheresis and immunosuppression (see later in this article). The presence of the associated gene deletions provides additional supportive evidence, but is not diagnostic because such mutations are relatively common in the general population. CFH levels are not low [26], and are thus not helpful in the diagnosis of this form of aHUS.

Diacylglycerol kinase ε

Diacylglycerol kinase ε (DGKE) normally prevents activation of protein kinase C, which promotes thrombosis. aHUS develops in patients with homozygous or compound heterozygous mutations in *DGKE* in this autosomal recessive disorder [12]. There is no evidence of a role of the complement system in TMA due to *DGKE* mutations; 2 patients had relapses despite treatment with plasmapheresis or eculizumab [12]. Penetrance appears to be high, and all cases described to date presented before 1 year [12]. Patients with *DGKE* mutations are more likely than other patients with aHUS to have persistent hematuria and proteinuria between TMA episodes and develop nephrotic syndrome [12].

Variable penetrance and modifying genes

Most cases of aHUS are associated with heterozygous mutations and autosomal dominant inheritance, but with a penetrance of approximately 50% in the genes that affect the complement system (*CFH, CFI, C3,* thrombomodulin, and *MCP*) [2]. Variable penetrance may be partially related to the whether a patient is exposed to a triggering event (see Box 3 and later in this article). For example, some patients may have their first episode of aHUS following surgery or during pregnancy [17]. Nevertheless, most aHUS episodes are triggered by fairly mild infections, and thus the variable penetrance is not easily attributed solely to differences in exposure to environmental triggers.

It is now clear that many patients with aHUS have other genetic risk factors that increase the likelihood of aHUS episodes. Unaffected heterozygote carriers are less likely to have these additional genetic predispositions to develop episodes of aHUS. There are specific polymorphisms in the *MCP, CFH,* and *CHFHR1* genes that increase the risk of aHUS and influence the severity of the disease among patients with aHUS [17,36,37]. Some patients have deficiency of CFHR3, which has a role in inhibiting the C3 convertase [38]. In addition, some patients have mutations in multiple complement genes (eg, *C3* and *MCP*) [17,18,37]. There are even patients with heterozygous mutations in 3 genes [2,17,18,37].

There is also evidence that some patients with aHUS and underlying abnormalities of the complement system have decreased levels of ADAMTS13 due to genetic polymorphisms [39]. This may lead to increased susceptibility to episodes of TMA [39]. Similarly, mutations in genes regulating the coagulation system may increase the likelihood of developing aHUS [13].

It thus appears that aHUS occurs in patients who have a genetic predisposition and an environmental trigger. Susceptibility varies depending on the underlying genetic predisposition, and aHUS episodes are more likely if there are multiple predisposing genetic abnormalities. This is perhaps not surprising given the duplicative mechanisms for regulating the alternative pathway of complement.

GENETICS AND GENOTYPE-PHENOTYPE INTERACTION
In a large registry report, more than 70% of patients have a gene mutation, a disease-associated *CFH* polymorphism, or CFH autoantibodies [2]. In another large series, more than 65% of patients had complement gene mutations or anti-CFH antibodies [17]. Detection of mutations is higher in familial cases than in sporadic cases [2]. For example, *CFH* mutations occur in 40% of familial cases,

Box 3: Atypical HUS triggers

Infection (upper respiratory infection or gastroenteritis)

Pregnancy

Oral contraceptives

Surgery

Medications

Transplant (no pretransplant aHUS)

but in only 16% of sporadic cases [2]. However, anti-CFH antibodies are less common in familial cases [17]. Only approximately 20% of patients have a family history of aHUS.

The clinical features of the disease correlate with the specific etiology (Table 1). Very early onset tends to occur most commonly in patients with *DGKE, CFH,* or *THBD* mutations [2]. Extrarenal involvement rarely occurs in patients with *MCP* mutations. Death or end-stage renal disease is more common in patients with *CFH* mutations than in patients with *MCP* mutations [2], although the risk increases in patients with an *MCP* mutation and a second mutation [37]. The outcome is worse in patients with defined genetic mutations, family history of aHUS, or diagnosis as adults [2].

CLINICAL PRESENTATION
Epidemiology
Patients may have their first episode of aHUS as young infants or as adults, and adult-onset cases were more common than childhood cases in a recent publication of the French experience [17]. The age of onset is partially related to the underlying etiology (see previously in this article). Most pediatric cases present before age 2 years [17]. The role of pregnancy as a clinical trigger (see the next section) at least partially explains the higher numbers of women among adult patients (not seen in children) [4,17].

Clinical triggers
It is clear that there are a variety of environmental factors that may initiate an episode of aHUS (see Box 3) [2]. Infections, usually minor, are the most

Table 1
Genotype-phenotype correlations

Abnormality	aHUS cases, % [17,18,82]	Risk of ESRD or death at 5 y (pre-eculizumab), % [17]	Response to plasmapheresis	Recurrence risk after transplantation, %
CFH mutation	24–28	66	Variable	80
MCP mutation	6–9	35	No	<20
CFI mutation	4–8	72	Variable	>80
C3 mutation	2–8	55	Variable	40–70
CFB mutation	<4	Limited data	Variable	>90
THBD mutation	<5	Limited data	Variable	Limited data
Anti-CFH antibodies	3–6	Limited data	Variable	Depends if antibodies still present
DGKE mutation	Limited data	Limited data	No	0
No mutation or autoantibodies	30–35	43	Variable	30

Abbreviations: aHUS, atypical hemolytic uremic syndrome; CF, complement factor; DGKE, diacylglycerol kinase; ESRD, end-stage renal disease; MCP, membrane cofactor protein; THBD, thrombomodulin.

common trigger, and diarrhea is very common at presentation in children [2,17,40]. In adults, pregnancy is an important trigger [4,17]. It is believed that an episode of aHUS occurs because the triggering event tips the balance in favor of complement activation and endothelial cell injury.

Signs and symptoms

Most patients with aHUS have the classic triad of microangiopathic hemolytic anemia, thrombocytopenia, and AKI (Box 4). Signs and symptoms of anemia may include pallor, fatigue, a systolic murmur, and tachycardia. Despite thrombocytopenia, spontaneous bleeding and petechiae are uncommon. AKI may cause evidence of fluid overload, including edema, hypertensive symptoms (headaches, seizures), and other uremic symptoms (decreased energy, anorexia, and emesis). Hypertension, a frequent finding, is often severe [40]. Hematuria and proteinuria are common; some patients may have nephrotic syndrome [41]. There are patients who do not have all of the classic findings, and even thrombocytopenia is not a universal finding [41].

Extrarenal involvement occurs in approximately 25% of patients [2]. The central nervous system and heart are most commonly affected [17]. Neurologic manifestations may be directly related to TMA, but may be secondary to hypertension or electrolyte abnormalities caused by renal failure [42].

Laboratory

A microangiopathic hemolytic anemia causes an elevated lactate dehydrogenase (LDH), which is released from ruptured red blood cells, and a low haptoglobin due to haptoglobin binding with released hemoglobin and removal by the reticuloendothelial system. The peripheral smear demonstrates schistocytes, helmet cells, and a paucity of platelets. Along with an elevated blood-urea-nitrogen and creatinine, there may be other findings of AKI, including hyperkalemia, metabolic acidosis, and hyperphosphatemia.

Box 4: Clinical manifestations of atypical hemolytic uremic syndrome

Classic Triad

   Microangiopathic hemolytic anemia

   Thrombocytopenia

   Acute kidney injury

Other Manifestations

   Brain injury

   Myocardial infarction

   Pancreatitis

   Skin necrosis

DIAGNOSIS

The diagnosis of aHUS is a 2-step process (Box 5). First, demonstrate that a patient has TMA. Second, determine that aHUS is the cause of the TMA. In children, TMA is often suspected when a patient has the triad of AKI, micro-angiopathic hemolytic anemia, and thrombocytopenia. Other potential causes of AKI, anemia, and thrombocytopenia (lupus, sepsis with DIC) are easily investigated. Confirmation of a microangiopathic hemolytic anemia is via demonstration of an elevated LDH, depressed haptoglobin, or schisto-cytes on peripheral smear. A negative Coombs test is helpful to eliminate an alternative cause of a hemolytic anemia, although it is generally positive in *S pneumoniae* HUS. Some patients may have limited renal involvement and

---

Box 5: Diagnosis of atypical HUS

Establish the Presence of Thrombotic Microangiopathy (TMA)

Microangiopathic hemolytic anemia

Elevated lactate dehydrogenase

Decreased haptoglobin

Peripheral smear with schistocytes

Thrombocytopenia

Acute kidney injury

Elevated creatinine

Evaluation for other causes of TMA

Shiga-toxin–producing *E coli* hemolytic uremic syndrome

Stool culture

Shiga toxin or shiga toxin genes

Lipopolysaccharide serology

Thrombocytopenic purpura

ADAMTS13 level

Presence of ADAMTS13 inhibitor

Lupus

Antinuclear antibody

Cobalamin metabolism

Urine and serum homocysteine and methylmalonic acid

Secondary

Review medications

Pregnancy testing

HIV serology

Antiphospholipid antibodies

thus ischemic injury to another organ may be the dominant clinical manifestation.

After TMA is confirmed, the etiology must be determined (see Box 5). In children, STEC-HUS is the most common cause of TMA, with most patients having a history of bloody diarrhea. Because a diarrheal illness also may trigger an episode of aHUS, it is important to confirm that the TMA is shiga-toxin mediated, especially in cases in which the diarrhea is not bloody or there is not a documented exposure to shiga-toxin–producing *E coli* as part of an outbreak. Testing should include culture and other methodologies (see Box 5), as culture is negative in a significant minority of patients, especially when testing is delayed. Stool testing is necessary in all patients with new-onset TMA because the classic diarrheal prodrome is not always present [43].

Although rare in young children, acquired TTP is an important consideration in the teenager with TMA. The diagnosis is established by finding low activity of the von Willebrand factor–cleaving protease, ADAMTS13. An activity level less than 5% to 10% of normal is diagnostic, and is associated with the presence of an autoantibody (inhibitor) in patients with acquired disease. Measurement of ADAMTS13 activity and the inhibitor should be done before plasma infusions or plasmapheresis. All patients should have measurement of ADAMTS13 levels because a congenital deficiency of functional ADAMTS13 may also cause TMA [11]. No inhibitor is present in the congenital form of the disease. With congenital TTP, there may be a relapsing course, and some patients have a history of neonatal hemolysis causing hyperbilirubinemia requiring an exchange transfusion [10,11].

Patients with defects in cobalamin metabolism causing HUS are most likely to present as infants, although late-onset cases have been described [6,7]. Clues to the diagnosis include clinical manifestations (hypotonia, lethargy, neurologic abnormalities, poor feeding, failure to thrive) and laboratory findings (megaloblastic anemia and leukopenia). Plasma homocysteine levels are elevated, as are methylmalonic acid levels in urine despite normal levels of plasma vitamin B_{12}. Genetic analysis provides confirmatory evidence of this disorder, most commonly due to mutations in the *MMACHC* gene, which causes methylmalonic aciduria and homocystinuria cblC type. Early diagnosis is important because there is specific therapy (intramuscular hydroxocobalamin and oral carnitine, betaine, and folic acid) and patients do not respond to plasmapheresis or eculizumab.

The other causes of TMA are usually easily suspected by the patient history. *S pneumoniae* HUS tends to occur during the winter, and is most commonly associated with a large bacterial burden, as occurs with an empyema, sepsis, or meningitis, especially if associated with a subdural fluid collection. The secondary forms of TMA may necessitate specific testing (HIV, pregnancy), although most are suspected based on the patient history. Endothelial injury from severe hypertension may trigger an episode of TMA, but the hematologic involvement is usually less severe and resolves with correction of the hypertension. In addition, there is usually another cause of the severe hypertension.

The presence of recurrent episodes of TMA is supportive of a diagnosis of aHUS. Previous episodes may be subtle, so it is important to ask about previous episodes of anemia or thrombocytopenia. The clinical presentation of aHUS is often sudden and thus resembles STEC-HUS or *S pneumoniae* HUS. However, a more insidious presentation, with waxing and waning symptoms and laboratory findings, is more consistent with aHUS than STEC-HUS or *S pneumonia* HUS. A family history of TMA is quite suggestive of aHUS, but is not present in 80% of patients [17]. Familial cases in aHUS do not occur simultaneously, unlike in STEC-HUS, when a common exposure can lead to multiple cases in a family. TMA in an infant younger than 6 months is especially likely to be aHUS given the decreased risk of STEC-HUS.

Pregnancy and transplantation are considered secondary causes of TMA (see Box 1). However, a significant percentage of these patients have an underlying genetic abnormality in the complement system [2], and thus should be considered candidates for further diagnostic testing and treatment. Pregnancy is an important trigger for an initial episode of aHUS in adults [17]. Transplant recipients without a history of aHUS may have an initial episode of aHUS due to complement gene mutations after transplantation.

aHUS is ultimately a clinical diagnosis, based on the presence of TMA and the elimination of other potential etiologies. This is because approximately 40% of patients do not have a defined genetic etiology. Nevertheless, it is important to screen for the known causes of aHUS, because identifying a disease-causing mutation confirms the diagnosis and provides important prognostic information and may help guide therapy (see Table 1). Box 6 lists recommended diagnostic testing. A low C3 is present in approximately 35% of patients with aHUS [17], but the specificity of a low C3 in the setting of TMA is unknown. C3 is more likely to be low in patients with *CFH, CFB*, or *C3* gene mutations [2,17]. A low level of CFH is supportive of a diagnosis of aHUS, but many patients with *CFH* mutations have normal CFH levels because the protein is produced, but has diminished function due to point mutations. Identification of an autoantibody to CFH has important therapeutic implications (see later in this article).

Genetic testing is available for the known etiologies, but is not required to make a diagnosis of aHUS and it is not currently available in a time frame to influence initial treatment decisions. All genes should be studied because patients may have mutations in multiple genes and the specific mutations detected provides prognostic information and may influence treatment decisions [37].

CLINICAL COURSE

The clinical course of aHUS is challenging to describe with precision because of its rarity, diagnostic challenges, and variable treatment approaches. The availability of eculizumab (see later in this article) appears to have dramatically improved the prognosis [41], but most of the long-term data are based on the experience with plasma therapy.

In the era before plasmapheresis, mortality was common, and it continues to occur even with plasmapheresis [17,40]. Children have a higher mortality than

Box 6: Laboratory testing in patients with suspected aHUS

Protein levels

  C3

  Complement factor H (CFH)

  Complement factor I

Factor H autoantibody

Membrane cofactor protein (MCP) levels on mononuclear cells

Genetic testing

  Specific gene mutations

    CFH (including homologous recombination with CFH-related protein [CFHR] gene)

    Complement factor I

    MCP

    Thrombomodulin

    Complement factor B

    C3

    Diacylglycerol kinase ε

  Deletion of CFHR3 and CFHR1 genes

adults [17]. AKI requiring dialysis is present in most patients during the first episode of aHUS [17]. A large percentage of patients develop end-stage renal disease despite the use of plasmapheresis; others have chronic kidney disease (see Table 1) [17]. Most patients have multiple relapses [40].

TREATMENT
Supportive care
Anemia may be profound at diagnosis of aHUS and red blood cell transfusion is commonly necessary. Ongoing hemolysis may lead to multiple transfusions. Red blood cell transfusion is used if patients have significant symptoms or the hemoglobin is below 6 to 7 g/dL, with higher cutoffs indicated if hemolysis is brisk or a procedure (eg, catheter placement) is planned. Because of concerns that platelet transfusion may increase ischemic injury because of increased formation of microthrombi in blood vessels, platelet transfusion is avoided unless there is clinically significant bleeding or an invasive procedure is planned.

Dialysis and other supportive care for AKI are used based on the usual criteria. Hyperkalemia is more likely to be problematic because of ongoing hemolysis causing release of potassium from red blood cells and the potassium load from blood transfusion. Use of washed blood to decrease the potassium load is occasionally indicated when severe anemia and hyperkalemia are present. Hypertension, sometimes severe, is quite common, and frequently requires medication along with correction of volume overload [40].

Plasma therapy

Infusions of fresh frozen plasma or plasmapheresis are effective in approximately two-thirds of patients with aHUS, with higher response rates in children than adults [2,44]. The specific strategy and the likelihood of a response are dictated by the underlying etiology. Plasma therapy is potentially effective in patients with a loss-of-function mutation in a plasma protein (CFH, CFI) [44]. The plasma provides a normal protein that can replace the defective protein. In contrast, plasmapheresis is necessary when the pathophysiology is based on the presence of a protein that needs to be removed (an autoantibody to CFH or an overactive C3 or CFB due to a gain of function mutation). In addition, plasmapheresis is probably more effective than plasma infusions in patients with loss of function mutations because of the higher volume of plasma that can be delivered with plasmapheresis. Plasma infusions are typically 10 to 20 mL/kg; plasmapheresis provides 50 to 100 mL/kg of plasma depending on the volume of the exchange. Neither plasmapheresis nor plasma infusion is believed to be effective in patients with mutations in the transmembrane protein MCP, because plasma does not contain MCP and would therefore not correct the underlying defect [45,46]. Fortunately, patients with *MCP* gene mutations frequently have spontaneous remissions of aHUS episodes, although progression to kidney failure occurs in a subset of patients [2,45,46].

Plasmapheresis is preferred over plasma infusions at initial diagnosis because the underlying mutation or mechanism is seldom known (unless it is a familial case) and because of the greater likelihood of a rapid response due to the higher plasma delivery with plasmapheresis [47]. In patients who respond to plasmapheresis, the treatment is typically slowly tapered, with monitoring for evidence of recurrence (thrombocytopenia, hemolysis, or AKI). Evidence of recurrence should prompt resumption or intensification of plasmapheresis. In patients who cannot be weaned off of plasmapheresis, plasma infusions may serve as an alternative and less cumbersome treatment option [44]. Plasma infusions are only an option in patients with etiologies that do not require protein removal.

Immunosuppression

Immunosuppression combined with plasmapheresis has been used effectively in patients with CFH autoantibodies [29,31]. Patients generally respond to plasmapheresis, but usually relapse if plasmapheresis is stopped without institution of immunosuppression to stop production of the autoantibody. An occasional patient has had a sustained remission with only plasmapheresis [29,32]. Immunosuppressive medications have included corticosteroids, azathioprine, rituximab, cyclophosphamide, and mycophenolate mofetil [27,29,32]. Some patients have relapses despite immunosuppression, and thus require either ongoing plasmapheresis or eculizumab (see later in this article) [31]. Long-term follow-up data are not available to assess the risk for recurrence with this strategy. Periodic monitoring for CFH autoantibodies and evidence of TMA seems prudent [31], but a specific strategy remains undefined.

Liver transplantation

Liver transplantation is curative of aHUS due to *CFH* mutations because almost all CFH is synthesized in the liver. With liver transplantation, normal CFH is synthesized by the new liver. Early results with liver transplantation were disappointing, with mortality probably secondary to TMA because of activation of the alternative pathway of complement by the surgical procedure [48–50].

Subsequent liver transplantations have been performed with perioperative plasmapheresis to provide normal CFH and prevent activation of the alternative pathway of complement [50,51]. This has led to better outcomes and patients have not had recurrence of aHUS [50–53]. Liver transplantation is theoretically effective in any form of aHUS caused by proteins produced predominantly in the liver and a consensus conference recommended that it be considered in select patients with *CFH* or *CFI* mutations [50], although this was before the reports of the efficacy of eculizumab in aHUS. Although curative, liver transplantation requires a lifetime of immunosuppression and the morbidity and mortality associated with liver transplantation.

Kidney transplantation

Patients with aHUS have a high rate of developing permanent kidney failure and becoming dialysis dependent. Kidney transplantation is the preferred treatment for kidney failure, given the morbidity and mortality of dialysis. However, kidney transplantation has been associated with a high rate of disease recurrence [45,54]. This is not surprising, because the new kidney is equally susceptible to the disease, and the transplantation procedure is likely to trigger activation of the alternative pathway of complement. One exception is seen in patients with mutations in *MCP*, which is a transmembrane protein. The new kidney has normal MCP and thus there is no increased predisposition for local activation of complement. Kidney transplantation in patients with *MCP* mutations has a low rate of recurrence of aHUS [22,45], but the risk increases dramatically if a patient with an *MCP* mutation has a second complement gene mutation, emphasizing the importance of screening patients for mutations in all genes [37].

The rate of recurrence after kidney transplantation varies depending on the underlying gene mutation, and patients without an identified mutation have a better prognosis (see Table 1) [2,54]. Recurrence also may occur in patients with CFH autoantibodies [31]. A variety of strategies have been used to prevent recurrence, including perioperative plasmapheresis, plasma infusions, and avoidance of calcineurin inhibitors (tacrolimus and cyclosporin) because of the theoretical risk that these medications may trigger TMA. Some patients have traded chronic dialysis for chronic plasmapheresis or plasma infusions. Overall results were disappointing, and some considered aHUS due to a mutation in a gene associated with a high rate of recurrence as a relative contraindication to kidney transplantation. As described later in this article, the availability of eculizumab has dramatically changed the approach and outcome of kidney transplantation in aHUS [55].

Eculizumab

Eculizumab is a humanized monoclonal antibody that binds to C5, preventing its cleavage into C5a and C5b by the C5 convertase. By functioning as a terminal complement inhibitor, eculizumab prevents the deleterious consequences of uncontrolled complement activation in aHUS. Eculizumab was initially approved for the treatment of paroxysmal nocturnal hemoglobinuria (PNH), and it is highly effective in this complement-mediated disorder [56]. Long-term use of eculizumab has been effective in PNH [57]. Off-label use of eculizumab for aHUS was initially reported in 2009 [58,59], and there have been multiple subsequent case reports and case series [3,25,41,60–72]. Two clinical trials and a retrospective pediatric experience were used to obtain Food and Drug Administration approval for eculizumab for aHUS in 2011. The clinical trials demonstrated that eculizumab treatment in aHUS suppresses complement activation, corrects thrombocytopenia, improves quality of life, and results in significant improvement in renal function [73]. Earlier treatment is associated with greater improvement in renal function [55,73,74]. Eculizumab may rapidly reverse extrarenal manifestations of aHUS that are resistant to plasmapheresis [68,71,75].

There is no apparent difference in the efficacy of eculizumab in patients with or without identified genetic mutations [73]. Moreover, eculizumab is effective in patients who are resistant to plasma or plasmapheresis [73], young infants [66,70], and in patients with loss-of-function mutations, gain-of-function mutations [3,25,55,60], or CFH autoantibodies [41]. Patients who appear to be responding to plasmapheresis may have improvement in kidney function and other parameters after switching to ecuzlizumab [55,76].

Eculizumab has been well tolerated, with limited side effects [73]. However, complement has an important role in protection from meningococcemia, as evidenced by the predisposition to meningococcemia in patients with inherited complement deficiencies. Treatment with eculizumab increases the risk for meningococcal infection [77], and thus all patients receiving eculizumab should receive vaccination before receiving eculizumab and periodic vaccination per guidelines for patients with complement deficiencies during chronic therapy with eculizumab. Moreover, antibiotic prophylaxis (amoxicillin) is indicated until the vaccination is effective (2 weeks after the initial dose). In countries in which there is a significant risk of meningococcal infection with a strain not covered by the vaccine, ongoing antibiotic prophylaxis is indicated. Patients also should be provided with instructions to seek medical care if they develop symptoms that could indicate meningococcal infection. A card explaining the risk of meningococcal infection should be carried by patients and families so that emergency room physicians can initiate appropriate antibiotics promptly with suggestive symptoms.

Ongoing eculizumab treatment is usually recommended because of the high risk of recurrence and the concern that recurrent episodes and low-level TMA may cause irreversible injury to the kidneys and other organs. The risk of recurrence if eculizumab is discontinued is unknown. There is an obvious burden of ongoing eculizumab infusions, although even small patients may receive infusions at home through a port.

Eculizumab is effective in kidney transplant recipients with aHUS [55,60,62]. It has been used as rescue therapy in patients who have recurrence of aHUS following kidney transplantation [55,62] and in patients who are dependent on plasmapheresis, but no longer tolerating the side effects of plasmapheresis [60,61]. Eculizumab also has been use prophylactically given the high risk of recurrence [55,63,67,69,78,79]. In this strategy, eculizumab is initiated before transplantation and continued posttransplantation. An initial dose up to 1 week before transplantation may be helpful with a living donor transplant, with a subsequent dose immediately before transplantation and the day following transplantation. In contrast, for cadaveric kidney transplantation, patients have been given a dose before and immediately after the kidney transplantation (either the same day or the following day), again followed by ongoing treatment [55,67]. Extra doses at the time of transplantation are believed to be necessary because of activation of the complement system induced by surgery and graft reperfusion [80]. Discontinuation of eculizumab after transplantation has led to recurrence of aHUS, suggesting a need for long-term treatment [55].

Treatment recommendations

Until recently, plasmapheresis was recommended for the initial treatment for aHUS [47]; however, given the morbidity [76,81] and variable responsiveness to plasmapheresis, eculizumab has become the preferred initial treatment for aHUS, especially given the evidence that a delay in treatment may be associated with a worse outcome [74]. When compared with historical controls who received plasma therapy, eculizumab has led to a significant improvement in outcome [41]. In addition, some patients who initially respond to plasmapheresis may become resistant or no longer tolerate plasmapheresis [60,65]. The response to eculizumab is often rapid [62,66] and there is no apparent advantage to combining eculizumab with plasmapheresis or delaying eculizumab treatment based on the response to plasmapheresis. However, plasmapheresis should be initiated as soon as possible if TTP due to ADAMTS13 inhibitor is suspected. Similarly, plasma infusions or plasmapheresis are the optimal treatment for congenital ADAMTS13 deficiency. Neither eculizumab nor plasma therapy is believed to be effective in patients with *DKGE* mutations [12].

References

[1] Tarr PI, Gordon CA, Chandler WL. Shiga-toxin-producing *Escherichia coli* and haemolytic uraemic syndrome. Lancet 2005;365:1073–86.

[2] Noris M, Caprioli J, Bresin E, et al. Relative role of genetic complement abnormalities in sporadic and familial aHUS and their impact on clinical phenotype. Clin J Am Soc Nephrol 2010;5:1844–59.

[3] Cayci FS, Cakar N, Hancer VS, et al. Eculizumab therapy in a child with hemolytic uremic syndrome and CFI mutation. Pediatr Nephrol 2012;27:2327–31.

[4] Fakhouri F, Fremeaux-Bacchi V. Thrombotic microangiopathy: eculizumab for atypical haemolytic uraemic syndrome: what next? Nat Rev Nephrol 2013;9:495–6.

[5] Banerjee R, Hersh AL, Newland J, et al. *Streptococcus pneumoniae*-associated hemolytic uremic syndrome among children in North America. Pediatr Infect Dis J 2011;30:736–9.

[6] Sharma AP, Greenberg CR, Prasad AN, et al. Hemolytic uremic syndrome (HUS) secondary to cobalamin C (cblC) disorder. Pediatr Nephrol 2007;22:2097–103.

[7] Menni F, Testa S, Guez S, et al. Neonatal atypical hemolytic uremic syndrome due to methylmalonic aciduria and homocystinuria. Pediatr Nephrol 2012;27:1401–5.

[8] Coppo P, Veyradier A. Thrombotic microangiopathies: towards a pathophysiology-based classification. Cardiovasc Hematol Disord Drug Targets 2009;9:36–50.

[9] Levy GG, Nichols WC, Lian EC, et al. Mutations in a member of the ADAMTS gene family cause thrombotic thrombocytopenic purpura. Nature 2001;413:488–94.

[10] Lotta LA, Garagiola I, Palla R, et al. ADAMTS13 mutations and polymorphisms in congenital thrombotic thrombocytopenic purpura. Hum Mutat 2010;31:11–9.

[11] Camilleri RS, Scully M, Thomas M, et al. A phenotype-genotype correlation of ADAMTS13 mutations in congenital thrombotic thrombocytopenic purpura patients treated in the United Kingdom. J Thromb Haemost 2012;10:1792–801.

[12] Lemaire M, Fremeaux-Bacchi V, Schaefer F, et al. Recessive mutations in DGKE cause atypical hemolytic-uremic syndrome. Nat Genet 2013;45:531–6.

[13] Bu F, Borsa N, Gianluigi A, et al. Familial atypical hemolytic uremic syndrome: a review of its genetic and clinical aspects. Clin Dev Immunol 2012;2012:370426.

[14] Delvaeye M, Noris M, De Vriese A, et al. Thrombomodulin mutations in atypical hemolytic-uremic syndrome. N Engl J Med 2009;361:345–57.

[15] Sadler JE. Thrombomodulin structure and function. Thromb Haemost 1997;78:392–5.

[16] Warwicker P, Goodship TH, Donne RL, et al. Genetic studies into inherited and sporadic hemolytic uremic syndrome. Kidney Int 1998;53:836–44.

[17] Fremeaux-Bacchi V, Fakhouri F, Garnier A, et al. Genetics and outcome of atypical hemolytic uremic syndrome: a nationwide French series comparing children and adults. Clin J Am Soc Nephrol 2013;8:554–62.

[18] Maga TK, Meyer NC, Belsha C, et al. A novel deletion in the RCA gene cluster causes atypical hemolytic uremic syndrome. Nephrol Dial Transplant 2011;26:739–41.

[19] Jozsi M, Heinen S, Hartmann A, et al. Factor H and atypical hemolytic uremic syndrome: mutations in the C-terminus cause structural changes and defective recognition functions. J Am Soc Nephrol 2006;17:170–7.

[20] Venables JP, Strain L, Routledge D, et al. Atypical haemolytic uraemic syndrome associated with a hybrid complement gene. PLoS Med 2006;3:e431.

[21] Francis NJ, McNicholas B, Awan A, et al. A novel hybrid CFH/CFHR3 gene generated by a microhomology-mediated deletion in familial atypical hemolytic uremic syndrome. Blood 2012;119:591–601.

[22] Bresin E, Daina E, Noris M, et al. Outcome of renal transplantation in patients with non-Shiga toxin-associated hemolytic uremic syndrome: prognostic significance of genetic background. Clin J Am Soc Nephrol 2006;1:88–99.

[23] Goicoechea de Jorge E, Harris CL, Esparza-Gordillo J, et al. Gain-of-function mutations in complement factor B are associated with atypical hemolytic uremic syndrome. Proc Natl Acad Sci U S A 2007;104:240–5.

[24] Tawadrous H, Maga T, Sharma J, et al. A novel mutation in the complement factor B gene (CFB) and atypical hemolytic uremic syndrome. Pediatr Nephrol 2010;25:947–51.

[25] Gilbert RD, Fowler DJ, Angus E, et al. Eculizumab therapy for atypical haemolytic uraemic syndrome due to a gain-of-function mutation of complement factor B. Pediatr Nephrol 2013;28:1315–8.

[26] Dragon-Durey MA, Loirat C, Cloarec S, et al. Anti-factor H autoantibodies associated with atypical hemolytic uremic syndrome. J Am Soc Nephrol 2005;16:555–63.

[27] Dragon-Durey MA, Sethi SK, Bagga A, et al. Clinical features of anti-factor H autoantibody-associated hemolytic uremic syndrome. J Am Soc Nephrol 2010;21:2180–7.

[28] Zipfel PF, Mache C, Muller D, et al. DEAP-HUS: deficiency of CFHR plasma proteins and autoantibody-positive form of hemolytic uremic syndrome. Pediatr Nephrol 2010;25: 2009–19.

[29] Strobel S, Hoyer PF, Mache CJ, et al. Functional analyses indicate a pathogenic role of factor H autoantibodies in atypical haemolytic uraemic syndrome. Nephrol Dial Transplant 2010;25:136–44.

[30] Blanc C, Roumenina LT, Ashraf Y, et al. Overall neutralization of complement factor H by autoantibodies in the acute phase of the autoimmune form of atypical hemolytic uremic syndrome. J Immunol 2012;189:3528–37.

[31] Le Quintrec M, Zuber J, Noel LH, et al. Anti-factor H autoantibodies in a fifth renal transplant recipient with atypical hemolytic and uremic syndrome. Am J Transplant 2009;9: 1223–9.

[32] Lee BH, Kwak SH, Shin JI, et al. Atypical hemolytic uremic syndrome associated with complement factor H autoantibodies and CFHR1/CFHR3 deficiency. Pediatr Res 2009;66: 336–40.

[33] Uslu-Gokceoglu A, Dogan CS, Comak E, et al. Atypical hemolytic uremic syndrome due to factor H autoantibody. Turk J Pediatr 2013;55:86–9.

[34] Jozsi M, Licht C, Strobel S, et al. Factor H autoantibodies in atypical hemolytic uremic syndrome correlate with CFHR1/CFHR3 deficiency. Blood 2008;111:1512–4.

[35] Abarrategui-Garrido C, Martinez-Barricarte R, Lopez-Trascasa M, et al. Characterization of complement factor H-related (CFHR) proteins in plasma reveals novel genetic variations of CFHR1 associated with atypical hemolytic uremic syndrome. Blood 2009;114: 4261–71.

[36] Esparza-Gordillo J, Goicoechea de Jorge E, Buil A, et al. Predisposition to atypical hemolytic uremic syndrome involves the concurrence of different susceptibility alleles in the regulators of complement activation gene cluster in 1q32. Hum Mol Genet 2005;14:703–12.

[37] Bresin E, Rurali E, Caprioli J, et al. Combined complement gene mutations in atypical hemolytic uremic syndrome influence clinical phenotype. J Am Soc Nephrol 2013;24: 475–86.

[38] Fritsche LG, Lauer N, Hartmann A, et al. An imbalance of human complement regulatory proteins CFHR1, CFHR3 and factor H influences risk for age-related macular degeneration (AMD). Hum Mol Genet 2010;19:4694–704.

[39] Feng S, Eyler SJ, Zhang Y, et al. Partial ADAMTS13 deficiency in atypical hemolytic uremic syndrome. Blood 2013;122:1487–93.

[40] Fitzpatrick MM, Walters MD, Trompeter RS, et al. Atypical (non-diarrhea-associated) hemolytic-uremic syndrome in childhood. J Pediatr 1993;122:532–7.

[41] Fakhouri F, Delmas Y, Provot F, et al. Insights from the use in clinical practice of eculizumab in adult patients with atypical hemolytic uremic syndrome affecting the native kidneys: an analysis of 19 cases. Am J Kidney Dis 2014;63:40–8.

[42] Koehl B, Boyer O, Biebuyck-Gouge N, et al. Neurological involvement in a child with atypical hemolytic uremic syndrome. Pediatr Nephrol 2010;25:2539–42.

[43] Gerber A, Karch H, Allerberger F, et al. Clinical course and the role of shiga toxin-producing *Escherichia coli* infection in the hemolytic-uremic syndrome in pediatric patients, 1997-2000, in Germany and Austria: a prospective study. J Infect Dis 2002;186: 493–500.

[44] Licht C, Weyersberg A, Heinen S, et al. Successful plasma therapy for atypical hemolytic uremic syndrome caused by factor H deficiency owing to a novel mutation in the complement cofactor protein domain 15. Am J Kidney Dis 2005;45:415–21.

[45] Caprioli J, Noris M, Brioschi S, et al. Genetics of HUS: the impact of MCP, CFH, and IF mutations on clinical presentation, response to treatment, and outcome. Blood 2006;108: 1267–79.

[46] Davin JC, Buter N, Groothoff J, et al. Prophylactic plasma exchange in CD46-associated atypical haemolytic uremic syndrome. Pediatr Nephrol 2009;24:1757–60.

[47] Arieta G, Besbas N, Johnson S, et al. Guideline for the investigation and initial therapy of diarrhea-negative hemolytic uremic syndrome. Pediatr Nephrol 2009;24:687–96.

[48] Remuzzi G, Ruggenenti P, Codazzi D, et al. Combined kidney and liver transplantation for familial haemolytic uraemic syndrome. Lancet 2002;359:1671–2.

[49] Remuzzi G, Ruggenenti P, Colledan M, et al. Hemolytic uremic syndrome: a fatal outcome after kidney and liver transplantation performed to correct factor h gene mutation. Am J Transplant 2005;5:1146–50.

[50] Saland JM, Ruggenenti P, Remuzzi G, et al. Liver-kidney transplantation to cure atypical hemolytic uremic syndrome. J Am Soc Nephrol 2009;20:940–9.

[51] Jalanko H, Peltonen S, Koskinen A, et al. Successful liver-kidney transplantation in two children with aHUS caused by a mutation in complement factor H. Am J Transplant 2008;8: 216–21.

[52] Saland JM, Emre SH, Shneider BL, et al. Favorable long-term outcome after liver-kidney transplant for recurrent hemolytic uremic syndrome associated with a factor H mutation. Am J Transplant 2006;6:1948–52.

[53] Saland JM, Shneider BL, Bromberg JS, et al. Successful split liver-kidney transplant for factor H associated hemolytic uremic syndrome. Clin J Am Soc Nephrol 2009;4:201–6.

[54] Le Quintrec M, Zuber J, Moulin B, et al. Complement genes strongly predict recurrence and graft outcome in adult renal transplant recipients with atypical hemolytic and uremic syndrome. Am J Transplant 2013;13:663–75.

[55] Zuber J, Le Quintrec M, Krid S, et al. Eculizumab for atypical hemolytic uremic syndrome recurrence in renal transplantation. Am J Transplant 2012;12:3337–54.

[56] Hillmen P, Young NS, Schubert J, et al. The complement inhibitor eculizumab in paroxysmal nocturnal hemoglobinuria. N Engl J Med 2006;355:1233–43.

[57] Parker C. Eculizumab for paroxysmal nocturnal haemoglobinuria. Lancet 2009;373: 759–67.

[58] Gruppo RA, Rother RP. Eculizumab for congenital atypical hemolytic-uremic syndrome. N Engl J Med 2009;360:544–6.

[59] Nurnberger J, Philipp T, Witzke O, et al. Eculizumab for atypical hemolytic-uremic syndrome. N Engl J Med 2009;360:542–4.

[60] Chatelet V, Fremeaux-Bacchi V, Lobbedez T, et al. Safety and long-term efficacy of eculizumab in a renal transplant patient with recurrent atypical hemolytic-uremic syndrome. Am J Transplant 2009;9:2644–5.

[61] Davin JC, Gracchi V, Bouts A, et al. Maintenance of kidney function following treatment with eculizumab and discontinuation of plasma exchange after a third kidney transplant for atypical hemolytic uremic syndrome associated with a CFH mutation. Am J Kidney Dis 2010;55:708–11.

[62] Larrea CF, Cofan F, Oppenheimer F, et al. Efficacy of eculizumab in the treatment of recurrent atypical hemolytic-uremic syndrome after renal transplantation. Transplantation 2010;89:903–4.

[63] Zimmerhackl LB, Hofer J, Cortina G, et al. Prophylactic eculizumab after renal transplantation in atypical hemolytic-uremic syndrome. N Engl J Med 2010;362:1746–8.

[64] Al-Akash SI, Almond PS, Savell VH Jr, et al. Eculizumab induces long-term remission in recurrent post-transplant HUS associated with C3 gene mutation. Pediatr Nephrol 2011;26:613–9.

[65] Lapeyraque AL, Fremeaux-Bacchi V, Robitaille P. Efficacy of eculizumab in a patient with factor-H-associated atypical hemolytic uremic syndrome. Pediatr Nephrol 2011;26: 621–4.

[66] Arieta G, Arrizabalaga B, Aguirre M, et al. Eculizumab in the treatment of atypical hemolytic uremic syndrome in infants. Am J Kidney Dis 2012;59:707–10.

[67] Krid S, Roumenina LT, Beury D, et al. Renal transplantation under prophylactic eculizumab in atypical hemolytic uremic syndrome with CFH/CFHR1 hybrid protein. Am J Transplant 2012;12:1938–44.

[68] Vilalta R, Lara E, Madrid A, et al. Long-term eculizumab improves clinical outcomes in atypical hemolytic uremic syndrome. Pediatr Nephrol 2012;27:2323–6.

[69] Xie L, Nester CM, Reed AI, et al. Tailored eculizumab therapy in the management of complement factor H-mediated atypical hemolytic uremic syndrome in an adult kidney transplant recipient: a case report. Transplant Proc 2012;44:3037–40.

[70] Besbas N, Gulhan B, Karpman D, et al. Neonatal onset atypical hemolytic uremic syndrome successfully treated with eculizumab. Pediatr Nephrol 2013;28:155–8.

[71] Gulleroglu K, Fidan K, Hancer VS, et al. Neurologic involvement in atypical hemolytic uremic syndrome and successful treatment with eculizumab. Pediatr Nephrol 2013;28: 827–30.

[72] Ohanian M, Cable C, Halka K. Eculizumab safely reverses neurologic impairment and eliminates need for dialysis in severe atypical hemolytic uremic syndrome. Clin Pharmacol 2011;3:5–12.

[73] Legendre CM, Licht C, Muus P, et al. Terminal complement inhibitor eculizumab in atypical hemolytic-uremic syndrome. N Engl J Med 2013;368:2169–81.

[74] Zuber J, Fakhouri F, Roumenina LT, et al, French Study Group for a HCG/C3G. Use of eculizumab for atypical haemolytic uraemic syndrome and C3 glomerulopathies. Nat Rev Nephrol 2012;8:643–57.

[75] Malina M, Gulati A, Bagga A, et al. Peripheral gangrene in children with atypical hemolytic uremic syndrome. Pediatrics 2013;131:e331–5.

[76] Tschumi S, Gugger M, Bucher BS, et al. Eculizumab in atypical hemolytic uremic syndrome: long-term clinical course and histological findings. Pediatr Nephrol 2011;26: 2085–8.

[77] Struijk GH, Bouts AH, Rijkers GT, et al. Meningococcal sepsis complicating eculizumab treatment despite prior vaccination. Am J Transplant 2013;13:819–20.

[78] Nester C, Stewart Z, Myers D, et al. Pre-emptive eculizumab and plasmapheresis for renal transplant in atypical hemolytic uremic syndrome. Clin J Am Soc Nephrol 2011;6: 1488–94.

[79] Weitz M, Amon O, Bassler D, et al. Prophylactic eculizumab prior to kidney transplantation for atypical hemolytic uremic syndrome. Pediatr Nephrol 2011;26:1325–9.

[80] Koskinen AR, Tukiainen E, Arola J, et al. Complement activation during liver transplantation—special emphasis on patients with atypical hemolytic uremic syndrome. Am J Transplant 2011;11:1885–95.

[81] Madore F, Lazarus JM, Brady HR. Therapeutic plasma exchange in renal diseases. J Am Soc Nephrol 1996;7:367–86.

[82] Noris M, Remuzzi G. Genetics and genetic testing in hemolytic uremic syndrome/thrombotic thrombocytopenic purpura. Semin Nephrol 2010;30:395–408.

ADVANCES IN PEDIATRICS

INDEX

Note: Page numbers of article titles are in **boldface** type.

0065-3101/14/$ – see front matter

http://dx.doi.org/10.1016/S0065-3101(14)00027-9

© 2014 Elsevier Inc. All rights reserved.